Passing the USMLE: Clinical Knowledge

Passing the USMLE
Clinical Knowledge

Ahmad Wagih Abdel-Halim, MD

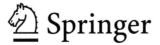 Springer

Ahmad Wagih Abdel-Halim, M.D.
Academic hospitalist and Internal medicine
faculty, McLaren Regional Medical Center,
Michigan; Clinical instructor of internal
medicine, Michigan State University (MSU)
College of human medicine, Lansing,
Michigan, USA
tommy48236@hotmail.com

Editors and Faculty Reviewers

Jami L. Foreback, M.D., Ph.D.
Internal Medicine Faculty
McLaren Regional Medical Center
Michigan State University
East Lansing, MI 48823
USA
jamif@mclaren.org

Trevor Banka, M.D.
Henry Ford Hospital
Detroit, MI 48202
USA
trbanka@gmail.com

ISBN: 978-0-387-68983-8   e-ISBN: 978-0-387-68984-5
DOI: 10.1007/978-0-387-68984-5

Library of Congress Control Number: 2008936884

Printed on acid-free paper

springer.com

Preface

Clinical medical science is an ocean of information. A good physician is one who can successfully figure out in which direction to swim when he faces a difficult medical problem. Acquiring that skill requires a strong grip on the basic facts behind each pathology, its most common presentation, what to look for during examination, and the best way to diagnose the pathology and treat your patient.

Preparing for the USMLE is a daunting and time-consuming task, and the exam is a difficult experience for most examinees. For many years, USMLE examinees have longed for a single source to prepare for the exam that could provide them with all the necessary details in just one concise book. This single source would be rich with information, figures and tables, yet be easy to memorize.

This book serves as a refresher on basic medical science facts and how best to apply these facts to the major specialties of clinical medicine. Enriched with key words, tables, figures and diagrams, this text will eliminate the need for any other books during your preparation for the USMLE. Simple vocabulary and straightforward prose ensure that the information you read will be easily stored in your memory for the longest period of time. The ocean of medical information was distilled down to a stream of only the most pertinent, high-yield facts, and the figures were carefully chosen to illustrate important concepts and maximize learning.

With this source as your guide, passing the USMLE will be just another step in your medical career.

MICHIGAN, USA   AHMAD WAGIH ABDEL-HALIM

Acknowledgments

I would like to express my gratitude to every person who helped and contributed to bring this work to life. I want to thank my mom and my dad for their love, support and encouragement; without them I would have never been who I am today.

I am deeply indebted to all my professors, colleagues and every single person who I have ever met who has helped add to my knowledge even with one word.

Special thanks to my amazing editors for their hard work; it was a pleasure working with them.

Finally, I am most grateful to Suzanne Stevens for her help, support and forbearance, and to all the staff at Springer for their support and cooperation.

MICHIGAN, USA   AHMAD WAGIH ABDEL-HALIM

Contents

Chapter 1
Internal Medicine

A.W.A. Halim, *Passing the USMLE*, DOI: 10.1007/978-0-387-68984-5_1,
© Springer Science+Business Media, LLC 2009

Endocrinology

Pituitary Gland

Parts and Actions

- *Anterior pituitary*: Releases FSH, LH, GH, TSH, ACTH and Prolactin (GH and prolactin are released from acidophil cells; everything else from basophil cells).
- *Posterior pituitary*:

  1. Supra-optic nucleus: Releases Anti-diuretic hormone (ADH) which acts on intercalated cells of the kidneys via *V2 receptors*, and on blood vessels via *V1*.
  2. Paraventricular nucleus: Releases *oxytocin*, which stimulates the contraction of the *uterus*, and *muscles surrounding the mammary glands' acini*.

Hyperprolactinemia

- *Introduction*:

  1. Prolactin release is inhibited by *dopamine* and dopamine agonists.
  2. *Normal serum prolactin level is less than 20 ng/mL (During pregnancy, a level up to 200 ng/mL is still considered normal)*.

- *Causes*:

  1. Physiological: *Pregnancy* and *lactation*.
  2. Pituitary: *Chromophobe* adenoma and Empty Sella Syndrome.
  3. Endocrinal: *Hypothyroidism* and Chronic renal failure.
  4. Drugs: Anti-Psychotics; via inhibition of dopamine.

- *Clinical picture*:

  1. *Amenorrhea* and infertility.
  2. *Galactorrhea: Milky nipple discharge.*
  3. Headache, vomiting and Bitemporal Hemianopia: Due to high intracranial pressure.

- *Diagnosis: Serum Prolactin level higher than 200 ng/mL. Also CT and MRI of brain to rule out pituitary adenoma and TSH to rule out hypothyroidism.*
- *Treatment: Dopamine agonists (First)*, e.g., Bromo-criptine, or hypophysectomy.

Acromegaly

- *Mechanism*: Caused by excess GH *after* closure of epiphysis. If it occurs before closure, it is called Gigantism.
- *Cause*: Acidophil cell adenoma. *In gigantism, it is mostly acidophil hyperplasia.*
- *Clinical picture*: Large head, hands and feet, gapping of teeth, and glucose intolerance. Refer to Fig. 1.1.

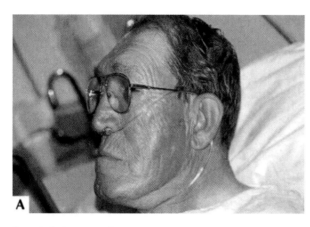

FIG. 1.1 Acromegaly

- *Diagnosis*:

  1. High serum insulin-like growth factor level (IGF): *Best next step.*
  2. Glucose suppression test is diagnostic: *For confirmation if IGF is elevated.*

- *Treatment*:

  1. Growth hormone antagonist, e.g., Somatostatin, bromocriptine.
  2. Surgery, i.e., Hypophysectomy.

Hypopituitarism

- *Causes*: Tumor or injury; however a very important cause is infarction of the anterior pituitary in the postpartum period a.k.a. *Sheehan's syndrome.*
- *Clinical picture*: In order of occurence Hypo-gonadism, -thyroidism, and lastly -adrenalism.
- *Diagnosis*: Low sex hormones, thyroid and cortisol levels, along with low FSH, LH, TSH and ACTH. *If the latter stimulatory hormones are elevated, this suggests polyglandular deficiency syndrome (Schmidt's syndrome).*
- *Treatment*: Hormone replacement. *Start with steroid replacement first.*
- *Notes*: Kallaman syndrome: Low GnRH, FSH and LH leading to anosmia, amenorrhea and associated with cleft lip/palate.

ADH Disorders

- *Syndrome of inappropriate ADH secretion (SIADH)*: Excessive ADH secretion leading to oliguria with a high urinary Na content and osmolality. Treatment: Fluid restriction and removing the underlying cause. Hypertonic saline, lithium and demeclocycline are used for severe non-resolving cases.

- *Diabetes insipidus*: Either due to decreased ADH secretion (Central diabetes insipidus) or decreased sensitivity (Nephrogenic diabetes insipidus). This leads to polyuria with low urinary Na content and osmolality. Central DI is treated with DDAVP, and nephrogenic DI is treated with thiazide diuretics.
- *Note*: Normal serum osmolality = 280 mosm/L.

Thyroid Gland

Thyroxine Synthesis

- Iodide is uptaken into the cells: This is inhibited by Thiocyanate, Perchlorate and high iodine levels (*Wolf Chaikoff effect*).
- Oxidation by peroxidase enzyme: Inhibited by Pro-pylthiouracil (PTU) and Methimazole.
- Organification and coupling: Inhibited by PTU and Methimazole.
- Deiodination: Performed by De-iodinase enzyme.
- T4 is converted to T3 (*T3 is 3 times more potent than T4*): Conversion is inhibited by PTU and Beta blockers.
- Binding to globulin: *Free (unbound) form is the active one.*

Regulation

- TRH from hypothalamus stimulates TSH release from pituitary.
- T3 performs negative feedback inhibition of TSH.

Actions of Thyroid Hormones

- *Mechanism*: Stimulate *Na/K ATPase* enzyme, which leads to increased oxygen consumption in all cells except the *brain, gonads* and the *spleen*.
- *CVS*: Increase stroke volume, heart rate and cardiac output.
- *CNS*: Maturation of the nervous system.
- *Metabolic*: Stimulate glycogenolysis, gluconeogenesis and lipolysis. *So, high thyroxin levels lead to low cholesterol levels and vice versa.*
- *Blood*: Increases 2,3 DPG, so increases O2 dissociation from hemoglobin.
- *Notes*:

  1. Calcitonin is released from parafollicular (C) cells of thyroid gland and it functions to decrease bone resorption, hence used to treat osteoporosis. *Medullary carcinoma of the thyroid originates from C cells, which are derived from the 4th pharyngeal pouch.*
  2. Thyroid and steroid hormones all act on *nuclear* receptors.

Thyrotoxicosis

- *Introduction*: Aka *Graves disease*, and is linked to *HLA-DR3* and *HLA-B8*.
- *Mechanism*: Thyroid stimulating immunoglobulins (*TSI*), also known as long acting thyroid stimulators (*LATS*).
- *Clinical picture*: *Heat intolerance, exophthalmia, sweating, tremors, increased appetite, weight loss* and *diarrhea*.
- *On exam*:

  1. Exophthalmia, lid retraction and lid lag. Refer to Fig. 1.2.
  2. Thyromegaly: *Moves up and down with deglutition*.
  3. Tremors of extremities, and excessive sweating.
  4. Tachycardia and arrhythmia, e.g., atrial fibrillation.

- *Diagnosis*: Low TSH, and high T3 and/or T4.
- *Next step*: *Thyroid ultrasound*, and *thyroid iodine uptake scan* revealing a *hot spot* (*Diffuse increased uptake is diagnostic of Grave's disease*).
- *Treatment*:

  1. Best is radioactive iodine: *Hypothyroidism is a common complication*.
  2. Surgery: Reserved for pregnant patients, or large compressive goiters.
  3. Medical: Methimazole or propylthiouracil. Beta blockers help alleviate the adrenergic symptoms, e.g., tachycardia, anxiety. *Note that methimazole is contraindicated during pregnancy as it can cause aplasia cutis*.

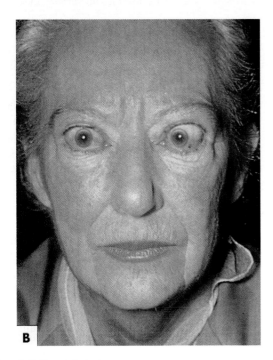

B

FIG. 1.2 Exophthalmia

- *Notes*:

  1. Exophthalmia occurs due to edema, fat and round cell infiltration, all behind the eye, along with weakness of extra-ocular muscles.
  2. Thyrotoxic crisis (Thyroid storm) is a fatal extreme hyperthyroidism characterized by altered mental status, fever, tremors and tachycardia. Treatment is urgent and includes all the following:

     - Cooling: Using ice. *Salicylates are contraindicated as they unbind thyroxine*.
     - PTU: Inhibits synthesis and peripheral conversion.
     - Beta blockers, e.g., Propranolol + Steroids: They both inhibit thyroxin release.

Hypothyroidism

- *Clinical picture*: *Cold intolerance, constipation, fatigue, weight gain* and *dry skin*.
- *On exam*: Delayed relaxation phase of deep tendon reflexes, and non-pitting edema on shin of tibia (*Myxedema*).
- *Diagnosis*: High TSH, and low T3 and/or T4.
- *Next step*: Check for *anti-thyroglobulin, anti-microsomal* and *anti-thyroperoxidase antibodies* to rule out *Hashimoto thyroiditis*.
- *Treatment*: Thyroxin replacement therapy.
- *Follow up*: Treatment takes 3–4 weeks to be completely effective. Follow up by measuring *TSH*. Recheck should be done 3–4 weeks after every dose adjustment.
- *Notes*:

  1. Cretinism is a neonatal form of hypothyroidism due to iodine deficiency during pregnancy. Newborn is *pale*, has *puffy face, pot belly* and *mental retardation*.
  2. Myxedemic coma is a fatal extreme hypothyroidism characterized by coma, hypothermia and muscle rigidity. Treatment: IV thyroxin.
  3. Hypothyroid female patients tend to have Fe deficiency anemia due to high susceptibility for menorrhagia.

Thyroiditis

- *De Quervain thyroiditis*: Due to giant cell infiltration triggered by a viral infection. This leads to painful enlargement of thyroid. Patient presents with sore throat radiating to the ears. On exam: Tender thyromegaly and normal oropharynx.
- *Hashimoto's thyroiditis*: Common in females and progresses to hypothyroidism. Commonly associated with autoimmune disorders, e.g., DM.

- *Diagnosis of thyroiditis*:
  1. Diffuse low iodine uptake on thyroid scan.
  2. Hashimoto's: Elevated *anti-thyroglobulin* and *anti-microsomal* antibodies.

- *Treatment*: Self resolving. Thyroxin therapy for Hashimoto's patients might be needed.

Thyroid Cancer

- *Papillary: Most common*. Metastasize through lymphatics. Treatment: Surgery.
- *Follicular*: Metastasize through blood. Most common site for mets is the skull. So when you see a patient in the USMLE with thyroid cancer and red hot mass on his skull, it is mostly follicular thyroid cancer. Treatment: Surgery and radioactive iodine. Note: Hurthle cell carcinoma is a subtype of follicular carcinoma.
- *Anaplastic*: Big firm tumor common in the elderly, with poor prognosis. Treatment: Surgery and radiation therapy.
- *Medullary*: Arise from *C cells* and secretes *calcitonin*. Microscopy shows amyloid stroma. Treatment: Surgery. *This tumor is radioresistant.*

Solitary Thyroid Nodule

- *If palpable*: Fine needle aspiration (FNA) and biopsy is always needed.
- *If not palpable*: FNA should only be done if nodule is bigger than 1.5 cm.
- *Note:* Hot nodules are mostly toxic, and cold nodules are mostly malignant.

Thyroglossal Cyst

- *Mechanism*: Non-obliteration of a part of the thyroglossal duct.
- *Clinical picture*: Midline cystic neck swelling that *moves up with tongue protrusion*.
- *Complication*: Rupture leaving a thyroglossal *fistula*.
- *Treatment*: Excision via *Sistrunk operation*.

Parathyroid Gland
Actions of PTH (Released by Chief Cells)

- *Bone*: Increase activity of *both osteoblasts and osteoclasts*, with an end result of bone destruction to increase serum calcium.
- *Kidney*:
  1. Increases *reabsorption of Ca* and *excretion of P*.

  2. Stimulates hydroxylation of vitamin D, which also increases calcium absorption via *Calbindin D-28*.
- *Intestine*: Increase calcium absorption, and decrease P absorption.
- *Note*: Vitamin D is hydroxylated once in the liver (25-OH) then the kidneys (1-OH), in order to increase *both* serum Ca and P by stimulating intestinal absorption and bone resorption.

Regulation

- Serum calcium regulates release or inhibition of PTH.
- 1,25-OH vitamin D causes feedback inhibition on its own formation.
- Ultraviolet B light is essential for regulating the action of vitamin D. So, suspect vitamin D deficiency in patients living in prison or cold areas with not much sun.

Hyperparathyroidism

- *Causes*: Adenoma, hyperplasia or secondary to another cause (renal failure); the most common of all these is the *adenoma*.
- *Clinical picture (Bones, Stones and Abdominal groans)*:

  1. Hypercalcemia: Causing constipation, polyuria, stones and fatigue.
  2. Osteitis fibrosa cystica: Causing bone pains and fractures.
  3. CNS: Altered mental status and corneal band keratopathy.

- *Treatment: Calcium chelators*, and *surgery* in severe cases.
- *Treatment of symptomatic hypercalcemia: Infusing the patient with 3–4 L of normal saline then starting furosemide. Note that you have to fill the tank first.*
- *Notes*:

  1. Pseudohypoparathyroidism a.k.a. Albright hereditary osteodystrophy is an X-linked dominant syndrome where PTH is abundant but organs are resistant to it, due to a *defective Gs protein*.
  2. MEN I and II must be ruled out in any case of hyperparathyroidism.

Multiple Endocrine Neoplasia (MEN)

- *Type I* (Wermer syndrome): Involves *p*ituitary, *p*ancreas and *p*arathyroid glands (PPP).
- *Type IIa* (Sipple syndrome): know it as (TAP):

  1. *T*hyroid gland: Medullary carcinoma.
  2. *A*drenal glands: Pheochromocytoma.
  3. *P*arathyroid glands: Hyperparathyroidisim.

- *Type IIb*: Just like IIa except for parathyroid being replaced by *neuroma* (TAN).

Adrenal Gland

Parts and Actions

- *Zona glomerulosa*: Aldosterone, which increases *Na absorption* and *K excretion*.
- *Zona fasiculata*: Cortisol, acts like aldosterone, plus being anti-inflammatory by stimulating lipocortin and *decreasing interleukin 2, eosinophils and lymphocytes*.
- *Zona reticularis*: Dehydroepiandrosterone (DHEAS) and Androstenedione.
- *Note: Cortisol stimulates gluconeogenesis and inhibits glycogenolysis, while glucagon stimulates both processes.*

Regulation

- CRH from hypothalamus stimulates ACTH release from pituitary. ACTH stimulates cholesterol desmolase in the adrenal glands.
- Renin converts angiotensinogen to angiotensin I, which later converts to angiotensin II via Angiotensin Converting Enzyme (ACE). Angiotensin II is then converted to Aldosterone, which performs a negative feedback on renin.

Cushing Syndrome

- *Causes*:

  1. Cushing disease: Excessive secretion of ACTH.
  2. Adrenal adenoma or hyperplasia: Excessive secretion of cortisol (low ACTH).
  3. Ectopic ACTH secretion, e.g., Small cell cancer of the lung.

- *Clinical picture*: refer to Fig. 1.3.

  1. *Moon face, buffalo hump* and *truncal obesity*.
  2. *Striae rubrae* and *thin limbs*.
  3. *Polycythemia and hirsutism*.

- *Diagnosis: Dexamethasone suppression test.*
- *Treatment: Ketoconazole.*

Conn's Syndrome

- *Introduction*: a.k.a. primary hyperaldosteronism.
- *Clinical picture: Resistant hypokalemic hypertension and metabolic alkalosis.*
- *Diagnosis: High serum aldosterone/renin activity ratio* and *salt loading test*.
- *Treatment*: Anti-aldosterone agent, e.g., Spironolactone.
- *Note*: These patients normally have polyuria, but at a certain aldosterone level, the kidneys do not respond to aldosterone anymore (Aldosterone escape phenomenon).

Pheochromocytoma

- *Introduction*: A rare *neural crest remnant* tumor arising from *chromaffin tissue*.
- *Rule of 10 s*: 10% are extra-adrenal, 10% bilateral, 10% malignant.
- *Clinical picture: Panic attack-like picture* (Palpitations, chest pain, sweating) and *labile resistant hypertension*.
- *Diagnosis*: Elevated 24-h urine concentration of vanillylmandelic acid (VMA), metanephrines and free catecholamines.

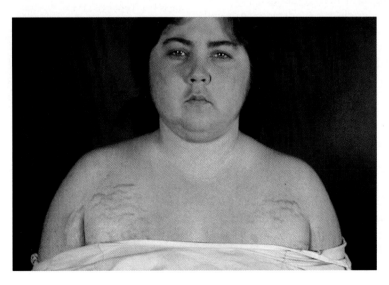

Fɪɢ. 1.3 Cushing syndrome

- *Next step*: Tumor must be localized by performing a *CT of the abdomen* and/or a *Metaiodobenzylguanidine (MIBG)* scan if CT failed to localize the tumor.
- *Treatment*:

  1. Drug of choice is alpha blockers, e.g., *Phenoxybenzamine*.
  2. Surgical resection of the tumor.

- *Note*: A similar tumor in children is *neuroblastoma*, which arises from the sympathetic chain and is diagnosed just like pheochromocytoma. Suspect this in any child presenting with *orbital ecchymosis* and *opsiclonus* (eyes jumping into different directions persistently). Biopsy of this tumor shows *Homer-Wright pseudo-rosettes*; treatment is surgical.

Adrenal Insufficiency

- *Types*:

  1. Primary: Due to adrenal cortex dysfunction
  2. Secondary: Due to pituitary dysfunction.

- *Clinical picture*:

  1. *Resistant hypotension* and *hypoglycemia*.
  2. Primary cases may also have *hyperpigmentation of mucous membranes* due to *high melanocyte stimulating hormone levels* (MSH) as a response to elevated ACTH. Note that secondary cases do not have this feature.

- *Diagnosis: Cosyntropin stimulation test.*
- *Treatment*: Systemic steroids.
- *Notes*:

  1. Addisonian crisis: Fatal extreme hypoadrenalism that occurs due to severe stress, or sudden stoppage of long term steroid therapy.
  2. Waterhouse Friderichson syndrome: Adrenal insufficiency that occurs due to adrenal hemorrhage. Caused by *Neisseria meningitidis*. So, when you see a patient in the USMLE with meningitis who suffers sudden severe hypotension, you know what to think!

Congenital Adrenal Hyperplasia

- *Mechanism*: *21-alpha* or *11-beta hydroxylase* enzyme deficiencies, *which are necessary for cortisol production*. Some cases are linked to *HLA BW47*.
- *Clinical picture*: Hirsutism, virilization and *precoccious puberty* due to increased ACTH-induced androgen production.
- *Diagnosis*: High serum *17-hydroxyprogesterone* levels.

- *Note*: This should be your first suspicion when you see a newborn with ambiguous genitalia. The next step after confirming the diagnosis would be to *check the patient's electrolytes* as they might have life threatening mineralo- or glucocorticoid deficiency.

Pancreas

Introduction

- Has exocrine and endocrine functions, the latter being regulated with:

  1. Alpha cells: Release *glucagon*.
  2. Beta cells: Release *insulin*.
  3. Delta cells: Release *somatostatin*.

Diabetes Mellitus (DM)

- *Definition*: Impaired glucose tolerance, which has 2 types as seen in Table 1.1.
- *Clinical picture*: Polyuria, Polydypsia, Polyphagia and weight loss.
- *Complications*:

  1. Neuropathy, Nephropathy and *lastly Retinopathy*. The mechanism here is *small vessel atherosclerosis* due to *non-enzymatic glycosylation and excessive conversion of glucose into sorbitol*.
  2. DM can also cause large vessel atherosclerosis leading to stroke and Coronary Artery Disease (CAD).
  3. Oculomotor nerve III palsy affecting the action of extraocular muscles.

TABLE 1.1 Types of DM.

	DM-1	DM-2
Mechanism	Viral destruction of beta cells leading to absence of insulin secretion. Underlying mechanism is anti-insulin and anti-islet cell antibodies	Insulin resistance
Genetics	Weak, but linked to HLA DR3 and HLA DR4	Strong genetic predisposition but it is not HLA linked
Insulin level	Very low or absent	Normal
Obesity	Not common	Very common
Complications	Very common	Not common
Treatment	Insulin	Oral hypoglycemics or insulin

- *Diagnosis*: High fasting glucose above *126 mg* is the test of choice.
- *Follow up*: HbA1C gives an idea about control of blood sugar over the last *3 months* (Target is below 6.5%). Fructosamine gives an idea about control of blood sugar over the last *3 weeks*.
- *Notes*:

  1. Major risk factor for complications in DM is *duration of disease*.
  2. Neuropathic leg ulcers occur mainly in the sole, caused by different organisms, but never by Clostridium. Treatment: Debridement.
  3. Note: Most common cause of death in patients with DM-I is:

     - First decade of life: DKA.
     - Second decade: Renal failure.

  4. Hypoglycemia is a common complication in patients with DM especially those patients:

     - On *sulfonylureas, e.g., Glyburide.*
     - *Excessive exogenous insulin injection: High insulin and Low C-peptide serum levels.*
     - Alcoholism: Due to *impaired gluconeogenesis. Mechanism here is high NADH, converting pyruvate to lactate, and oxaloacetate to malate.*

  5. Glucagonoma: Malignant tumor which presents with hyperglycemia and migrating erythematous skin lesions. So when you see a patient in the USMLE with high blood sugars and unexplained fleeting rash, you know what to suspect!

Insulin

- Insulin is secreted from beta cells of the pancreas.
- Upon eating, glucose blocks K channels and open Ca channels in the beta cells, which leads to insulin secretion in a *pulsatile fashion; an early big phase followed by a smaller one.*
- Diabetic pancreas either *does not release any insulin (DM Type I),* or it releases it in *one small phase (DM Type II).*
- Insulin secreted in response to oral glucose is more than that in response to injected glucose; *the secret lies in stimulation of GI enzymes by oral glucose.*
- *Actions of insulin*:

  1. Increase cellular uptake of glucose everywhere *except brain, kidney tubules and RBCs.*
  2. Increase cellular uptake of amino acids and K, and increase lipogenesis.

- *Types of insulin*:

  1. *Rapid and Short acting*: Crystalline insulin. Used in emergencies.Onset of action = 1 h. Duration of action = 6 h.
  2. *Intermediate*: Lente, Semilente, Neutral Protamine Hagedorn (NPH).Onset of action = 1×2 = 2 h. Duration of action = 6×2 = 12 h.
  3. *Long acting*: Ultralente, Protamine Zinc Insulin (PZI). Onset of action = 2×2 = 4 h. Duration of action = 12×2 = 24 h.

- *Side effects of insulin*:

  1. Skin allergy and *lipodystrophy*: Common at site of injection.
  2. *Somogyi phenomenon*: High early morning blood sugar as a rebound, due to a preceding drop of blood sugar. Treated by *decreasing* the evening insulin dose.
  3. *Dawn phenomenon*: High early morning blood sugar which is *not* preceded by any drop. Occurs due to early morning catecholamine surge. Treated by *increasing* the evening insulin dose.

Oral Hypoglycemics

1. *Sulfonylureas.*
   - *Mechanism*: Increase insulin release and tissue sensitivity. *This is achieved by blocking K channels and opening Ca channels in the beta cells of pancreas.*
   - *Metabolism*: Takes place in the *liver*, and excretion is in the *urine*.
   - *Examples and side effects*:

     1. Glyburide: High risk of *hypoglycemia.*
     2. Chlorpropramide: *Disulfiram like action* and syndrome of inappropriate ADH (*SIADH*).
     3. Others: Glipizide, Tolbutamide.

2. Biguanides.

   - *Mechanism: Inhibit hepatic gluconeogenesis.*
   - *Example*: Metformin.
   - *Side effects and contraindications*:

     1. Alcoholism or IV dye + Metformin: High risk of *lactic acidosis.*
     2. Renal failure: Contraindication for using Metformin.

3. Thiazolidinediones.

   - *Mechanism: Decrease insulin resistance.*
   - *Examples*: Rosiglitazone, Pioglitazone.

4. Alpha glucosidase inhibitors.

   - *Mechanism: Inhibit carbohydrate absorption.*
   - *Side effects*: GI upset and flatulence.
   - *Examples*: Acarbose.

Diabetic Ketoacidosis (DKA)

- *Clinical picture*: Diffuse *abdominal pain and vomiting* with no obvious explanation.
- *Diagnosis*:

  1. High blood glucose and *high anion gap metabolic acidosis*.
  2. *Ketones* in urine and serum.

- *Treatment*: Aggressive *hydration, insulin* and *potassium* replacement.
- *Complications during treatment*:

  1. Rapid dropping of blood glucose causes *cerebral edema*.
  2. Insulin therapy leads to *hypophosphatemia*, which causes muscles paralysis.

- *Hyperosmolar coma: Presents and looks just like DKA, minus the high anion gap, the acidosis and the ketones. Treated similarly.*

Others

- *Thymoma*: Diseases associated with this *benign tumor* are Myasthenia Gravis, pure red cell aplasia, Systemic Lupus Erythematosus (SLE), mediastinal syndrome, polymyositis and neutrophilic agranulocytosis.
- *Pinealoma*: Germ cell tumor that presents with high intracranial pressure (Headache, nausea, vomiting, blurry vision), and treated by surgical resection and radiation therapy. Clinical picture: 3 (P)s: *P*recoccious puberty, *P*apilledema and *P*arinaud syndrome (Paralysis of *upward gaze* of the eyes).

Drug Induced Endocrinal Disorders

- *Iodine and Thyroxin*: Hyperthyroidism.
- *Lithium*: Hypothyroidism and Diabetes insipidus.
- *Amiodarone*: Hypothyroidism or Hyperthyroidism.
- *Carbamazepine and Chlorpropramide*: SIADH.
- *Ketoconazole*: Adrenal insufficiency.
- *Metoclopramide*: Hyperprolactinemia.
- *Steroids*: Hyperglycemia and cushinoid features.

Endocrinal Causes of Excessive Sweating

1. Hypoglycemia: Also *palpitations* and *confusion*.
2. Acromegaly/Gigantism.
3. Hyperthyroidism.
4. Pheochromocytoma.

Gastrointestinal System

Musculature and Nerve Supply

- *Musculature*: The entire GI is made up of smooth muscles except the (*UPS*) which are made up of skeletal muscles: *U*pper third of esophagus, *P*harynx and External anal *S*phincter.
- *Local GI nerve plexuses*:

  1. *Submucous* Meissner plexus: Regulates *Secretions*.
  2. *Myenteric* Auerbach plexus: Regulates *Motility*.

Digestion

- Swallowing center is located in *medulla oblongata* and it initiates peristalsis in the pharynx, which goes through 2 phases:

  1. *1ry peristalsis*: Mediated by gravity pushing food down the esophagus.
  2. *2ry peristalsis*: Active peristalsis that follows to clear food remains left behind in the esophagus.

- Lower esophageal sphincter relaxation is mediated by contact with the food bolus, and this process is regulated by Vasoactive Intestinal Peptide (*VIP*).
- Once food reaches the stomach, receptive relaxation takes place, which is mediated by *cholescystokinin (CCK)*.
- The stomach performs *3 slow waves/min*; also *motilin* initiates *migratory myoelectric complex* every 60–90 min to clear the gastric food remains.
- Gastric emptying process is hastened by *isotonic food,* and is slowed down by *CCK* and presence of *fat* or *excess hydrogen ions in the duodenum.*
- The small intestine works in a magical way; the reason is that ileum starts performing peristalsis and the ileocecal valve relaxes once the food reaches the stomach. This is know as the *Gastro-ileal reflex.*
- Na and glucose pass from intestinal lumen into intestinal cells by *co-transport* mechanism; then they pass into the circulation by *facilitated diffusion*.
- Amino acids and peptides are also absorbed by Na-cotransport. *Fructose is the only monosaccharide absorbed in the intestine by facilitated diffusion without co-transport.*

Hormones and Mediators

- *Gastrin*: Secretion is stimulated by *Phenylalanine* and *tryptophan* and has these actions:

  1. Stimulates HCL secretion.
  2. Hypertrophy of gastric and intestinal mucosa.

- *Cholecystokinin (CCK)*: Secreted by *I cells* of duodenum and jujunum, which are stimulated by *free fatty acids* and *monoglycerols*, and has these actions:

1. Contracts gall bladder and relaxes sphincter of Oddi.
2. Stimulates pancreatic *enzymes* secretion.
3. Delays gastric emptying, and stimulates growth of exocrine pancreas.

- *Secretin*: Secreted by S cells of duodenum, and it stimulates *pancreatic bicarbonate* secretion.
- *Somatostatin*: Secreted by D cells of pancreas, and it inhibits *all* GI hormones.
- *Histamine*: Stimulates *HCL secretion* (Remember H2 blockers?).
- *Gastro-Intestinal Peptide (GIP)*: Stimulates pancreatic *insulin* secretion. *That is the reason why oral glucose stimulates insulin secretion in big amounts compared to IV glucose.*
- *Vasoactive Intestinal Peptide (VIP)*: Mediator of *pancreatic cholera*, stimulates gastric HCL and pancreatic bicarbonate secretion, and also regulates relaxation of lower esophageal sphincter.

Secretions

Saliva

- *Hypotonic* solution that is rich in *K and HCO₃*, and *deficient in Na and Cl.*
- *Aldosterone* regulates the Na/K transfer in and out of salivary ducts.
- Parasympathetic stimulation via cranial nerves *VII* and *IX* causes the saliva to be *abundant and watery.*
- Sympathetic stimulation via *cAMP* system causes saliva to be *scanty and viscid.*
- Lingual lipase cleaves triglycerides to monoglycerols and free fatty acids.
- Lingual amylase (Ptyalin) is responsible for *starch* digestion. Works on *alpha 1-4* bonds.

Gastric Secretions

- Parietal cells of stomach secrete *HCl* and *intrinsic factor*. Intrinsic factor binds to vitamin B12 all the way to the ileum where *only B12* gets absorbed (Without intrinsic factor). Ileal resection leads to *vitamin B12 deficiency, steatorrhea* and *recurrent oxalate stones.*
- In pernicious anemia, there is autoimmune destruction of parietal cells and intrinsic factor and higher risk of developing *gastric adenocarcinoma.*
- Low HCl content of the stomach puts it at risk of infection with *Salmonella.*
- Chief cells secrete *pepsinogen, which further breaks down to pepsin.*

- G cells secrete gastrin, which stimulates HCl secretion by parietal cells.

Pancreatic Secretions

- It is *isotonic* fluid with *high HCO₃* and *low Cl content.*
- Pancreatic amylase: For *starch* digestion to *oligosaccharides and maltose.*
- Pancreatic lipase: For *fat* digestion. *Elevated in pancreatitis.*
- Pancreatic proteases, e.g., Elastase, Trypsin and Chemotrypsin: For *protein* digestion.
- Trypsinogen, which is then converted to trypsin by duodenal enterokinase.
- Trypsin (as well as Thrombin) acts on the *arginine-glycine* bond.
- Bentiromide is used to assess the pancreatic function by measuring the duodenal chemotrypsin and its ability to cleave Para-Amino Benzoic Acid (PABA).
- Note: All pancreatic enzymes are released in an inactive form to protect the pancreas from digesting itself.

Bile

- *Secreted by the liver* and *stored in the gall bladder.*
- Composition: Mainly *water*, plus bile salts, cholesterol and bilirubin.
- Bilirubin can cause jaundice of the skin and sclera and is of 2 types:

  1. Direct (Conjugated): Passes in the urine and stools.
  2. *In*direct (Unconjugated): *In*capable of passing into urine or stools, but can cross blood brain barrier. *That is the bilirubin form that causes kernicterus in neonatal jaundice.*

- *Note*: Amount of secretions:

  1. Salivary: *1.5 L/day.*
  2. Gastric: *2.5 L/day.*
  3. Pancreatico-biliary: *1 L/day.*
  4. Succus entericus: *3 L/day.*

Dysphagia

- *Causes*: Internal obstruction, e.g., tumor, or external compression, e.g., tumor, enlarged left atrium or lymph nodes.
- *First thing to do*: Barium swallow, then esophago-gastroduodenoscopy (EGD) if the barium swallow was inconclusive. Why not EDG to begin with? Risk of perforation.

- *Note*: Oropharyngeal dysphagia usually occurs after a major cerebrovascular accident (CVA) and is evaluated by *Videoesophagography*.
- *Keywords for dysphagia*:

  1. Dysphagia mainly to liquids: *Achalasia*.
  2. Dysphagia mainly to solids: *Tumor*, e.g., Malignancy.
  3. Dysphagia + regurgitation of undigested food: *Zenker's diverticulum*.
  4. Dysphagia + long standing GERD: *Esophageal strictures*.
  5. Dysphagia + tight shiny skin: *Scleroderma*.

Esophageal Varices

- *Definition*: Dilated porto-systemic shunts between *left gastric* and *azygos veins*, mostly due to portal hypertension.
- *Clinical picture*: Patient *with liver cirrhosis vomiting bright red blood*.
- *Treatment*: *Sandostatin*, and EGD to perform *banding* or *sclerotherapy*.
- *Note*: Balloon tamponade is only used if above measures fail.

Achalasia

- *Definition*: *Abnormal peristalsis* and *incomplete relaxation* of lower esophageal sphincter, due to loss of Auerbach plexus.
- *Clinical picture*: Intermittent dysphagia, more to liquids, and regurgitation of meals.
- *Diagnosis*:

  1. Barium swallow shows *Bird's beak sign*. Refer to Fig. 1.4.
  2. Esophageal manometry shows high intra-esophageal pressure (>25 mmHg).

- *Treatment*: Myotomy (*best*), dilatation or botulinum toxin injection.
- *Postmortem*: Brown spots of digested hemoglobin could e seen in the esophageal wall, a.k.a. *Leopard spots*.

Diffuse Esophageal Spasm

- *Clinical picture*: Chest pain, related to meals. *Often confused with angina*.
- *Diagnosis*: Barium swallow shows *corkscrew esophagus*.
- *Treatment*: Calcium channel blockers to relax the smooth muscles.

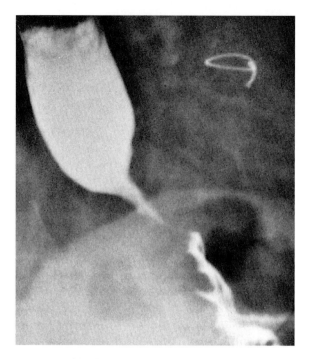

Fig. 1.4 Bird beak sign of Achalasia

Plummer Vinson Syndrome

- *Clinical picture*: Esophageal webs, atrophic glossitis, iron deficiency anemia.
- *Complication*: Esophageal *squamous cell cancer*.
- *Treatment*: Dilatation and iron therapy.

Peptic Ulcer Disease (PUD)

- *Mechanism and location*:

  1. Gastric: *Lesser curvature*, due to *impaired protective layer*.
  2. Duodenum: Dudenal *bulb*, due to *hyperacidity* or *Helicobacter Pylori infection; which is a Gram negative rod normally residing in the antrum*.

- *Clinical picture*:

  1. Gastric ulcer: Epigastric pain that increases immediately after eating.
  2. Duodenal ulcer: Epigastric pain that gets better with eating, but gets worse an hour later.

- *Complications*:

  1. Perforation of an ulcer in the posterior duodenal wall leads to injury of the *gastroduodenal artery*, so suspect in any patient with Duodenal ulcer who suddenly develops severe abdominal pain and becomes hemodynamically unstable.

2. Perforation: Presents with severe abdominal pain. Patient has *tympanic abdomen* on percussion and upright abdominal X-ray shows *air under diaphragm*.

- *Treatment*:

1. Proton pump inhibitor (PPI) for 6 weeks; if no improvement perform EGD and test for H. Pylori by *antral biopsy (Clo test), urease breath test or stool antigens*. Clo test depends on a urea rich medium that changes its color once the H. pylori's urease cleaves the urea into ammonia.
2. Surgery: Vagotomy or gastrectomy, e.g., Billroth surgery. Complications of Billroth include *abdominal distention and hypotension* followed by *reactive hypoglycemia* induced by meals aka *Dumping syndrome*.

- *Treatment of H. Pylori*:

1. Amoxicillin, clarithromycin, and proton pump inhibitor for 2 weeks.
2. *If the patient has penicillin allergy, the second preferred combination is Tetracycline, Metronidazole and Bismuth for 2 weeks.*

- *GERD*: Long standing Gastro-esophageal Reflux Disease (GERD) may result in replacement of the distal esophageal *stratified squamous epithelium* with gastric *columnar* epithelium. This is known as *Barrett's esophagus* and is associated with high risk of *adenocarcinoma*. Any other carcinoma in the esophagus is a *squamous cell carcinoma*, where smoking and alcohol are 2 major risk factors. Patients with esophageal cancer have dysphagia, more to *solids* (unlike achalasia).
- *Notes*:

1. Barrett's esophagus treatment: Cisapride + Proton pump inhibitor.
2. Barrett's esophagus with no dysplasia: Annual EGD. Low grade dysplasia: EGD every 6 months. High grade dysplasia: Esophagectomy.
3. *Zollinger Ellison syndrome*:

   - It is hypergastrinemia due to either *antral G cell hyperplasia* or a *gastrinoma in the pancreas*.
   - Clinical picture: *Recurrent peptic ulcers and Chronic diarrhea*.
   - Diagnosis: *Elevated fasting serum gastrin + Positive secretin stimulation test*.
   - Treatment: *Somatostatin* + PPI + Surgical resection of the gastrinoma.

4. *Vitamin C inhibits reduction of nitrite to nitrosamine, which decreases the risk of atrophic gastritis and stomach cancer.*
5. *In duodenal ulcers, there is hypertrophy of Brunner glands.*

6. Acute gastritis shows *erosions*, while chronic ones show *atrophy and infiltration with mononuclear cells*.
7. *Patients with long standing GERD may develop esophageal strictures and webs causing dysphagia. They are known as Schatzki rings.*
8. Severe repeated vomiting and retching can lead to a tear in the gastric mucosa near gastro-esophageal junction. This tear is known as *Mallory-Weiss tear*. Presents as patient having *severe repeated non bloody vomiting*, and ends up with *episodes of hematemasis. If esophageal perforation happens, it is known as Boerrhaave esophagus*.

Celiac Sprue

- *Mechanism*: Gluten associated disease that causes *atrophy of the small intestinal villi* and malabsorption.
- *Inheritance*: HLA DQ2 associated.
- *Clinical picture*:

1. *Chronic osmotic diarrhea* and *low albumin, iron* and *calcium* levels in blood.
2. Vesiculo-papular skin lesions known as *Dermatitis Herpetiformis*.

- *Diagnosis*:

1. Abnormal D-Xylose test.
2. High serum level of *IgA anti-endomysial and Anti-gliadin antibodies* (Most sensitive test) and Tissue Transglutaminase antibodies (TTG).
3. Confirm diagnosis by *small intestine biopsy*.

- *Complication*: If an elderly patient with celiac sprue who has been stable for a long time deteriorates suddenly, suspect *T cell lymphoma of small intestine*.
- *Treatment*: *Gluten free diet*.

Inflammatory Bowel Disease IBD (refer to Table 1.2, Figs. 1.5 and 1.6)
Irritable Bowel Syndrome (IBS)

- *Introduction*: Common in middle-aged patients with stressed personalities.
- *Clinical picture*: *At least 3 months* of unexplained abdominal pain with diarrhea or constipation or both, *mainly associated with eating*, and *relieved by bowel movements*.
- *Diagnosis*: The key here will be the *stressed out personality* and *normal workup*.
- *Treatment*:

1. Constipation predominant form: *Tegaserod*.
2. Diarrhea predominant form: *Alosetron* Note: Tegaserod and Alosetron are falling out of favor currently due to life threatening adverse

Table 1.2 Inflammatory bowel diseases.

	Crohn's Disease	Ulcerative Colitis
Location	Anywhere except the rectum; most common in ileocecal segment	Anywhere in the colon; most common in the rectum
Extent of lesions	Skip lesions and cobblestoning	Diffuse
Depth of lesions	Deep, causing fistulas and abscesses	Superficial
Effect of smoking	Worsens symptoms	Improves symptoms
Symptoms	Abdominal pain, diarrhea and mass in the RLQ of abdomen	Abdominal pain and bloody diarrhea
Barium enema	String sign	Loss of colonic haustrations
Treatment	Sulfasalazine, mesalamine or steroids Fistula: Treated by Metronidazole or Infliximab. If failed, perform fistulotomy	Sulfasalazine, mesalamine or steroids
Malignant transformation	High, need annual colonoscopy	High, need annual colonoscopy
Extra-intestinal manifestations	Possible, but not as common as in ulcerative colitis.	Arthritis, Scleritis, uveitis, pyoderma gangrenosum and sclerosing cholangitis. If any patient with IBD develops jaundice, do ERCP to rule out sclerosing cholangitis
Microscopy	Non-caseating granuloma	Crypt abscesses and ulcers

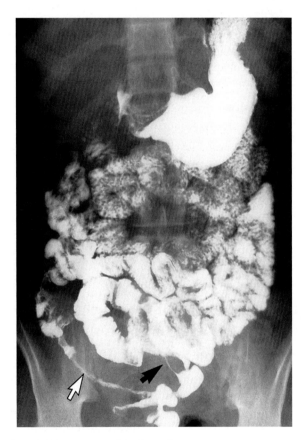

Fig. 1.5 String sign of Crohn's disease

effects, so treatment of IBS is back to be entirely symptomatic, i.e.: laxatives and anti-diarrheals.

Diarrhea

- *Definition*: Increase in amount or frequency of bowel movements of a person compared to his usual habit.

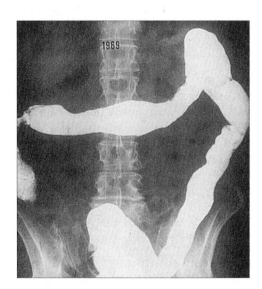

Fig. 1.6 Ulcerative colitis

- *Types*:

  1. *Osmotic*: *Related to meals*, and does not occur if the patient is fasting. Indicates a malabsorption or motility disorder.
  2. *Secretory*: Mediated by toxins, thus not related to meals, and *not resolved by fasting.*

- *Giardiasis*: Targets the duodenum and upper jujunum. Causes *watery diarrhea with excessive mucus*. Diagnosis: Stool analysis for ova and parasites to identify Giardia Lamblia trophozites and/or cysts. Treatment: Metronidazole.
- *Rotavirus*: Most common cause of diarrhea in children. Most common during the winter months and causes *watery diarrhea*.

- *Campylobacter jejuni*: Causes bloody diarrhea. Treatment: Erythromycin Note: Infection is highly associated with subsequent Guillain-Barre syndrome.
- *Cryptosporidium parvum*: Causes watery diarrhea in patients with HIV.

Colon Cancer

- *Introduction*: Polyps suggestive of malignancy are bigger than 1 cm and have a *villous component*, e.g., villous, tubulovillous. A benign polyp can turn malignant due to mutation of *DDC* and *p53* genes.
- *Risk factors*:

  1. Old age, low fiber and high fat diet.
  2. IBD.
  3. FAP and HNPCC.
  4. High risk polyps: If bigger than *1 cm* in diameter, or has a *villous* component.

- *Screening*:

  1. Starting age 40 by performing annual digital rectal exam.
  2. Starting age 50 by checking for *occult blood in stools annually* along with *colonoscopy every 10 years (or sigmoidos copy every 5 years)*. Start earlier in high risk groups.

- *Location*: Most common site is the *rectosigmoid area*.
- *Metastases*: Most common site of metastasis is the *liver*.
- *Clinical picture*:

  1. Asymptomatic or altered bowel habits, e.g., Constipation, bleeding per rectum.

  2. Anemia and weight loss. *Any elderly with unexplained iron deficiency anemia must get a colonoscopy to rule out colon cancer.*

- *Diagnosis*:

  1. Colonoscopy and biopsy is diagnostic.
  2. Barium enema shows *apple core sign*. Refer to Fig. 1.7.
  3. Elevated serum *Carcinoembryonic antigen (CEA)*. It is used mainly for the purpose of following up on the tumor response to treatment and to detect recurrence.

- *Treatment*: Surgery, radiation and chemotherapy.

Familial Adenomatous Polyposis (FAP)

- *Mechanism*: FAP is an autosomal dominant disease that occurs due to mutation of *APC* gene on *chromosome 5*. Polyps in this disease get *bigger due to mutation in the ras gene.*
- *Clinical picture*: Lower abdominal pain and bleeding per rectum.
- *Diagnosis*: Colonoscopy or barium enema with double contrast.
- *Treatment*: Total proctocolectomy by age 20, as it has a 100% potential of transformation into colon cancer.
- *Notes*:

  1. *Peutz Jeger syndrome: Colonic polyps + Lips and oral hyperpigmented lesions.*
  2. *Gardner's syndrome: FAP + Sebaceous cysts + Osteomas + Desmoid tumor.*
  3. *Turcot's syndrome: As Gardner's + neurovascular tumors.*

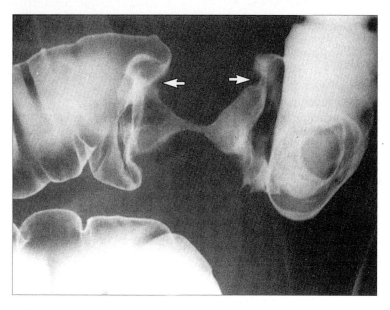

FIG. 1.7 Apple core sign of colon cancer

Diverticular Disease

- *Definition*: It is an outpouching of *mucosa* and *submucosa* in the colon, mostly in the sigmoid portion, *never in the rectum.*
- *Clinical picture*: *LLQ abdominal pain* and *bleeding per rectum.*
- *Diagnosis*: Barium enema, CT abdomen or colonoscopy. They show the *saw tooth appearance.*
- *Complications*:

  1. Painless bright red bleeding per rectum: Diverticular disease is the most common cause of lower GI bleeding in the elderly. *Bleeding stops spontaneously.*
  2. Diverticula can become infected, leading to *diverticulitis.* It is best treated by ciprofloxacin and metronidazole.

- *Notes*:

  1. Bleeding in diverticular disease occurs due to rupture of a blood vessel around the neck of a diverticulum. *Again, this bleeding stops spontaneously.*
  2. Surgery, e.g., *Sigmoidectomy* is indicated only in severe complicated cases of diverticular disease, e.g., Recurrent attacks, perforation, abscess formation.
  3. AV malformations are another common cause of painless bright red bleeding per rectum. They are most common in the *cecum and ascending colon.* Diagnosis: Angiography or colonoscopy. Treatment: Electrocoagulation, vasopressin, or segmental colectomy in severe resistant cases.
  4. GI bleeding as a rule is either upper (*Proximal to ligament of Treitz*) causing *melena* (Black tarry stools), or lower (*Distal to ligament of Treitz*) causing *bright red bleeding per rectum.*

Acute Pancreatitis

- *Causes* in descending order: *Alcohol, gall stones* or *hypertriglyceridemia.* Other less common causes are mumps and pancreas divisum. In pancreas divisum. The *accessory duct* becomes the main duct of the pancreas as the primary (main) duct is very small.
- *Clinical picture*: Epigastric abdominal pain *radiating to the back*, and is decreased by *leaning forwards.*
- *Physical exam*: Not conclusive except for hemorrhagic types, which may show bruising around the umbilicus (Cullen's sign) or in the left flank (Grey Turner sign). *Remember Cullen's by imagining a bruise Curving around the belly button.*
- *Diagnosis*:

  1. High serum lipase (specific) and amylase (non specific).

  2. CT of the abdomen: Shows edema of the pancreas with stranding of its fat.
  3. Abdominal X-ray shows *Sentinel loop* or *Colon cutt-off* signs.
  4. Ultrasound of the gall bladder if gall stones are the suspected cause.

- *Complications*: Hypocalcemia, DIC and Pseudocyst formation. Pseudocyst presents as an *epigastric* fixed *cystic* swelling which is easily visualized by ultrasound or CT scan. Barium meal in lateral view shows *semilunar stomach* with *widened vertebrogastric space.* Treatment of pseudocyst is conservative, and internal drainage is indicated only if >6 cm in diameter or if it lasts *>6 months.*
- *Treatment*: Bowel rest, aggressive hydration and pain control.
- *Note*: Persistent fever and toxemia after treatment is suggestive of pancreatic abscess and repeat CT of the abdomen should be the next step.

Chronic Pancreatitis

- *Introduction*: Occurs due to repeated attacks of pancreatitis.
- *Diagnosis*:

  1. X-ray of the abdomen shows *calcifications.*
  2. ERCP pancreatogram shows *chain of lakes* appearance of pancreatic duct.

- *Clinical picture*:

  1. Recurrent attacks of abdominal pain and acute pancreatitis.
  2. *Malabsorption*: Steatorrhea and vitamin A, D, E and K deficiency.
  3. *Hyperglycemia.*
  4. *Vitamin B12 deficiency.*

- *Treatment*: Pancreatic enzymes replacement.
- *Note*: In both acute and chronic pancreatitis, D-xylose test is *normal.*

Pancreatic Cancer

- *Introduction*: Very aggressive malignancy, not curable even with chemotherapy. Lifetime expectancy is *less than 6 months* in most cases.
- *Clinical picture*:

  1. Epigastric pain radiating to the back, decreased by leaning forwards.
  2. *Painless obstructive jaundice* and *weight loss.*
  3. Palpable gall bladder a.k.a. *Courvoisier sign.*

- *Diagnosis*: CT of abdomen and high level of serum CA 19-9; confirmed with biopsy.
- *Complications*: Migratory thrombophlebitis aka *Trousseau syndrome*.
- *Treatment*: Palliative surgery, best is pancreatico-duodenectomy (Whipple's).

Hepatology

Introduction

- Liver is the body's heaviest visceral organ (1000–1500 g).
- Main blood supply is through *portal vein*, and to a lesser extent the hepatic artery.
- Glancing at the hepatic lobule, the space of Disse is located between the blood sinusoids and hepatocytes. It contains *Ito (stellate) cells*, which serves for *synthesizing collagen* and *storing vitamin A*.
- Also in the walls of sinusoids lie the *Kupffer cells* which serve as the liver *macrophages*.
- *Functions of liver*: Storage of energy in the form of glycogen, and synthesizing plasma proteins, fat and bile salts (*for absorption of fat*).
- *Liver function tests*:

  1. *AST (SGOT)*: *Inside mitochondria*, has a *short* half life and is not specific.

  2. *ALT (SGPT)*: *In the cytoplasm*, has a *long* half life and is liver specific.
  3. *Alkaline phosphatase*: Present in hepatocytes membranes and in bones. *Elevation is suggestive of biliary obstruction*.
  4. *Gamma Glutamyl Transferase (GGT)*: Specific to the liver, especially alcoholic liver disease.
  5. *Bilirubin*: Indirect is the majority (0.8 mg) and it *cannot pass in the urine or stools*, but it *can cross blood brain barrier*. Direct (0.2 mg) can pass into urine and stools but cannot cross the BBB, and is more suggestive of biliary obstruction.
  6. *Albumin* (4–5 g): Best indicator of the *chronicity* of liver disease.
  7. *Prothrombin time (PT)*: Best indicator of the *severity* and *prognosis* of liver disease.
  8. *Globulins* (2–3 g): *IgG is elevated in chronic hepatitis, IgA in alcoholic liver disease and IgM in biliary cirrhosis*.
  9. *Alpha fetoprotein* (Normal <25 ng/ml): Hepatoma marker, but can also rise in pregnancy.

Hepatitis

- *Definition*: Inflammation of the hepatic tissue.
- *Causes*: Hepatitis virusus A, B, C, D, E, F, G, CMV, EBV, Alcohol.
- Refer to Table 1.3 for Hepatitis A, B and C viruses. Note that hepatitis D and E are weak viruses.

TABLE 1.3 Hepatitis A, B and C.

	Hepatitis A	Hepatitis B	Hepatitis C
Type	RNA Picornavirus	DNA Hepadnavirus	RNA Flavivirus
Incubation period	2–6 weeks	2–6 months	Variable
Transmission	Feco-orally	Parenterally	Parenterally
Carrier state	No	Yes	Yes
Chronicity	No	Yes	Yes
Malignancy	No	Yes	Yes
Serology	• HA IgM: Recent infection • HA IgG: Old infection	• HBs antigen: Active infection • HBs antibodies: Old infection or vaccination (Patient is Immune) • HBc antigen: Present only in hepatocytes; not serum • HBc IgM: Active inection (Patient is in window gap) • HBc IgG: Old infection • HBe antigen: Active viral replication and high contagiousity • HBe antibody: Old infection	• HC antibodies: Not measurable in the serum consistently, even during an active infection • Polymerase Chain Reaction (PCR): It is the best measure to detect hepatitis C
Prevention	• Vaccine available • Immunoglobulin can be given within 72 hours after exposure	• Vaccine (Inactivated HBs antigens) is available (Given at 0, 1 and 6 months) • Immunoglobulin can be given within 7 days after exposure	No vaccine or immunoglobulin

Hepatitis D can cause superinfection in a patient already infected with Hepatitis B. Hepatitis E can cause fulminant infection *only during pregnancy*.

- *Clinical picture*:

  1. Fever, headache and generalized fatigue.
  2. Right upper quadrant pain: Mild tender hepatomegaly on exam.
  3. Jaundice: Best seen in *sclera* and *palate*. Sclera stays jaundiced for a while after disease resolution. *The reason being the high affinity of collagen fibers of the sclera to bilirubin.*

- *Complications*:

  1. Chronicity, fulmination or relapse.
  2. Immune mediated due to *HBs* antigens: Glomerulonephritis and vasculitis, e.g., Polyarteritis nodosa.

- *Pathology*: *Lymphocytic infiltration* of the liver (Centrizonal and portal tract).
- *Treatment*:

  1. Hepatitis A: Supportive and bed rest.
  2. Hepatitis B: *Interferon* and *Lamivudine*.
  3. Hepatitis C: *Interferon* and *Ribavirin*.

- *Notes on treatment*:

  1. Interferon causes flu-like symptoms and immune disorders, e.g., Thyroiditis, Bone marrow depression, hemolytic anemia and Guillain Barre syndrome.
  2. Sudden rise of AST and ALT after starting treatment is a sign of successful therapy. *This occurs due to destruction of the virally infected hepatocytes.*

- *Other forms of hepatitis*:

  1. *Chronic active hepatitis*: Pathology shows *piecemeal* and *bridging necrosis*, and *rosette formation* in the hepatocytes.
  2. *Autoimmune hepatitis*: Diagnosed by positive ANA and *Anti-smooth muscle antibodies*. Treatment: *Steroids*, if fail, *add Azathioprine*.
  3. *Alcoholic hepatitis*: Pathology shows *perivenular ballooning* and *necrosis* along with *Mallory bodies*. Labs shows *AST:ALT ratio of more than 2, elevated IgA* and *elevated GGT*.
  4. *Acute fatty liver of pregnancy*: Severe hepatitis and liver failure during pregnancy, could be caused by hepatitis E virus infection.
  5. *Cholestasis of pregnancy*: Benign condition presenting with *pruritis* during the *3rd trimester* and it resolves spontaneously after delivery. There is high Alkaline phosphatase and direct bilirubin.

6. *HELLP*: A pregnancy associated disease. H: Microangiopathic hemolysis. EL: Elevated liver enzymes. LP: Low platelets.
7. *Reye's syndrome*: Treatment of viral illness in children with *aspirin* causes this disease; manifested by hepatomegaly, jaundice, hypoglycemia and hyperammonemia.

Liver Cirrhosis

- *Definition*: *Fibrosis and nodule formation of the liver* as a sequel of a primary disease, mostly hepatitis.
- *Pathologically*: divided into 2 types:

  1. Micronodular (<3 mm): as in alcoholism ($AST:ALT >2$).
  2. Macronodular (>3 mm): as in hepatocellular carcinoma.

- *Other causes*:

1. *Hemochromatosis*:

   - *Mechanism*: Congenital (*HFE gene AR mutation*) or acquired iron overload, e.g., Repeated blood transfusions.
   - *Clinical picture*: Liver cirrhosis, Bronze-colored skin in exposed areas, Cardiomyopathy and hyperglycemia, hence the term *Bronze diabetes*.
   - *Diagnosis*: High iron, *ferritin* and *transferrin*. Biopsy of the liver stains with *Prussian blue* due to high iron content.
   - *Treatment*: Phlebotomy and iron chelation therapy.

2. *Wilson's disease*:

   - *Mechanism*: Genetic *ceruloplasmin deficiency* (AR).
   - *Clinical picture*: Liver cirrhosis, Renal tubular damage, *Kayser-Fleischer rings in corneas* (Refer to Fig. 1.8) and *basal ganglia injury* causing *wing beating tremors* and *extra-pyramidal* symptoms.
   - *Diagnosis*: Low serum ceruloplasmin, and high copper levels in liver and urine. These patients also have glucosuria and amino aciduria.
   - *Treatment*: Copper chelating agents, e.g., *Penicillamine* (Causes B6 deficiency).
   - *P.S.*: Think of Wilson's in a patient suffering recurrent attacks of hepatitis with negative hepatitis serology.

- *Clinical picture of liver cirrhosis and failure*: *Hepatosplenomegaly* and:

  1. Wasting of temporalis muscles.

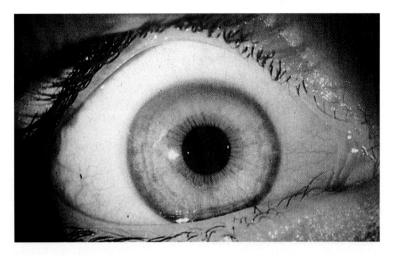

FIG. 1.8 Kayser-Fleisher ring

2. Parotid enlargement.
3. Jaundice and Fetor hepaticus (Malodorous breath due to mercaptans).
4. Gynecomastia: Unilateral and tender enlargement of breast *glandular tissue.*
5. Palmar erythema and flapping tremors (Asterixis).
6. Spider angiomata.
7. Female hair distribution: Due to androgen deficiency.
8. Hyperdynamic circulation: Due to vasodilator effect of toxins.
9. Pancytopenia: Due to hypersplenism.

- *Portal hypertension*: Patients with cirrhosis are at risk of portal hypertension (>20 mmHg), which leads to *hepatosplenomegaly, gastropathy, ascites* and opening of proto-systemic shunts:

  1. *Esophageal varices*: Shunting of *left gastric veins* with *azygos* veins.
  2. *Hemorrhoids: Superior and middle rectal veins* with *inferior rectal* veins.
  3. *Caput medusae: Para-umbilical veins* with *inferior epigastric* veins.

- *Pathology*: Liver shows *Mallory bodies*, fatty change, intrahepatic cholestasis and fibrosis around the central vein.

- *Treatment*: Correcting cause of cirrhosis, plus *beta blockers for portal HTN.*
- *Notes*:

  1. Cirrhotic patients have *low serum albumin* and *high beta and gamma globulin.*
  2. *Child's classification of liver diseases.* Refer to Table 1.4.

Hepatic Encephalopathy

- *Definition*: Neuropsychiatric complication of liver cell failure.
- *Clinical picture*: A cirrhotic patient with *reversed sleep rythm* and confusion, progressing to lethargy and stupor and may be coma and death.
- *Diagnosis*: Elevated serum *ammonia* level.
- *Treatment*:

  1. Lactulose and enemas: To wash out intestinal contents. *Lactulose is preferred as it is a non-absorbable disaccharide.*
  2. *Neomycin* or metronidazole: To kill intestinal flora metabolizing proteins.

Ascites

- *Definition*: Accumulation of fluid in the peritoneum.
- *SAAG*: Serum/ascitic albumin gradient (SAAG) *>1.1 is indicative of cirrhosis*, while <1.1 is indicative of TB, malignancy or pancreatitis.
- *Nature*: How to know if the fluid is exudate or transudate? Refer to Table 1.5.

TABLE 1.4 Child's classification.

	Class A	Class B	Class C
Nutrition	Excellent	Good	Poor
Ascites	None	Mild	Large
Serum Albumin	>3.5 g	3–3.5 g	<3 g
Serum Bilirubin	<2 mg	2–3 mg	>3 mg
Encephalopathy	None	Mild	Severe
Operative mortality	2%	10%	50%

TABLE 1.5 Exudate and transudate diagnostic criteria.

Criteria	Exudate	Transudate
Ascitic protein: Serum protein	>0.5	<0.5
Ascitic LDH:Serum LDH	>0.6	<0.6
Specific gravity	>1018	<1018

- *Treatment*:

  1. Salt and fluid restriction, Spironolactone and Furosemide. In huge symptomatic ascites, paracentesis should be performed.
  2. In case of recurrent ascites refractory to medical treatment, Transjugular Intrahepatic Porto-Systemic Shunt (*TIPSS*) should be performed. It is also indicated for recurrent bleeding esphageal varices.

Spontaneous Bacterial Peritonitis (SBP)

- *Definition*: A complication of ascites due to *E. coli* or less likely Klebsiella.
- *Clinical picture*: Ascites, *plus diffusely red warm and tender abdomen*.
- *Diagnosis*: Paracentesis, showing neutrophil count of $>250/mm^3$ is diagnostic.
- *Treatment*: Drug of choice is 3rd generation cephalosporin, e.g., Cefotaxime.

Biliary Cirrhosis

- *Prevalence*: Common in *middle-aged females*.
- *Causes*: Primary, or secondary to biliary obstruction.
- *Clinical picture*: *Middle-aged female* with:

  1. Liver cirrhosis, itching, dark urine and clay colored stools, and *negative past history for hepatitis or alcoholism*.
  2. Vitamin *K* and Vitamin *D* deficiency.

- *Diagnosis*:

  1. Primary: High levels of *anti-mitochondrial antibodies*.
  2. Secondary: Ultrasound of liver, if that shows dilatation of intrahepatic ducts, *ERCP* should be done next to manage the extrahepatic obstruction.

- *Treatment*: Ursodiol, *and relieving the obstruction if any. The only curative treatment is* liver transplant.

Hepatocellular Carcinoma (Hepatoma)

- *Definition*: Highly malignant tumor that might be predisposed by hepatitis virus B or C, cirrhosis, hemochromatosis or aflatoxins from Aspergillus flavus.

- *Clinical picture*: Patient with cirrhosis or hepatitis with *sudden deterioration*, flare up of symptoms and weight loss of unexplained reason.
- *Diagnosis*:

  1. Definitive diagnosis is established by *liver biopsy*.
  2. Elevated serum *alpha-fetoprotein*.
  3. CT and MRI shows the hepatic lesions.

- *Treatment*: Surgery, radiation and chemotherapy.
- *Notes*:

  1. Fibrolamellar carcinoma is a liver cancer with good prognosis that occurs in young age. The trick here is that alpha-fetoprotein will be within normal values.
  2. Cavernous hemangioma is a benign vascular swelling in the liver, more common in females using oral contraceptive pills (OCPs). Complication: Rupture and bleeding. Diagnosis: Angiography. Treatment: Stop OCPs and observe.

Jaundice

- *Definition*: Yellowish discoloration of skin and mucous membranes due to hyperbilirubinemia.
- *Causes of indirect hyperbilirubinemia*: Hemolysis, and congenital as discussed below. Indirect bilirubin is elevated, *so urine and stool color is normal*.
- *Causes of direct hyperbilirubinemia*: Biliary obstruction, and congenital as below. Direct bilirubin is elevated, *so urine is tea colored and stools are clay colored*.

  1. First thing to do in obstructive jaundice is hepatobiliary ultrasound. If there is dilatation of intrahepatic and/or extrahepatic biliary tree, that means there is extrahepatic biliary obstruction and Endoscopic Retrograde Cholangiopancreatography (ERCP) should be the next step.
  2. Palpable gall bladder in obstructive jaundice is suggestive of malignancy (Courvoisier sign).

- *Hepatocellular jaundice* occurs due to 2 defects; defective uptake and conjugation resulting in *high indirect bilirubin*, and defective excretion resulting in *high direct bilirubin*. This leads to *dark urine and dark stools*.

Congenital Hyperbilirubinemia

- *Criggler Najjar syndrome*: Occurs due to *deficiency* of UDP glucuronyl transferase. The bilirubin elevated is mainly *indirect*, so kernicterus is a risk.
- *Gilbert syndrome (AR)*: Occurs due to *presence of only a small amount* of UDP glucuronyl transferase plus *defective uptake*, so *indirect* bilirubin rises only

if the patient fasts or experiences severe stress or exercise.

- *Dubin Johnson syndrome (AR)*: Occurs due to defective hepatic *excretion*. The bilirubin elevated here is *direct* bilirubin, and macroscopically the liver is brown or black. There is a high coproporphyrin I/coproporphyrin III ratio.
- *Note*: Last place for jaundice to disappear is the sclera, the reason being its high *elastin* content, which has high affinity to bilirubin.

Drug Induced Hepatotoxicity

- *Cholestatic picture* (High Alk.Phos, High direct bilirubin): Anabolic steroids, OCP.
- *Hepatitis like picture*: INH, Halothane, Phenytoin and Alpha methyl dopa. Confirmed by the presence of *anti-histone antibodies*.
- *Acute hepatic necrosis*: Acetaminophen (*Treated with N-acetylcysteine*).
- *Adenomas*: Oral Contraceptive Pills (OCP).

Hematology

Red Blood Cells (RBCs)

- *RBCs*: Biconcave with no nucleus, and their half life is around *120 days*. RBCs count is 5–6 million/mm^3 in males and 4–5 million/mm^3 in females.
- *Hemoglobin*: In adults is HbA (2 alpha and 2 beta chains) and its normal values are 13–17 g/dL in males and 12–16 g/dL in females.
- *Hematocrit*: Also known as the Packed Cell Volume (PCV). It is the volume of packed RBCs in 100 cc of blood and is around 40–50% on average, and of course slightly less in females (*Females lose blood in menstruation*).
- *Erythrocyte Sedimentation Rate (ESR)*: Rate of sedimentation of RBCs in a tube due to rouleaux formation. It is normally below 20 mm/h. ESR above 100 mm/h indicate severe *infection, malignancy* or *connective tissue disease* or *multiple myeloma*.
- *Mean Corpuscular Volume (MCV)*: Volume of a red blood cell = 78–100 fL.
- *Mean Corpuscular Hemoglobin (MCH)*: Amount of Hb per cell = 27–32 pg.
- *Mean Corpuscular Hemoglobin Concentration (MCHC)* = Hb concentration/Hematocrit = 33%.
- *Anemia*: Hb <13 in males, <12 in females, <11 in pregnant. Anemia is associated with increase in pulse pressure.
- *Abnormal forms of hemoglobin*: Detected by *multiple wavelength co-oximetry*, most common toxicities are:

1. *Carboxyhemoglobin: Common in old houses with fireplaces, treated with 100% or hyperbaric oxygen.*
2. *Methemoglobinemia*: Common in *Lidocaine toxicity* and is treated with *methylene blue*.

- *Abnormal cell forms*:

1. Reticulocytes: 0.2–2% of RBCs. They are the immature form of RBCs and *the first cell to rise after starting iron therapy in iron deficiency anemia*.
2. Microcytosis: MCV <78 fL. Common in iron deficiency anemia.
3. Macrocytosis: MCH >100 fL. Common in megaloblastic anemia.
4. Basophilic stippling: Common in *lead poisoning*. Refer to Fig. 1.9.
5. Tear drop RBCs: Common in *myelofibrosis*.
6. Burr cells: Common in renal diseases.
7. Schistocytes: Common in *hemolysis*. Refer to Fig. 1.10.
8. Acanthocytes: Common in *abetalipoproteinemia*.
9. Auer rods: Seen on peripheral smear in *acute myelogenous leukemia (AML)*. Refer to Fig. 1.11.
10. *Howell Jolly bodies*: Common in patients with *absent or non-functioning spleen*.

White Blood Cells (WBCs)

- *Normal count*: 4,000–11,000/mm^3.
- *Embryology*: Develop from blast cells (N <3% in the blood).

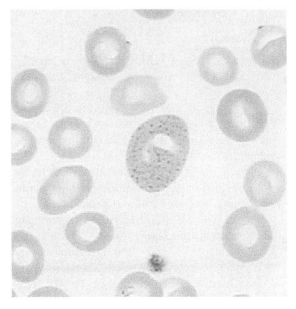

Fɪɢ. 1.9 Basophilic stippling of RBCs

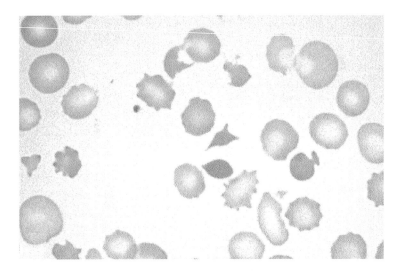

Fɪɢ. 1.10 Schistocytes

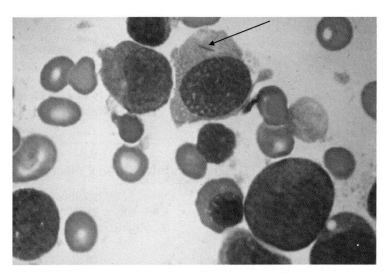

Fɪɢ. 1.11 Auer rods of AML

- *Neutrophils*: 70% of WBCs and perform phagocytosis and chemotaxis and contain *azurophilic granules*.
- *Lymphocytes*: 20% of WBCs and are divided into T and B cells.
- *Eosinophils*: 5% of WBCs and are elevated in allergic and parasitic conditions.
- *Basophils*: 2% of WBCs and are linked to IgE, hence elevated in allergic conditions. They contain *h*eparin and *h*istamine within their granules.
- *Monocytes*: 3% of WBCs and convert to macrophages once they reach any tissue.
- *Note*: Neutrophils and monocytes exist vessel walls by a process known as *Diapedesis*, which is usually preceded by sticking to the blood vessel wall through a process known as *Pavementation*.

Platelets

- *Normal count*: 150,000–400,000/mm^3.
- *Embryology*: Develop from megakaryocytes in the bone marrow.
- *Function*: Coagulation and as *antigen recognition cells*.
- *Hemostasis*: Upon blood vessel injury, vasoconstriction occurs due to effect of Thromboxane A2. Also release of Von Willebrand factor (vwf) causes *platelet adhesion*. Platelets release ADP to induce *platelet aggregation* and a platelet plug is formed.
- *Notes*:

1. First thing to do in low platelet count is to *repeat the test*, then examine a peripheral smear.
2. Alcohol inhibits Thrombopoeitin in the liver and causes transient thrombocytopenia that lasts

around 7 days. However, alcoholism can also cause hypersplenism which causes permanent pancytopenia.

Coagulation Cascade

- *Extrinsic*: Rapid, starts with tissue injury and release of tissue thromboplastin (Factor VII), which activates factor X in the presence of calcium. *Reflected by prothrombin time (PT) which is normally 10–15 seconds.*
- *Intrinsic*: Starts with contact with a foreign object. Factors activated in order are: XII → XI → IX → X. *Reflected by activated partial thromboplastin time (APTT) which is normally 30–40 seconds.*
- *Common pathway*: Starts with factor X activating conversion of prothrombin to thrombin. Thrombin converts fibrinogen to fibrin and platelet plug forms.
- *Platelet abnormalities*: Lead to petechiae and purpura.
- *Clotting factors abnormalities*: Lead to big bleeds, e.g., Joints, Intracranial etc.
- *Causes of isolated high PT*: Warfarin.
- *Causes of isolated high PTT*: Hemophilia, Von Willebrand disease and Antiphospholipid antibody syndrome.
- *Causes of elevated PT and PTT*: DIC, Liver disease and Vitamin K deficiency.
- *When blood clots inside a test tube*, the supernatant contains mainly plasma rich in vitamin K dependant clotting factors (II, VII, IX and X).
- *Assessment of intra-operative bleeding risk*: Best way is to ask the patient if he had any previous prolonged bleeding episodes during any procedure, e.g., Tooth extraction.

Iron Deficiency Anemia

- *Introduction*: Normal iron requirement is *10 mg/day*, out of which only *1 mg is absorbed* in the *ferrous* form. Absorption occurs in the *duodenum* and is stimulated by *vitamin C* and inhibited by *phosphates*.
- *Causes*: Decreased intake or increased loss, e.g., Bleeding or *Ankylostoma* infection.
- *Clinical picture*: Fatigue, pallor and craving for ice (*Pica*).
- *On exam*: Spooning of the nails aka *Koilonychia*.
- *Diagnosis*: Low iron, ferritin, MCV and MCH and High Total iron binding capacity (TIBC). Refer to Fig. 1.12.
- *Treatment*: Iron therapy.
- *Follow up on response*: *Reticulocytes* are the first cells to be elevated (*after around one week*) and are a marker of response to therapy which should be continued for *at least 6 months*.
- *Notes*:

  1. Iron deficiency anemia is the most common form of anemia in females.
  2. Side effects of iron therapy: *GI upset*, constipation and *black stools* (not melena).
  3. *Any elderly with iron deficiency anemia must get a colonoscopy to rule out colon cancer.*
  4. Ferritin is an active phase reactant, so in inflammatory conditions, it will be elevated, *even in patients with iron deficiency anemia*.
  5. *Anemia of chronic disease: Normocytic normochromic with low iron and normal ferritin. However, 25% of cases have microcytic hypochromic picture.*
  6. Sideroblastic anemia is an X-linked recessive microcytic hypochromic anemia that leads to deposition of iron studded normoblasts in the

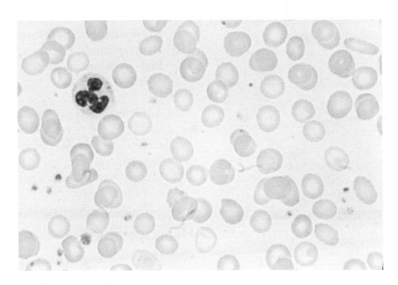

Fɪɢ. 1.12 Microcytic hypochromic anemia

bone marrow. Diagnosis: Prussian blue stain of bone marrow. Treatment: *Vitamin B6*.

Megaloblastic Anemia

- *Introduction*: Due to Folic acid or Vitamin B12 deficiency. *Normal requirement of folic acid is 50 mcg/day*, while that of *B12 is 1 mcg/day*.
- *Causes*: Decreased intake, intrinsic factor deficiency or *Diphylobothrium latum infection (fish tapeworm)*. The latter causes B12 deficiency.
- *Clinical picture*: Fatigue, pallor and possibly neurological symptoms.
- *Diagnosis*:

  1. High MCV and MCH, Low B12 and/or Folic acid.
  2. Folic acid deficiency: Positive *Fromiminoglutamic acid (FIGLU) test*, done using Histidine.
  3. B12 deficiency: Positive *Schilling test, Hypersegmented neutrophils* on peripheral smear (Refer to Fig. 1.13), and elevated serum *homocysteine and methylmalonic acid*.

- *Treatment*: Replacement therapy.
- *Notes*:

  1. Liver stores of B12 last for *3–5 years*, so B12 deficiency is not common.
  2. Vitamin B12 is abundant in meat products, so deficiency of B12 is more common among *vegetarians*. Meat-eaters (who eat no vegetables), on the other hand, are more likely to suffer from *vitamin C deficiency*.
  3. B12 deficiency can lead to *pancytopenia* and *neurological manifestations*. Look up Subacute Combined Degeneration in neurology.
  4. *Pernicious anemia* is a form of B12 deficiency that occurs due to antibodies against intrinsic factor and gastric parietal cells, and is associated with other immunological diseases.

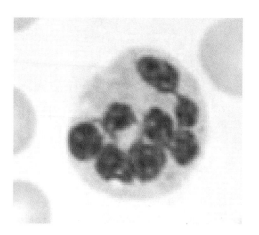

FIG. 1.13 Hypersegmented neutrophil

5. *Folic acid deficiency is the most common type of anemia in the US.*

Hemolytic Anemia

- *Clinical picture*: Fatigue, jaundice of skin and sclera, and *normal colored urine*.
- *Diagnosis*:

  1. High *indirect bilirubin* and *Low haptoglobin*.
  2. Peripheral smear: *Schistocytes*.
  3. Coombs test: positive in autoimmune hemolytic anemia as follows:

     - *Ig G*: Positive *direct* Coomb's test due to SLE, Lymphoma or Lupus (LLL).
     - *Ig M*: Positive *Indirect* Coomb's test due to viral infections, e.g., Mycoplasma.

- *Notes*:

  1. Drugs, e.g., Amphotericin B and penicillin can cause hemolysis.
  2. Intravascular hemolysis causes increased *urinary hemosiderin*.

Aplastic Anemia

- *Causes*: Bone marrow destruction, e.g., Benzene, chemotherapy or radiation, or infection with *parvovirus B19*.
- *Clinical picture:*:

  1. Anemia: Fatigue and pallor.
  2. Leukopenia: Repeated infections.
  3. Thrombocytopenia: Bleeding.

- *Diagnosis*: Bone marrow biopsy reveals *empty marrow*.
- *Treatment*: Treat the cause, *bone marrow transplantation*, and rule out 2 diseases that present similarly:

  1. B12 deficiency: Severe cases lead to pancytopenia.
  2. Hypersplenism: Occurs with liver cirrhosis and leads to pancytopenia.

- *Note*:

  1. Antilymphocyte or antithymocyte globulins could be used to treat aplastic anemia; however, *serum sickness* is always a concern during therapy.
  2. Most common cause of acquired aplastic anemia is *drug-induced*.

Hypersplenism

- *Definition*: Pancytopenia that is reversible by splenectomy.
- *Clinical picture*: Fatigue, infections and bleeding.

- *Diagnosis*:

  1. Low hemoglobin, WBCs and platelets.
  2. *Chromium 51 labelled RBCs*: Shows excessive spleen uptake.

- *Treatment*: Splenectomy.

Thalassemia

- *Mechanism*: Absent alpha or beta chains of hemoglobin, and is common in *Mediterranean* population, and that is a key in the USMLE.
- *Defect in alpha chain*: Alpha thalassemia could be due to defect in 1 locus causing alpha thalassemia trait, 2 loci (alpha th. Minor), 3 loci (Hemoglobin H) or all the 4 loci (Hemoglobin Barts) which causes *hydrops fetalis. Common in asians.*
- *Defect in Beta chain* causes Beta thalassemia minor, intermedia or major aka Cooley's anemia.
- *Clinical picture and diagnosis*:

  1. *Microcytic hypochromic* anemia.
  2. *Target cells* on peripheral blood smear. Refer to Fig. 1.14.
  3. Hb electrophoresis: Hemoglobin F in Cooley's anemia (*Hgb A2 in Beta thalassemia minor*).
  4. *Chipmunk facies*, and *hair on end appearance* on bone X-rays due to extramedullary hematopoeisis.

- *Treatment*: Blood transfusion, folic acid and bone marrow transplantation.

Sickle Cell Disease

- *Mechanism*: Replacement of *glutamic acid* with *valine* in *position 6 of beta chain of Hb*.

- *Risk factors*: Patients present in sickle cell crisis *usually induced by infections* or hypoxia.
- *Clinical picture*:

  1. Diffuse dactylitis, abdominal pain and shortness of breath, mostly due to microinfarctions by sickle cells.
  2. Multiple infections due to functional asplenia: So these patients have to be vaccinated against *H.influenza B, Strept. Pneumococci* and *Neisseria Meningitidis.*
  3. Normocytic normochromic anemia.
  4. Sickle cells on peripheral smear. Refer to Fig. 1.15.
  5. Hb electrophoresis: Hemoglobin S.

- *Complications*:

  1. Aplastic anemia: Due to *parvovirus B19* infection.
  2. Osteomyelitis: Salmonella is more common in this population, but the most common organism is still *Staphylococcus aureus.*

- *Treatment*:

  1. Supportive: Warming, fluids, analgesics and oxygen if needed.
  2. Exchange transfusion: Only if there is severe *dyspnea* or *priapism.*
  3. Hydroxyurea: It increases HbF and decreases HbS.

- *Notes*:

  1. Sickle cell deficiency is a predisposing factor for *folic acid deficiency.*
  2. Sickle cell patients are resistant to infection by *Plasmodium falciparum.*

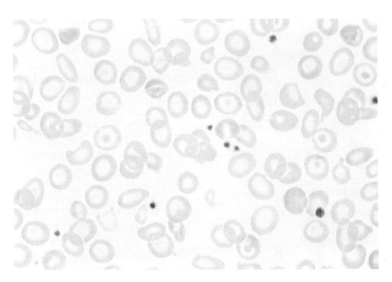

FIG. 1.14 Target cells

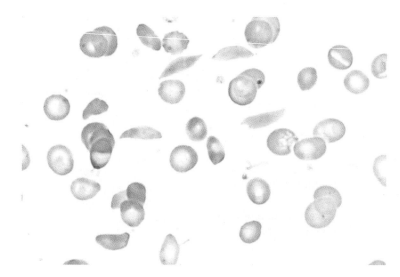

FIG. 1.15 Sickle cells

Spherocytosis

- *Mechanism*: Defect in RBC membrane, namely *spectrin*.
- *Clinical picture and diagnosis*:

  1. *Extravascular* hemolytic normocytic normochromic anemia.
  2. *Spherocytes* on peripheral smear (MCHC >33%). Refer to Fig. 1.16.
  3. Positive *osmotic fragility test*.
  4. Gall stones and splenomegaly.

- *Treatment*: Splenectomy.
- *Notes*:

  1. Remember 3 vaccines before surgery: H. Influenza B, Streptococcus pneumoniae and Meningococci. *Also remember that pneumococci is the most fatal.*

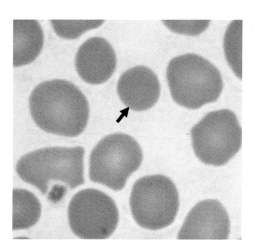

FIG. 1.16 Spherocytes

  2. Postsplenectomy patients have chronic low Immunoglobulin *M* levels.

G6PD Deficiency

- *Mechanism*: Absent RBC membrane enzyme; common in *African Americans*.
- *Clinical picture and diagnosis*:

  1. Hemolysis after ingestion of fava beans, sulfa or antimalarial medications.
  2. Low G6PD levels in RBCs few days after the hemolysis episode.
  3. *Heinz bodies* and *Bite cells* in the peripheral smear.

- *Treatment*: Supportive and avoiding the inducing agent.

Paroxysmal Nocturnal Hemoglobinuria (PNH)

- *Mechanism*: Absent Decay Accelerating Factor (DAF) in the RBC membrane, which leads to activation of complement *C3* to attack the RBCs (*Intravascular hemolysis*).
- *Clinical picture*:

  1. Blood in the urine *only upon awakening in the morning*, but not throughout the day (That is the key for the whole case).
  2. Leukopenia: Recurrent infections.
  3. Platelets: Decreased count, yet increased aggregation leading to thromboembolic events.

- *Diagnosis*: *Ham test* and *sucrose lysis test*: Hemolysis occurs at pH of <6.2. Recently, we check for *CD55* and *CD59* levels.
- *Treatment*: Steroids.

Hemophilia

- *Mechanism*: *XLR* disease due to deficiency of clotting factors VIII (A) or IX (B).
- *Clinical picture*:

  1. Bleeding since birth, e.g., Cephalhematoma, bleeding after circumcision.
  2. Multiple ecchymosis and big joints hemorrhagic effusion.
  3. Retroperitoneal hematoma: Patients can only present with femoral neuropathy (*Unilateral leg pain, weakness and numbness*).

- *Diagnosis*: Prolonged PTT, Normal PT, and Low factor VIII and/or IX.
- *Treatment*: Desmopressin DDAVP (Factor VIII rich substance).

Idiopathic Thrombocytopenic Purpura (ITP)

- *Mechanism*: Immunologically generated antibodies *IgG* against platelets, mostly following a recent flu like illness.
- *Clinical picture*: Repeated prolonged bleeding episodes.
- *Diagnosis*: Low platelet count, and elevated IgG against platelets.
- *Treatment*: Steroids, if failed, consider *rituximab* or *splenectomy*.
- *Note*:

  1. *Evans syndrome*: *ITP + Autoimmune hemolytic anemia*.
  2. Most cases in children – unlike adults – resolve spontaneously.

Von Willebrand Disease (VWD)

- *Mechanism*: *Autosomal dominant disorder* that affects the platelets *adhesion* process, while the platelet count and aggregation are both normal.
- *Clinical picture*: Repeated *easy bruising* and prolonged bleeding after injuries.
- *Diagnosis*: *Prolonged PTT*, normal PT, prolonged bleeding time, *Low vwf and defective vwf activity on ristocetin platelet study*.
- *Treatment*: Desmopressin (DDAVP) or factor VIII (*Both rich in vwf*).

Disseminated Intravascular Coagulopathy (DIC)

- *Mechanism*: It is a process that involves *consumption of the clotting factors* to end up with bleeding.
- *Causes*: Sepsis, Malignancy, Leukemia or pulmonary embolism. Most common DIC associated leukemia is *Acute progranulocytic leukemia*.
- *Clinical picture*: Extensive bleeding or thrombosis.
- *Diagnosis*:

  1. Low platelets and elevated LDH.
  2. Prolonged *PT and PTT*.
  3. Low fibrinogen and elevated Fibrin degradation products (FDP).

- *Treatment*: Treat the cause. If the patient is actively bleeding, transfuse with fresh frozen plasma (FFP).

Antiphospholipid Antibody Syndrome

- *Mechanism*: Immunologically derived antibodies against enzymes of the coagulation pathways.
- *Clinical picture*:

  1. Multiple unprovoked thromboembolic events, e.g., Deep venous thrombosis, myocardial infarction, cerebrovascular accidents.
  2. *Recurrent unprovoked abortions* (This is the key for the case).
  3. *Livedo reticularis*: *Net shaped* violaceous rash on extremities.

- *Diagnosis*:

  1. Prolonged PTT, normal PT.
  2. Elevated antibodies: Lupus anticoagulant, Anti-cardiolipin, Glycoprotein B1.

- *Treatment*: Life long anti-coagulation, e.g., warfarin.

Thrombotic Thrombocytopenic Purpura (TTP)

- *Mechanism*: Lack of ADAM-TS13; which is a vwf cleaving factor.
- *Clinical picture*: Pentad:

  1. Microangiopathic hemolytic anemia: Diagnosed by *schistocytes*.
  2. Thrombocytopenia.
  3. Renal failure.
  4. Neurological symptoms.
  5. Fever.

- *Diagnosis*: Schistocytes on the peripheral blood smear.

- *Treatment*: Life threatening disease, urgent plasma-pharesis is required.
- *Note*: Hemolytic uremic syndrome (HUS): Caused by *E. coli-0157-H7*, which causes *bloody diarrhea* followed by TTP like picture *minus the fever and neurological symptoms*. Diagnosis and treatment is the same as TTP. *Chemotherapy combinations containing Mitomycin can also induce HUS.*

Myeloproliferative Disorders

Introduction

- Biggest complication of following disorders is transformation into *leukemia*.

Polycythemia

- *Definition*: It is excessive RBCs causing *hyperviscosity syndrome*.
- *Causes*: Primary (*Polycythemia vera*), or secondary to hypoxia, smoking or erythropoietin secreting tumor, e.g., Renal cell cancer.
- *Clinical picture*:

  1. Plethora, facial flushing and itching: *Gets worse after a warm shower.*
  2. Elevated B12, basophils and uric acid levels.
  3. Splenomegaly.

- *Diagnosis*:

  1. High RBC mass and hematocrit *(>48 in females and >52 in males)*.
  2. Erythropoietin level: *Low in 1ry cases* and *high in 2ry ones*.

- *Treatment*: Treat the cause, phlebotomy and Hydroxyurea.

Myelofibrosis

- *Definition*: Fibrosis of the bone marrow.
- *Clinical picture*: Pancytopenia and hepatosplenomegaly.
- *Diagnosis*: *Dry bone marrow tap*, and *tear drop RBCs on peripheral smear*. Refer to Fig. 1.17.
- *Treatment*: Hydroxyurea and bone marrow transplant.

Thrombocytosis

- *Causes*: Could be primary, i.e., *Count >1,000,000*, or reactive to *iron deficiency* or infection (*<1,000,000*).
- *Clinical picture*: Thrombosis or bleeding.
- *Treatment*: Treat the cause and Hydroxyurea.

Henoch Schonlein Purpura

- *Mechanism*: *Post-streptococcal* vasculitis that is more common in children.
- *Clinical picture*:

  1. Abdominal pain.
  2. Hematuria: Due to glomerulonephritis.
  3. Purpuric rash on buttocks and lower extremities. Refer to Fig. 1.18.

- *Diagnosis*: Skin biopsy show *IgA deposits*.
- *Treatment*: *Self resolving*.

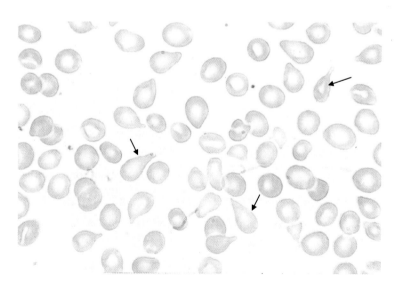

Fɪɢ. 1.17 Tear drop RBCs

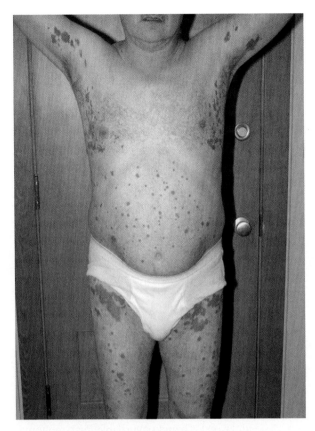

FIG. 1.18 Henoch-Schonlein purpura

Multiple Myeloma

- *Mechanism*: Plasma cell malignancy leading to *IgG spike* on protein electrophoresis.
- *Clinical picture*:

  1. Bone pains: *The key symptom*. If you hear about any elderly complaining of bone pains in the USMLE, look for multiple myeloma. It occurs due to osteolytic "*punched out*" bone lesions, which develop due to release of Osteoclast Activating Factor (*OAF*).
  2. Anemia and Thrombocytopenia.
  3. *Hypercalcemia* and *renal failure resulting in nitrogen retention*.

- *Diagnosis*:

  1. High serum protein, mainly IgG (*Monoclonal spike*).
  2. High urine protein, a.k.a. *Bence Jones proteinuria*.
  3. High serum calcium.
  4. *Rouleaux formation of RBCs* on peripheral smear.
  5. Plasma cell content of the bone marrow >10%. *Plasma cells have a "Cartwheel" or "Clockface" nucleus, and are basophilic due to their high content of rough endoplasmic reticulum and golgi apparatus. Refer to Fig. 1.19.*

- *Treatment*: Chemotherapy (Melphalan) or bone marrow transplant.
- *Note:* Bone lesions in multiple myeloma are *osteolytic* lesions, so they are best visualized by a *skeletal survey* and not a bone scan (Misses lytic lesions)

Leukemia

- *Definition*: Abnormal uncontrolled proliferation of WBCs.
- *Causes*: Genetic, *benzene*, alkylating agents and Human T-cell leukemia virus (HTLV).
- *Clinical picture*:

  1. Low RBCs and Hb: Fatigue and pallor.
  2. Low platelets: Bleeding.
  3. High WBCs:

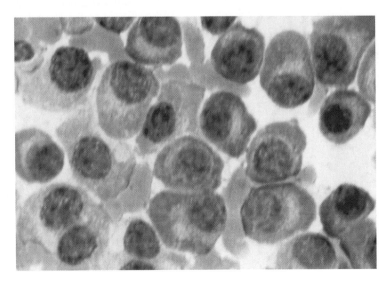

FIG. 1.19 Plasma cells

- Hepatosplenomegaly and lymphadenopathy: Through infiltration of white pulp in all types, *except hairy cell leukemia targeting red pulp*.
- Skin: *Greenish nodules* in acute myeloid leukemia (AML).
- Bones: Fractures.
- CVS: Cardiomyopathy and effusion.
- Renal: Acute Tubular Necrosis (ATN).

- *Diagnosis*:

  1. High WBC count with *>90% blasts*.
  2. Low RBCs and low platelets.

- *Treatment*:

  1. AML: Cytosine arabinoside (ara-c) and Doxorubicin.
  2. ALL: Prednisone, Vincristine and Doxorubicin.
  3. CML: Imatinib (Tyrosine kinase inhibitor).
  4. CLL: *No need to treat* unless symptomatic. Treatment: Fludarabine.
  5. Hairy cell leukemia: 2-chlorodeoxyadenosine (2-CdA).

- *Notes*:

  1. *Auer rods* are specific to AML. *t15:17* is associated with a good prognosis in AML (M3 subtype).
  2. Positive Common Acute Lymphoblastic Leukemia (CALLA) antigen and Terminal Transferase Detection (TdT) favor the prognosis of ALL and vice versa.
  3. Philadelphia chromosome *t9:22* is a poor prognostic indicator for ALL and is a good one for CML.
  4. CML is associated with *high basophil, uric acid and B12 levels*, and low leukocyte alkaline phosphatase levels.

5. *Smudge (Smear) cells* can be seen on the peripheral smear of CLL. Refer to Fig. 1.20.
6. CLL is associated with high incidence of *autoimmune hemolytic anemia*.
7. Bone marrow in hairy cell leukemia shows *Fried-egg shaped cells*.
8. Leukamoid reaction: High WBC count due to a severe infection, it's not leukemia because blast cells are less than 5% and there is elevated leukocyte alkaline phosphatase.

Lymphoma

- *Clinical picture*:

  1. Painless enlargement of lymph nodes (Discrete and rubbery), hepatosplenomegaly, fever and pruritis.
  2. *B symptoms*: Night fever, night sweats, loss of weight and loss of appetite.

- *Types*:

  1. *Hodgkin's*:

     - *Bimodal* age distribution (20 s and 60 s).
     - Best prognosis is *lymphocyte predominance* and worst is lymphocyte depletion lymphoma. The latter has the highest amount of Reed Sternberg cells.
     - Diagnosis: Lymph node biopsy; *Reed Sternberg cell* is diagnostic. Refer to Fig. 1.21.
     - Treatment: *ABVD* (Adriamycin, Bleomycin, Vinblastine, Dacarbazine).
     - Note: Treatment of lymphomas can cause Tumor lysis syndrome characterized by high serum (*KUP*): *K*, *U*ric acid and *P*hosphorus and low Calcium. Aggressive fluid and bicarbonate infusion and allopurinol during therapy is essential to prevent renal failure.

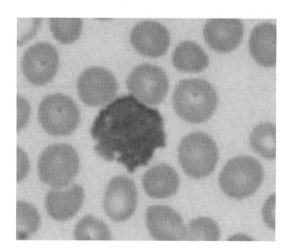

Fig. 1.20 Smudge (Smear) cells of CLL

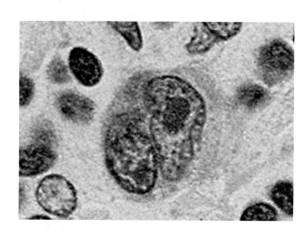

Fig. 1.21 Reed Sternberg cell

2. *Non-Hodgkin's*:

- More common in the elderly.
- Most common type is *large B cell lymphoma.*
- Burkitt lymphoma is a non-Hodgkin lymphoma caused by Epstein Barr virus (*EBV*) and it causes *mandibular tumor* in african children population. *American Burkitt's lymphoma (t8:14) presents with intestinal obstruction, especially in young adult females with breast cancer.*
- Treatment: *CHOP* (Cyclophosphamide, Hydroxydaunomycin "Doxorubicin", Oncovin "Vincristine", Prednisone).
- Note: Hemorrhagic cystitis caused by cyclophosphamide can be prevented by MESNA.

Common Blood Transfusion Reactions

- *Hemolysis*: Due to *ABO incompatibility.*
- *Febrile non-hemolytic reaction*: Due to antibodies against *WBCs or HLA.*
- *Treatment: Stop the transfusion* and send the blood for typing and cross matching, plus supportive therapy with acetaminophen and Diphenhydramine.
- *Note*:

1. Banked blood is deficient in clotting factors *V* and *VIII,* and it shifts the O2-Hemoglobin dissociation curve to the *left.*
2. Most common virus transmitted by blood transfusion: *CMV.*

Renal System

Introduction

- *Function*: Kidneys filter the blood, secrete erythropoietin, activate vitamin D by adding the *1-hydroxyl group* and regulate the renin angiotensin aldosterone system. Renal blood flow constitutes around *25%* of the cardiac output.
- *Autoregulation*: Between *80 and 200 mmHg* is accomplished by changing the renal vascular resistance, which is regulated by *Lacis cells of the macula densa* in the distal convoluted tubules.
- *Glomerular basement membrane*: Formed of (*FFF*) as follows: Foot processes of podocytes, Fenestrated endothelium of glomerular capillaries, Fused basement membrane (*This is the charged part of the membrane*).
- *TBW: Total body water constitutes 60% of total body weight, intracellular fluid constitutes 40% and extracellular fluid 20%.*

- *Threshold of glucosuria*: Plasma concentration of glucose at which it starts to appear in the urine. It is equal to *250 mg.*
- *Tm for glucosuria*: Represents full nephron saturation for glucose (N = *350 mg*).
- *Renal clearance*: It is the volume of plasma from which a certain substance is cleared in a certain period of time. If clearance of a substance is less than GFR, there is net reabsorption of that substance, and vice versa.
- *GFR depends on 4 factors*: High glomerular hydrostatic pressure, high Bowmann oncotic pressure, normal renal blood flow and normal capillary permeability.
- *Loop of Henle*:

1. *Proximal convoluted tubule (Rich in mitochondria)*: Performs *obligatory water absorption,* and it also absorbs 2/3 of sodium, most of the glucose and amino acids in the tubular fluid.
2. *Descending limb of loop of Henle: Counter current effect* leading to increased concentration of the fluid by at least 3 times.
3. *Ascending limb of loop of Henle: NA/K/2CL co-transport* takes place. *Loop diuretics act here.*
4. *Distal convoluted tubule*:

   1. *Na/Cl co-transport. Thiazide diuretics act here.*
   2. *Calcium excretion through the action of parathyroid hormone.*

5. *Collecting duct*:

   1. *Principal cells*: Na/K exchange through action of *Aldosterone.*
   2. *Intercalated cells*: H/K exchange through action of *ADH on V2 receptors.*

Fluid Measurements

- *Extracellular fluid*: Using *mannitol.*
- *Plasma*: Using *Evans blue.*
- *Glomerular filtration rate (GFR)*: Using *creatinine or inulin clearance* = 125, calculated by the famous equation $C = U \times V/P.$
- *Effective renal plasma flow*: Using *Paraaminohippuric acid,* which normally has a very high clearance.

Acid-base Balance

- Main acid base buffers are:

1. Carbonic acid-Bicarbonate system.
2. Chloride shift phenomenon: K-HCO3 exchange.
3. Lungs: Acidosis causes hyperventilation to wash away CO2, and vice versa.

4. Kidneys: Control absorption and excretion of H and HCO_3.

- K and H follow each other, so *hypokalemia* causes *alkalosis* and vice versa.
- Major extracellular buffer is *HCO3*, while the major intracellular one is *Hemoglobin*.
- *Anion gap = Na − (Cl + HCO₃) = 8 − 16.*
- *Know this equation by heart: pH = HCO₃/CO₂.*

Metabolic Acidosis (Low pH, Low HCO3, Low CO2)

- *Normal anion gap*: Diarrhea and Renal tubular acidosis (RTA).
- *High anion gap*:

    1. Salicylate toxicity: Starts with respiratory alkalosis first.
    2. Alcohol toxicity: Mainly ethylene glycol (Antifreeze) and methanol (Wood alcohol). *The former is converted to oxalate crystals in the kidneys*, while the latter is converted into *formaldehyde and formic acid, causing blindness.*
    3. Renal failure.
    4. Ketosis: Diabetic Ketoacidosis (DKA), Alcoholic Ketoacidosis and Lactic acidosis.

- *Clinical picture*: Hyperventilation and *Hyperkalemia.*
- *Treatment*: HCO_3 and treatment of the cause. Note that in DKA, fluids and insulin therapy are enough to correct the pH; the only indication to give HCO_3 is *pH <7.*
- *Note*: Oil of wintergreen is a rich source of salicylates.

Metabolic Alkalosis (High pH, High HCO₃, High CO₂)

- *Causes*:

    1. Loss of fluids to the point of dehydration aka *contraction alkalosis.*
    2. Loss of acid, e.g., Vomiting, or ingestion of excessive HCO_3.

- *Clinical picture*: Hypokalemic alkalosis, which results in *tetany,*
- *Treatment: Normal saline* and treatment of the cause. In resistant cases, acetazolamide could be used (*Causes metabolic acidosis and alkaline urine*).

Respiratory Acidosis (Low pH, High HCO₃, High CO₂)

- *Causes*: *Slow* breathing, e.g., Respiratory failure, COPD.

- *Clinical picture*: High CO_2 causing lethargy (CO_2 narcosis), full bounding pulse and tremors.
- *Treatment*: O_2 + CO_2, as pure O_2 will cause further respiratory center depression.

Respiratory Alkalosis (High pH, Low HCO₃, Low CO₂)

- *Causes*: *Fast* breathing, e.g., Salicylate poisoning, Mid brain lesion.
- *Clinical picture*: Hyperventilation leading to tetany and seizures.
- *Treatment*: Rebreathing mask, e.g., Paper bag.

Electrolytes

- Refer to Table 1.6 for electrolytes imbalance.

Nephrotic Syndrome

- *Pathology*: Heavy proteinuria (>3.5 g/day), hyperlipidemia and - lipiduria.
- *Causes*: DM, HTN and Amyloidosis.
- *Clinical picture*: Generalized edema that starts from the face downwards.
- *Types of nephrotic syndrome*:

    1. *Minimal change disease (Lipoid nephrosis)*: *Foot processes effacement*. Responds to steroids. It is the most common form of idiopathic nephrotic syndrome in *children and young adults.*
    2. *Membranous glomerulonephritis (GN)*: *Spike and dome* appearance. High risk of malignancy and DVT, so if you get a nephrotic patient in the USMLE having DVT, renal vein thrombosis or malignancy, it is most likely membranous GN. It is the most common form of idiopathic nephrotic syndrome in *Caucasians.*
    3. *Focal segmental sclerosis*: Shows *segmental sclerosis*. Common in *HIV*. It is the most common form of idiopathic nephrotic syndrome in *African Americans.*
    4. *DM*: *Kimmelstiel-Wilson* syndrome. First sign of diabetic nephropathy is glomerulosclerosis, which is detected by checking for *microalbuminuria.*
    5. *SLE*: *Wire loop lesions with subendothelial deposits.*
    6. *Amyloidosis*: Diagnosed by *Congo red staining of abdominal pad of fat or peripheral nerve*. Treatment: *Colchicine.*
    7. *Familial Mediterranean Fever* (Fever + Serositis + Nephrotic): Treatment: *Colchicine.*

TABLE 1.6 Electrolyte imbalance.

Electrolyte imbalance	Effect
Hypocalcemia	• Neuromuscular hyper-excitability, twitching and seizures • *Peroneal sign*: Flexion of foot on tapping of peroneal nerve • *Chvostek sign*: Contraction of facial muscles on tapping of facial nerve • *Trousseau sign*: Carpal spasm on occlusion of the brachial artery with the sphygmomanometer cuff • EKG: Q-T prolongation • Treatment: Replacement and treat the cause
Hypercalcemia	• Causes: Hyperparathyroidism or malignancy, which increases serum calcium either via osteolytic metastases or release of PTH-related peptide (Treatment of malignancy induced hypercalcemia: Mithramycin or Bisphosphonates) • Polyuria and constipation • Altered mental status and hyporeflexia • Tissue calcification • Osteitis fibrosa cystica • EKG: Short Q-T interval • Treatment: *Fluid loading first*, then diuresis using furosemide (*HCTZ causes hypercalcemia*). Treat cause
Hypokalemia	• Causes: Diarrhea and Diuretics are the most common • Muscle cramps and weakness • Cardiac arrhythmia • EKG: Depressed S-T segments and flat or inverted T waves + *prominent U waves* • Treatment: Replacement and treat the cause

Hyperkalemia	• Causes: Acidosis, ACEI, Spironolactone, Hypoadrenalism
	• Cardiac arrhythmia
	• EKG: Wide QRS and *tall peaked T waves*
	• Treatment:
	   1. If there is EKG changes, give calcium gluconate to protect the heart
	   2. Kick K outside of the body: K exchange resins, e.g., Kayexelate
	   3. Shift K inside the cells: Glucose + insulin, bicarbonate injection
	   4. If no response: Urgent hemodialysis

Hypomagnesemia	• Neuromuscular hyper-excitability • Common to see in *malnourished patients, patients on Total Parenteral Nurtition (TPN)* and *alcoholics* • EKG: Wide P-R, QRS and Q-T • Treatment: Replacement

Hyponatremia	• Altered mental status and seizures
	• Common in postoperative patients, and due to diuretics
	• Treatment:
	   1. Fluid restriction
	   2. If failed or the patient developed neurological manifestations, give hypertonic
	
	• Rapid correction of hyponatremia leads to *central pontine myelinolysis*
	• Rapid correction of hypernatremia leads to *brain edema*.

Nephritic Syndrome

- *Clinical picture and pathology*: Proteinuria (<3 g/day), Hematuria and HTN.
- *Causes*: Mostly infectious, e.g., Group A beta hemolytic streptococcus.
- *Types of glomerulonephritis*:
  1. *Acute post-streptococcal*: *Lumpy bumps deposits* and *subepithelial humps*.
  2. *Goodpasteur*: *Linear deposits*. Discussed in Rheumatology.
  3. *Rapidly progressive*: *Crescent moon-shaped* deposits.
  4. *Membranoproliferative*: *Tram track* deposits.
  5. *IgA nephropathy (Berger disease)*: *Mesangial Ig A deposits*.

- *Note*: GN with low serum complement levels are (*PMS*): *P*ost-streptococcal, *M*embranoproliferative and *S*LE.
- *Note*: One of the markers of any GN is the presence of *RBC casts* in the urine.

Urinary Tract Infection (UTI)

- *Cause*: Most commonly caused by *E. Coli* and *Klebsiella*.
- *Clinical picture*: Dysuria, urinary frequency, urgency, and even *hematuria*.
- *On exam*: Costovertebral angle tenderness is alarming for pyelonephritis.

- *Diagnosis*: Urine analysis showing more than 5 WBCs/ hpf with bacteria is diagnostic of UTI, however if it shows more than 5 WBCs/hpf without any bacteria, this is known as sterile pyuria. *Causes of sterile pyuria: Interstitial nephritis, TB or nephrolithiasis.*
- *Treatment*:

  1. Complicated UTI, e.g., Pyelonephritis: *IV ampicillin and gentamycin.*
  2. Uncomplicated UTI: Oral ciprofloxacin or SMX/TMP (Bactrim).

- *Notes*:

  1. UTI in polycystic kidney is best treated with SMX/TMP or tetracycline due to their *high lipid solubility.*
  2. Chronic or recurrent UTI in females could occur due to colonization of the vaginal introitus by fecal material.
  3. UTI during pregnancy occurs without symptoms, however it must be treated or pyelonephritis would be a sequel in *40% of cases.*
  4. UTI in diabetic patients can trigger *acute papillary necrosis.*
  5. Upper UTI (Pyelonephritis) could be differentiated from lower UTI (Cystitis, Urethritis) by presence of WBC casts in the urine in the former. Upper UTI is caused by organisms releasing *Hemolysin*, and is treated for *10–14 days*, while lower UTI treatment course is *3 days* long.
  6. Treatment failure of UTI: Caused by non-compliance or resistance to treatment. *Next thing to do: Urine culture and sensitivity.*

Interstitial Nephritis

- *Definition*: Inflammation mediated infiltration of interstitial tissues with neutrophils.
- *Causes*: Mostly drugs, e.g., Ampicillin, *methicillin*, cephalosporins.
- *Clinical picture*: Fever, rash and acute renal insufficiency.
- *Diagnosis*: Elevated creatinine, sterile pyuria and most importantly *eosinophiluria.*
- *Treatment*: Stop the offending drug.

Polycystic Kidney Disease (PKD)

- *Mechanism*: Genetic disease due to mutation of *PKD1 gene.* Inherited as AD in adults and AR in children.
- *Clinical picture*: Patients, children or adults, might present with hematuria, proteinuria, HTN or even chronic kidney disease.

- *Diagnosis*:

  1. Ultrasound: Polycystic kidneys.
  2. IVP: Shows *spider leg deformity.*

- *Treatment*: Supportive, the *drug of choice for treating HTN is an angiotensin-converting enzyme inhibitor (ACEI).*
- *Note*: These patients also tend to have *polycystic liver* and *Berry aneurysms*, so when you face a case in the USMLE about a patient with some form of congenital kidney disease who is presenting with subarachnoid bleeding, you know what to think!

Acute Renal Failure

- *Pre-renal*: e.g., Hypovolemia, congestive heart failure: *BUN/Cr ratio of more than 20* and *fractional excretion of sodium FeNa <1%.*
- *Renal*: e.g., Intravenous contrast, rhabdomyolysis or toxic drugs as aminoglycosides: *BUN/Cr <20* and *FeNa >2%. Urine shows epithelial or granular muddy casts indicating Acute Tubular Necrosis (ATN).*
- *Postrenal*: e.g., Obstructive uropathy. *Note that post-obstructive diuresis results in dilute and alkaline urine.*
- *Note*:

  1. ATN starts with an oliguric phase for 2–4 weeks, followed by polyuric phase (*Low serum Na and K*) and finally a post-diuretic phase.
  2. Rhabdomyolysis is diagnosed by elevated serum CPK (*In thousands*) and elevated urine myoglobin. Treatment: Fluids and bicarbonate drip.

Chronic Kidney Disease (CKD)

- *Causes*: Most common causes are *DM* and *HTN.*
- *Clinical picture*:

  1. Anemia, increased capillary fragility, platelet and lymphocyte dysfunction.
  2. GI: Nausea, vomiting and ammonia-like odor in the breath.
  3. CVS: Hypertension, cardiomyopathy and uremic pericarditis.
  4. Endocrine: Hypothyroidism, hypocalcemia and hyperkalemia.
  5. Renal osteodystrophy: Osteitis fibrosa cystica + Osteomalacia + osteoporosis.
  6. CNS: Motor, sensory and autonomic neuropathy.
  7. Skin: Itching, and earthy colored skin. Due to calcium deposition in skin.

8. Urine: Oliguria (<400 cc/day) or anuria (<100 cc/day), and low fixed urine specific gravity (Isothenuria).

- *Pathology*: Urine shows *waxy* casts.
- *Treatment*:

  1. Treat the cause, electrolyte and hormonal imbalance.
  2. Calcium replacement.
  3. Prepare the patient for hemodialysis once the glomerular filtration rate is *less than 15*. Peritoneal dialysis is not preferred due to high risk of infection and visceral injury.

Nephro- and Uretero-Lithiasis

- *Types*:

  1. The most common are *calcium oxalate stones* which *are radiopaque* and *recurrent*
  2. Magnesium ammonium phosphate (MAP) stones, a.k.a. *struvite* stones, are common in females with recurrent UTI secondary to urea-splitting organisms such as *Proteus mirabilis*.

- *Clinical picture*: Colicky flank pain radiating to the groin and inner thigh, dysuria and even *hematuria*.
- *Diagnosis*: Test of choice is *Spiral CT of the abdomen and pelvis*. Abdominal X-ray KUB view; however, shows most urinary stones. Refer to Fig. 1.22.

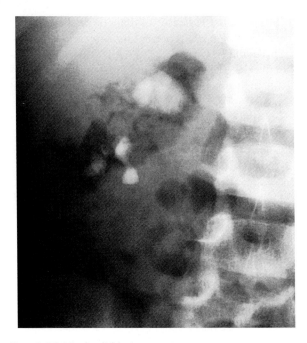

FIG. 1.22 Nephrolithiasis

- *Treatment*:

  1. Stone <4 mm: Increase fluid intake and stone will pass spontaneously.
  2. Stone >4 mm: Admit to the hospital and consult urology for extraction or extra-corporal shock wave lithotripsy (ESWL).
  3. Recurrent calcium stones are treated with *thiazide diuretics*.
  4. Recurrent oxalate stones are treated with *cholestyramine* (Oxalate chelator) and *magnesium citrate* (Decreases intestinal oxalate absorption).
  5. Alkalinization of the urine with $NaHCO_3$ is used to manage all types of stones, except for *phosphate stones* (Acidify urine with vitamin C).

- *Notes*:

  1. A stone in the uretro-vesical junction is the most common cause for ureteral dilatation.
  2. Uric acid stones are common after the use of uricosuric drugs or in case of tumor lysis syndrome. They are *radiolucent*.
  3. Cystine stones can form in *cystinuria*, which is screened for by nitroprusside test and treated with *penicillamine*.

Renal Tubular Acidosis (RTA)

- Refer to Table 1.7.

Renal Artery Stenosis (RAS)

- *Causes*: *Fibromuscular dysplasia in youngs*, and *atherosclerosis in elderly*.
- *Clinical picture*: Resistant hypokalemic hypertension.
- *On exam*: Continuous systolic *and* diastolic bruit on ausculatation to epigastrium.
- *Screening*: Captopril provocation test.
- *Diagnosis*: Gold standard is *angiography*, however practically we use Magnetic Resonance Angiography (MRA) or duplex ultrasound.
- *Treatment*: Significant stenosis is corrected by stent placement.
- *Notes*:

  1. ACEI is the drug of choice to control HTN in cases of *unilateral* RAS.
  2. ACEI are absolutely contraindicated in bilateral RAS, and in unilateral stenosis in one kidney when the other kidney absent or non-functioning.
  3. The kidney whose artery is stenosed is smaller in size compared to the healthy kidney.
  4. Renal vein of the stenosed side has *higher renin* level than the healthy side.

TABLE 1.7 Renal Tubular Acidosis (RTA).

Type	Mechanism	Acid base	Serum K	Urine pH
Type I (Distal)	Due to decreased H secretion in the distal tubules	Normal anion gap metabolic acidosis	Low	>5.5
Type II (Proximal)	Due to decreased HCO3 absorption in the proximal tubules	Normal anion gap metabolic acidosis	Low	<5.5
Type IV	Due to decreased cation exchange in the distal tubules, mostly due to low aldosterone level	Normal anion gap metabolic acidosis	High	<5.5

5. Fibromuscular dysplasia mainly affects the *media* of the blood vessel.

Urinary Incontinence

- *Introduction*: Pathological process, *even in the elderly*.
- *First step*: First thing to order in a patient with urinary incontinence is *urine analysis* to rule out infection.
- *Types*: Has 3 main types:

  1. *Urge incontinence*:

     - The *most common* form of incontinence.
     - Occurs mainly due to *detrusor overactivity*.
     - Treatment: Frequent, scheduled voiding and antimuscarinic medication, such as oxybutynin or imipramine.
     - Always ask about history of sexual abuse in these patients.

  2. *Stress incontinence*:

     - Occurs due to defect in the urinary outlet, whether a *sphincter problem* or *hypermobile bladder neck*.
     - Incontinence occurs with any increase in intraabdominal pressure, such as coughing or laughing.
     - Treatment: Pelvic floor exercises and topical steroids into the external meatus; also alpha blockers such as phentolamine.
     - In stress incontinence the flow rate, residual volume and bladder compliance are all *normal*.

  3. *Overflow incontinence*:

     - Occurs due to an obstruction (e.g., Benign prostatic hypertrophy) or anticholinergic medication overuse.
     - Normal urge to urinate is lost and small amounts of urine leak spontaneously on intermittent basis.
     - More common among elderly males.
     - Treatment: Identify and correct the underlying cause.

Neurogenic Bladder

- Refer to Table 1.8.

Drug-Induced Nephropathy

- *Acute renal failure*: Diuretics, antibiotics causing interstitial nephritis.
- *Chronic kidney disease*: Analgesics (Cause glutathione and prostaglandin depletion).
- *Nephrotic syndrome*: NSAIDs, Gold, Penicillamine.
- *ATN*: Aminoglycosides, IV contrast.

Nephrology Notes

- *Causes of hematuria*: SHITTT: *S*tones, *H*ematological disease, *I*nfection, *T*umor, *T*rauma, *T*reatment (Anticoagulants, Cyclophosphamide).
- *Blood Urea Nitrogen*: Not as specific as creatinine for the kidney function. BUN is elevated in upper GI bleeding, steroids or after a high protein diet.
- *DM*: The first indicator of diabetic nephropathy is *microalbuminuria* representing *glomerulosclerosis*. This could be treated by *ACEI*. If you see a patient in the USMLE on ACEI and urine microalbumin is still high, increase the ACEI dose. If the patient

TABLE 1.8 Neurogenic bladder.

	Spastic neurogenic bladder	Atonic neurogenic bladder
Lesion	Upper motor neuron lesion	Lower motor neuron lesion
Bladder wall	Thick	Thin and dilated
Detrusor muscle	Hyperreflexic	Hyporeflexic
Symptoms	Urinary frequency and urgency	Overflow incontinence
Treatment	Antimuscarinic medications + Urinary catheterization	Treat the cause, e.g., spinal cord injury + Urinary catheterization

cannot tolerate the ACEI (*e.g., due to cough caused by bradykinins accumulation in the lungs*), switch to Angiotensin Receptor Blocker (ARB).

- *Bartter syndrome*: Also known as *Juxta-glomerular hyperplasia*. There is resistance to angiotensin, accordingly, hyponatremia ensues. The low Na stimulates the renin-angiotensin-aldosterone system which leads to hypokalemia. Treatment: Prostaglandin blockage, e.g., Indomethacin. (PG stimulates renin).
- *Urethral Diverticulum*: Suspect it in any female patient presenting with a (DDD) triad: *D*ysuria, *D*ribbling and *D*yspareunia.
- *Indications of urgent hemodialysis*: Fluid overload, resistant hyperkalemia, resistant metabolic acidosis and uremic pericarditis.

Rheumatology

Rheumatoid Arthritis

- *Mechanism*: Immunologically mediated *T lymphocyte* inflammatory synovitis. Linkage to *HLA-DR4* has been suggested.
- *Clinical picture*:

  1. *Symmetrical small joint* pains: Mainly metacarpophalengeal (MCP) and proximal interphalengeal (PIP), *never the distal ones*.
  2. *Morning stiffness for at least 1 h*, that gets better towards the end of the day (Osteoarthritis gets worse with exercise; not better).
  3. Systemic: Serositis, fever, pulmonary rheumatoid nodules.

- *Diagnostic criteria* (*At least 4 criteria for at least 6 weeks duration*):

  1. Morning stiffness for *at least 1 h*.
  2. Symmetrical involvement of joints.
  3. Arthritis of 3 or more joints.
  4. Arthritis of the hand joints.
  5. Positive Rheumatoid factor.
  6. Rheumatoid nodules.
  7. X-ray changes, e.g., Erosions, Loss of joint space.

- *Complications*:

  1. Joint deformities: *Ulnar deviation* and *Swan neck deformity*. Refer to Fig. 1.23.
  2. Joint sublaxation: Most dangerous is *atlanto-axial joint*. So when you get a patient with RA in the USMLE having any neurological issues in his neck or upper extremities, you know what to think!

- *Diagnosis*:

  1. Positive rheumatoid factor (RF): An *IgM* directed against serum *IgG*.
  2. Positive *antineutrophil cytoplasmic antibody (ANA)* and *anti-cyclic citrullinated peptide antibody (Anti-CCP)*.
  3. Low *synovial complement* with normal serum complement levels.

- *Treatment*:

  1. NSAIDs, e.g., *acetaminophen, phenacetin, salicylates* and *indomethacin*.
  2. Steroids: Provide relief and may slow the progression of the disease.
  3. Anti-Tumor Necrosis Factor (TNF): e.g., Infliximab, Adalimumab and Etanercept. Side effects: Overwhelming infections, so *annual PPD is necessary*.
  4. Disease modifying anti-rheumatoid drugs (DMARDs): Now the first line of therapy once there is any X-ray changes in the joint:

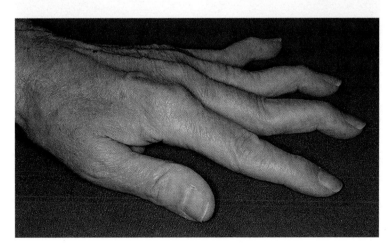

Fɪɢ. 1.23 Swan neck deformity

- Methotrexate: *Immunosuppressant and folic acid antagonist.* Side effects: *Bone marrow depression* and *elevated liver enzymes.*
- Hydroxychloroquine: *Antimalarial drug that acts by stabilizing the lysosomes.* Side effects: *R*etinopathy, *R*enal failure and hemolysis in G6PD deficiency.
- Sulfasalazine: Works through the *sulfapyridine* portion, *whereas in inflammatory bowel disease it works through the 5-aminosalicylic portion.* Side effects: *Reversible infertility in males.*
- Gold salts: Taken up by macrophages and lysosomes and *stop bone destruction.* Side effects: Rash and stomatitis. Antagonist: *Dimercaprol.*
- Penicillamine: *Analogue of cysteine.* Also used in *Wilson disease as a copper chelator.*

- *Notes:*

  1. *Psoriatic arthritis:* Occurs in patients with psoriasis; is characterized by *DIP involvement* (Sausage digits) and (*Pencil in cup appearance*) on hands X-ray.
  2. *Sjogren syndrome:* A subtype of RA in which patients have arthritis plus *dry secretions,* i.e., Dry eyes, dry mouth, etc. Diagnosis: Anti-Ro (Anti-SSA), anti-La Anti-SSB and anti-salivary duct antibodies. Complication: Lymphoma.
  3. *Juvenile rheumatoid arthritis:* Occurs in children and is associated with fever, rash, irido-cyclitis, pericarditis and negative RF. Treatment: NSAIDs.
  4. *Felty syndrome:* RA + Hypersplenism due to lymphocyte infiltration. Suspect it when you see

a patient in the USMLE with RA and pancytopenia.

Osteoarthritis

- *Mechanism: Wear and tear*
- *Clinical picture:*

  1. Morning stiffness: *Lasts less than 30 min.*
  2. Arthritis gets *worse* by exercise towards the end of the day.
  3. The distal interphalengeal joints (DIP) *are commonly involved* here.
  4. Deformities: Proximal interphalengeal joints can swell up and form *Bouchard* nodes, while the DIP can form *Heberden* nodes (*Genetically determined*).

- *Diagnosis:* X-ray of joints shows *subchondral bone formation* and *osteophytes.*
- *Treatment:* Physical therapy, NSAIDs, glucosamine and chondroitin sulfate.

Systemic Lupus Erythematosus (SLE)

- *Introduction:* A systemic connective tissue disease, mainly in females (*F:M = 9:1*). It is more common in females due to alleles existing on *class II MHC.*
- *Clinical picture:*

  1. Photosensitivity and rash: Could be discoid or the famous *butterfly malar rash.* Refer to Fig. 1.24.
  2. Painless oral ulcers.

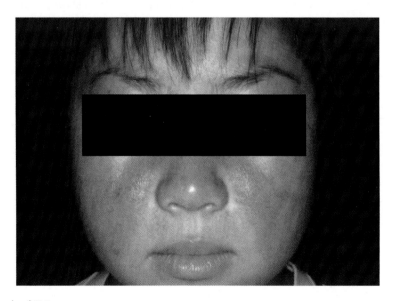

FIG. 1.24 Butterfly rash of SLE

3. -itis: Serositis, arthritis and *wire loop glomerulo-nephritis due to immune complex deposition*.
4. *Anemia, lymphopenia and thrombocytopenia (RA does not cause that!)*.

- *Complications*:

  1. *Libman Sacks endocarditis*, where vegetations *do not embolize*.
  2. Lupus nephritis: It has 5 types; the most aggressive is type IV (Diffuse proliferative GN). Treatment: Steroids + Cyclophosphamide.

- *Diagnosis*:

  1. Positive ANA, *anti-double stranded DNA antibodies (dsDNA)* and *anti-smith antibodies*.
  2. Low serum complement factors *C3* and *C4*.
  3. *False positive work up for syphilis*, e.g., VDRL and RPR.

- *Notes*:

  1. Markers of SLE activity: *Elevated ESR and CRP*, and *low C3 and C4*.
  2. Most common cardiac manifestation of SLE is *pericarditis*.
  3. Most specific ocular manifestation of SLE is *retinal cytoid bodies*.
  4. Drugs, e.g., INH, Hydralazine and Procainamide can cause lupus-like syndrome, and is diagnosed by *positive anti-histone antibodies*.
  5. Neonatal lupus can cause *heart block* and is diagnosed by positive *anti-Ro* antibodies, so keep your eyes open in the USMLE for this neonate with heart block whose mother has been having this weird rash and joint pains.
  6. Kidney biopsy in lupus nephritis shows *C3* and *fibrinogen* deposits.

- *Treatment*: NSAIDs and steroids.

Polyarteritis Nodosa (P.A.N.)

- *Mechanism*: Necrotizing vasculitis affecting *medium sized vessels*, causing *fibrinoid necrosis* and *tiny aneurysms* formation.
- *Causes*: Multiple, most common being *hepatitis B* infection.
- *Clinical picture*:

  1. Skin: Purpura and skin ulcers.
  2. Joints: Arthralgias and arthritis.
  3. Renal: Renal hypertension due to involvement of *arcuate artery*, and *crescentic necrotizing glomerulonephritis*.
  4. CVS: Coronary artery disease (CAD).
  5. CNS: Cerebrovascular accidents (CVA).

- *Diagnosis*: Kidney biopsy and positive *P-ANCA*.
- *Treatment*: Steroids.
- *Note*:

  1. Suspect P.A.N. if you see a *young patient* in the USMLE with *hepatitis B* and multiple elderly diseases (CAD, CVA, Renal failure).
  2. Churg Strauss vasculitis is another necrotizing vasculitis characterized by AAA: *A*sthma, *A*llergic rhinitis and eosinophili*A*.

Ankylosing Spondylitis

- *Mechanism*: Inflammatory arthropathy that is linked to *HLA-B27, usually following a prostate infection especially with Klebsiella*.
- *Clinical picture*: Back pain due to sacroiliitis, uveitis and *pulmonary fibrosis*.
- *X-ray of the back*: Bamboo spine.
- *P.S.*: If you hear a murmur in this patient, it is mostly a diastolic murmur for *aortic regurgitation*.
- *Treatment*: Similar to RA.

Reiter's Syndrome

- *Mechanism*: Rheumatologic disease that follows *non-gonococcal infections*.
- *Clinical picture*: Uveitis, *circinate balanitis* and big joint fleeting *arthritis*.
- *Diagnosis*: Elevated ESR, negative rheumatoid factor and positive HLA-B27.
- *Notes*:

  1. These patients might also have *aortic regurgitation murmur* and *lung fibrosis*.
  2. Reactive arthritis: Common after infection with salmonella, shigella, campylobacter, gonococci and chlamydia. It affects big joints, is fleeting in nature and associated with tenosynovitis, e.g., DeQuervain tenosynovitis.

Temporal Arteritis

- *Mechanism: Giant cell vasculitis* that mainly affects the elderly.
- *Clinical picture*:

  1. *Temporal headache* with *tender, palpable and pulseless* temporal artery.
  2. *Jaw claudications, especially upon eating*.

- *Complications: Blindness* due to *ischemic optic neuropathy* secondary to the involvement of *posterior ciliary branches of ophthalmic artery*.

- *Diagnosis*: *Elevated ESR* (>40 mm/hour). *Temporal artery biopsy* shows infiltration with *plasma cells* and *giant macrophages*.
- *Treatment*: High dose systemic steroids is the first next step (*Even before the biopsy*)

Wegener Granulomatosis

- *Mechanism*: *Focal necrotizing vasculitis* and *granuloma* formation.
- *Clinical picture*:

  1. Upper airway involvement, e.g., Sinusitis, epistaxis and saddle nose.
  2. Lower airway involvement, e.g., Cough, hemoptysis and lung cavitation.
  3. Renal involvement, e.g., Proteinuria and hematuria.

- *Diagnosis*: Positive anti-neutrophil cytoplasmic antibodies (*C-ANCA*).
- *Treatment*: Steroids and Cyclophosphamide.
- *Note*: *Goodpasteure's syndrome is a type II hypersensitivity disease that involves anti-glomerular basement membrane antibodies causing HH; Hematuria and Hemoptysis.*

Takayasau Disease

- *Mechanism*: Vasculitis affecting the big vessels, e.g., aorta and its major branches.
- *Clinical picture*: *Decreased pulse on one extremity* plus claudications.
- *Diagnosis*: Angiography.
- *Treatment*: Steroids.
- *Note*: Do not confuse this with Kawasaki disease, where patients have *mucocutaneous lesions, cervical lymphadenopathy and aneurysms of the coronary arteries*. Treatment here is *aspirin and immunoglobulin therapy*.

Behcet Syndrome

- *Clinical picture*: Disease of unknown etiology causing three major *recurrent* symptoms: *Recurrent* iritis, *Recurrent* painful oral ulcers and *Recurrent* painful genital ulcers.
- *Treatment*: Steroids.

Dermatomyositis

- *Mechanism*: Immune mediated infiltration of the connective tissue with inflammatory cells.
- *Clinical picture*:

1. Dermato-: *Heliotrope eyelids* (Purple rash) and *Gottron papules* over metacarpophalengeal and proximal interphalengeal joints. *Gottron papules is the most specific sign of Dermatomyositis.*
2. -myositis: Proximal bilateral symmetrical muscle weakness and tenderness.
3. Others: Arthralgia, cardiomyopathy and *malignancy*. If you see a patient in the USMLE with muscle pains, rash described above and any kind of cancer, think of dermatomyositis.

- *Diagnosis*: Elevated CPK, EMG and muscle biopsy are diagnostic.
- *Treatment*: Steroids, plus careful malignancy screening.
- *Notes*:

1. Polymyositis could exist alone, and is diagnosed by high *anti-Jo-1* antibodies.
2. Dermatomyositis is well known to be highly associated with malignancy, so when you see any patient with this disease, *you must screen him/her for malignancy.*

Gout and Pseudogout

Introduction

- Normally, 2/3 of the uric acid is excreted by the kidneys and 1/3 by GI tract.
- Hypouricemia can occur in pregnancy and in patients with Fanconi syndrome (Glucosuria, aminoaciduria, phosphaturia and uricosuria).

Gout

- *Mechanism*: Deposition of *monosodium urate* crystals. This could be idiopathic or secondary, e.g., Lesch Nyhan syndrome (Rypoxanthine guanine phosphoribosyl transferase enzyme "HGPRT" deficiency) or renal failure.
- *Clinical picture*:

1. Arthritis is an *asymmetrical*, painful, warm joints. The first metatarsophalangeal joint is a classic site, a.k.a. *Podagra*.
2. Chronic cases are associated with formation of *tophi* and renal failure.

- *Diagnosis*:

1. Joint aspiration showing *needle shaped strongly negative birefringent crystals*.
2. Serum uric acid more than 7 mg%. *Joint aspiration remains the test of choice.*

- *Prevention*: Low purine diet and avoidance of alcohol.

- *Treatment of acute gout*: Treatment of choice is *oral indomethacin*. You can also use Colchicine; It depolymerizes tubulin and decreases leukocyte entry into the cells. Side effects of colchicine are *diarrhea and GI upset*. *Long term use may cause aplastic anemia.*
- *Treatment of chronic gout*:

  1. *Allopurinol*: Converts inside the body to *Alloxanthine* which *inhibits xanthine oxidase*. Xanthine oxidase typically regulates the conversion of hypoxanthine to xanthine, and the conversion of xanthine to uric acid. Indications: *High serum* plus *high urinary* uric acid levels.
  2. *Probenecid*: *Blocks uric acid reabsorption* in proximal convoluted tubule. Indications: *High serum* plus *low urinary* uric acid level. Sulfinpyrazone is another drug that acts exactly like Probenecid.

Pseudogout

- *Mechanism*: Deposition of *calcium pyrophosphate*.
- *Clinical picture*: Same as gout.
- *Diagnosis*: Joint aspiration. Crystals are *rhomboid shaped with weakly positive birefringence*.
- *Treatment*: NSAIDs.

Scleroderma

- *Limited*: CREST: *C*alcinosis of the skin, *R*aynaud phenomenon, *E*sophageal diverticulae and dysmotility, *S*clerodactyly and *T*elangiectasis.
- *Diffuse*: Involves all systems.
- *Diagnosis*: Positive *Anti-Scl 70* and *Anticentromere antibodies*.
- *Treatment*: Supportive.
- *Notes*:

  1. *Suspect it in the USMLE when you see a patient with shiny tight skin and bad uncontrollable GERD and dysphagia.*
  2. Scleroderma renal crisis: If you see a patient in the USMLE with scleroderma and renal failure, *ACEI* is the treatment of choice.

Polymyalgia Rheumatica

- *Mechanism*: Giant cell vasculitis.
- *Clinical picture*: Disease of the elderly, who present with early morning pain and *stiffness of shoulders and hips*.
- *Diagnosis*: Elevated ESR (>40 mm/hour).
- *Treatment*: Steroids.

Osteoporosis and Osteomalacia

- *Osteoporosis*: Loss of bone mass, with the remaining bone being of normal density. Could be postmenopausal (type 1) or senile (type 2), and puts the patients at risk of fractures, e.g., Compression vertebral fracture, fracture neck of femur. *These patients have normal serum calcium and alkaline phosphatase.*
- *Osteomalacia*: Normal bone mass, but the bone density is significantly decreased. *These patients have low serum calcium and high alkaline phosphatase. Bone X-ray in these patients shows pseudofractures (Looser's zones).*
- *Diagnosis*: Dual Energy X-ray Absorptiometry (DEXA scan).
- *Treatment*: Calcium and vitamin D, Calcitonin and Bisphosphonates *which act by inhibiting the osteoclasts,* e.g., Alendronate.
- *Note*:

  1. Smoking and alcohol increase the risk of osteoporosis *twofold*.
  2. Most common side effect of Bisphosphonates is *Erosive esophagitis*.
  3. Raloxifen is a Selective Estrogen Receptor Modulator (SERM) that acts like estrogen on bones (*Prevents osteoporosis*), and acts as an estrogen blocker on breast and endometrium (Decreases risk of cancer). Ideal for *postmenopausal*.
  4. Osteopetrosis: Occurs due to *defective osteoclasts*. Patient presents with *bone fractures and facial nerve palsy*. Treatment: Steroids, and low calcium diet.

Paget's Disease of the Bone

- *Mechanism*: Rapid bone turnover, mostly due to infection, e.g., Paramyxovirus.
- *Clinical picture*: Presents in the USMLE with a patient having frequent bone fractures and deformities, and his *hat recently does not fit anymore* (Due to frontal bossing).
- *Diagnosis*:

  1. X-ray of bones: Thick bone cortex and trabeculae.
  2. High *serum alkaline phosphatase* and *urinary hydroxyproline*, everything else is within normal limits.

- *Treatment*: Bisphosphonates, e.g., Alendronate.

Septic Arthritis

- *Causes*: Staphylococci (*Most common*), Streptococci or H. Influenza B.

- *Clinical picture*: Red, warm, tender and swollen joint.
- *Diagnosis*:

    1. Arthrocentesis should be the first next step.
    2. High WBC in serum and synovial fluid, elevated ESR and CRP.

- *Treatment*: Arthrocentesis and systemic antibiotics.

Fibromyalgia

- *Introduction and clinical picture*: Syndrome of unclear etiology, with pain and tenderness in at *least 11 out of the following 9 × 2 = 18 points* (*all bilaterally*):

    1. Occiput: At insertion site of suboccipital muscles.
    2. Lower neck: At the level of C7.
    3. Trapezius muscle: In the middle of superior border of the muscle.
    4. Supraspinatus muscle: On the mid scapular region.
    5. 2nd rib: At the costo-chondral junction.
    6. Lateral epicondyle: Just distal to it.
    7. Upper outer quadrants of the buttocks.
    8. Greater trochanters.
    9. Knees: On the medial aspect just proximal to the joint.

- *Treatment*: TCAs or SSRI. Recently, drug of choice is *Duloxetine*.

Cardiovascular System

Introduction

- *Arteries*: Contain stressed volume of the circulation, and *arterioles is where there is maximal resistance to blood flow*.

- *Veins*: Contain the non-stressed volume of the circulation, and *most of our blood is contained within the venous system*.
- *Capillaries*: Have the largest surface area of the entire vascular system, and blood flow through them is regulated by *pre-capillary sphincters*.
- *The lower the surface area of a blood vessel, the faster the blood flow*, i.e., Capillary blood flow is very slow due to the large surface area.
- Adding resistance in parallel *decreases the peripheral resistance*, and *increases blood flow*.
- Turbulence is highest in big vessels with high blood velocity, e.g., Aorta.
- *Local autoregulation*: Done by the heart, brain and muscles. The most important vasodilator of cerebral circulation is CO_2.
- *Active Hyperemia*: Blood flow to organs is *directly proportional* to its metabolic activity.
- *Reactive hyperemia*: Increased blood flow to an organ after temporary occlusion of its circulation.
- *Pulse pressure*: Difference between systolic and diastolic blood pressure; determined by *stroke volume* and compliance of large arteries; that is the reason atherosclerosis causes wide pulse pressure.

Electrocardiogram Waves (Refer to Fig. 1.25)

- *P wave*: Atrial depolarization.
- *P-R interval*: Atrio-ventricular conduction.
- *QRS*: Ventricular depolarization.
- *S-T interval*: Isoelectric.
- *T wave*: Ventricular repolarization.
- *Notes*: Conduction a.k.a. Dromotropism is *fastest in purkinje fibers*, and is *slowest across the AV node*.

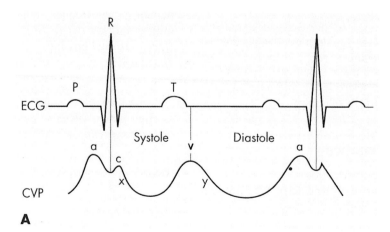

FIG. 1.25 Normal EKG and jugular vein waves

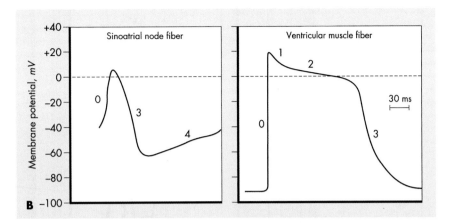

FIG. 1.26 Action potential of SA and purkinje

Action Potentials

Action Potential of Purkinje Fiber (Refer to Fig. 1.26)

- *Phase 0* (Depolarization): Due to *Na influx*. Inhibited by *Quinidine*.
- *Phase 1* (Partial repolarization): Due to *K efflux*.
- *Phase 2* (Plateau): Due to *K efflux* and *Ca influx*.
- *Phase 3* (Repolarization): Due to *K efflux*.
- *Phase 4* (Forward current): Due to *Na influx*.

Action Potential of Sinoatrial Node (Pacemaker) (Refer to Fig. 1.26)

- *Stage 4*: Mediated by *Na influx*.
- *Stage 0*: Mediated by *Ca influx*.
- *Stage 3*: Mediated by *K efflux*.

Cardiac Cycle (refer to Figs. 1.27 and 1.28)

- The following few points show how changing certain variables can shift the cardiac cycle curve shown on Fig. 1.28.
- *Increased Preload*, i.e., Venous return causes *right shift* of curve.
- *Increased Afterload*, i.e., Peripheral resistance causes *upward shift* of curve.
- *Increased Contractility*, i.e., Inotropy causes *left shift* of curve.
- *Note*: Preload = EDV, and Afterload = Diastolic BP.

Heart Sounds

- *S1*: Due to closure of AV valves, i.e., mitral and tricuspid.
- *S2*: Due to closure of semilunar valves, i.e., Aortic and pulmonary.

- *S3*: Due to ventricular filling. *Prominent in CHF*.
- *S4*: Due to high atrial pressure caused by atrial contraction. *Prominent in ventricular diastolic dysfunction*.

Heart Murmurs

- *Aortic stenosis*: Systolic *ejection diamond shaped* murmur on the base, *radiating to the carotids*.
- *Aortic regurgitation*: *Blowing diastolic* murmur on base, along with *wide pulse pressure, water hammer pulse and strong carotid and capillary pulsations*.
- *Mitral stenosis*: *Diastolic rumbling* murmur on the apex with *opening snap*.
- *Mitral regurgitation*: *Pansystolic murmur on the apex*.
- *Mitral prolapse*: *Midsystolic click* with *late systolic* murmur.
- *Notes*:

  1. *Mitral stenosis murmur that changes with position in a female patient who also has positional syncope are signs of left atrial myxoma*.
  2. Most common cause of valve lesions is *wear and tear*.
  3. *Valve replacement is done using tissue valves in elderly (Side effect: Calcification), and mechanical valves otherwise (Side effect: Thrombosis and hemolysis). Only patients with mechanical valves require life long anticoagulation with warfarin to a target INR of 2.5–3.5*.

Jugular Vein Waves (refer to Fig. 1.25)

- *A*: Due to atrial contraction.
- *C*: Due to right ventricle contraction, causing mitral bulge inside the atrium.
- *V*: Due to high atrial pressure.

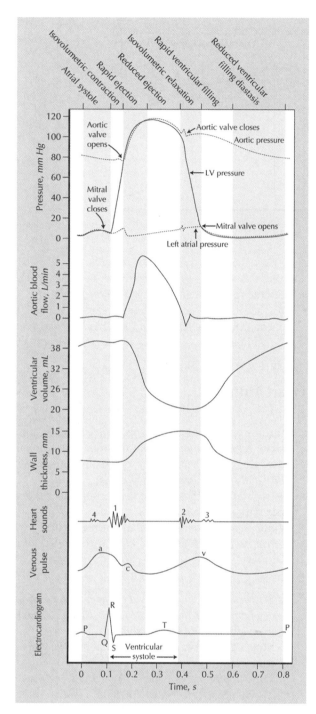

FIG. 1.27 Cardiac cycle

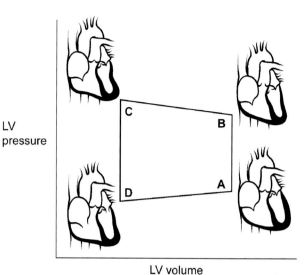

FIG. 1.28 Cardiac cycle.
A–B: Isovolumetric contraction phase.
B: Aortic and pulmonary valves open.
B–C: Ventricular ejection phase, i.e., Stroke volume.
C: Aortic and pulmonary valves close.
C–D: Isovolumetric relaxation phase.
D: AV valves open.
D–A: Ventricular filling phase.
A: AV valves close

- *Ejection Fraction (EF)* = SV/EDV = >50%.
- *Cardiac output (CO)* = Stroke Volume (SV) × Heart Rate (HR).
- *Fick equation*: CO = Rate of oxygen consumption/ Difference between arterial and venous oxygen contents.
- *Mean arterial pressure* = CO × Peripheral resistance (PR).

Hypertension

- *Definition*: Persistently elevated blood pressure beyond *140/90 on at least 3 separate occasions*.
- *Types*: Hypertension could be only *systolic,* e.g., thyrotoxicosis, *diastolic,* or *both*.
- *Cause*: HTN could be idiopathic (*essential*) or secondary to a cause, e.g., Pheochromocytoma, Hyperaldosteronism, Renal artery stenosis.
- *Physiology*: Blood pressure is controlled by baroreceptors in *aortic arch* and *carotid sinus*, signaling the CNS via *vagus* and *glossopharyngeal* nerves respectively.
- *Clinical picture*: Headache, blurry vision, nausea and vomiting.
- *Complications of HTN*: Left ventricular hypertrophy, CAD, CVA (Mostly Basal ganglia), Renal failure, Copper wiring and A-V nicking of retinal vessels.
- *Treatment*: Classes listed below in details.

- *Y descent*: Drop in atrial pressure during ventricular filling.
- *X descent*: Ventricular ejection phase.

Important Equations

- *Stroke volume* = End Diastolic Volume (EDV) – End Systolic Volume (ESV).

1. Diuretics

Hydrochlorothiazide

- *HCTZ is recommended as the first line of therapy for any HTN patient.*
- *Mechanism*:

  1. Decreases NaCl absorption at the level of distal convoluted tubules.
  2. Vasodilation through release of prostaglandins. This leads to a decrease in peripheral resistance (PR) and cardiac output (CO). *Note that blood pressure = CO × PR.*

- *Indications*:

  1. CVS: Hypertension, CHF.
  2. Renal: Nephrogenic diabetes insipidus. Metalo-zone is used in nephrotic syndrome.

- *Side effects*:

  1. *2 Hypos*: Hypotension and hypokalemia.
  2. *3 Hypers*: Hypercalcaemia, hyperuricemia and hyperglycemia.

- *Contraindications*: Severe recurrent gout attacks and hypercalcaemia.
- Beside HCTZ, other thiazides include Chlorthalidone and Indapamide.

Furosemide

- *Mechanism*: Loop diuretic that acts by inhibiting Na/K/2 Cl cotransport at the level of thick ascending limb of loop of Henle.
- *Indications*:

  1. Urgent HTN and fluid overload situations, e.g., Pulmonary edema.
  2. Hypercalcaemia.

- *Side effects*: *Ototoxicity, Nephrotoxicity,* Hypocalcemia and Hypokalemia.
- *Note: Bumetanide and Torsemide are stronger loop diuretics.*

K Sparing Diuretics

1. *Spironolactone*:

   - K sparing, *anti-aldosterone* diuretic that acts via *canrenone.*
   - Indications: *HTN secondary to hyperaldosteronism,* and *CHF.*
   - Side effects: *Gynecomastia* and hyperkalemia.

2. *Amiloride and Triametrene*:

   - Act by *blocking Na channels in collecting ducts.*
   - Side effects: Leg cramps and hyperkalemia.

Carbonic Anhydrase Inhibitors

- *Mechanism*: Inhibit reabsorption of HCO_3 in the proximal convoluted tubules. The result is *hyperchloremic metabolic acidosis with alkaline urine.*
- *Indications*:

  1. Open angle glaucoma.
  2. *Mountain sickness syndrome* (Cerebral and pulmonary edema and nausea).

- Examples: Acetazolamide aka *Diamox.*

2. Centrally acting medications

Alpha Methyl Dopa

- *Mechanism*: Decreases sympathetic outflow from the CNS.
- *Indication*: Hypertension during pregnancy.

Clonidine

- *Mechanism*: Decreases sympathetic outflow from the CNS.
- *Side effects*: Fluid retention.
- *Precautions*: Sudden stoppage leads to *rebound hypertension.*

3. Vasodilators

- *Hydralazine*: Also used in CHF. Side effects: Reflex tachycardia and lupus-like syndrome.
- *Minoxidil*: Notorious side effect is *hypertrichiosis.*
- *Sodium nitroprusside*: Used as a drip in hypertensive emergencies. Major side effect is *cyanide poisoning* which is treated by *nitrates and thiosulfate.*

4. Calcium Channel Blockers (CCB)

Nifedipine

- *Mechanism*: Coronary and peripheral vasodilator. *Does not have any inotropic or chronotropic actions.*
- *Side effects*: Hypotension, flushing and headache.

Verapamil

- *Mechanism*: Negative inotropy and chronotropy. *Its effects on the coronary arteries is very mild.*
- *Side effects*: *Constipation* and *increase risk of digoxin toxicity.*

Diltiazem

- *Mechanism*: Vasodilator, negative inotropy and chronotropy.
- *Indications*: Anti-angina, and rate control in arrhythmias, e.g., Atrial Fibrillation.
- *Note: Nifedipine causes reflex tachycardia, while verapamil and diltiazem cause bradycardia.*

5. Alpha blockers

Phenoxybenzamine

- *Introduction*: *Non-competitive irreversible* alpha blocker.
- *Mechanism*: Antagonizes the effect of epinephrine and NE on blood pressure.
- *Indications*: Treatment of hypertension secondary to pheochromocytoma.
- *Side effects*: Hypotension and tachycardia.
- *Contraindications*: Coronary artery disease.
- Phentolamine is another *reversible* alpha blocker used to *diagnose pheochromocytoma.*

Prazosin, Terazosin and Doxazosin

- Metabolites pass in the urine, except *doxazosin's which pass in stools.*
- *Indications*: Hypertension and benign prostatic hypertrophy.
- *Side effects*: Hypotension known as *first dose syncope*. Prevented by starting the patient on *only third of the dose and increasing it gradually*, also make sure that the patient *takes the pill at bedtime.*

Yohimbine

- Alpha-2 antagonist used to treat impotence.

6. ACEI and ARBs: Discussed later.

7. Beta Blockers: Discussed later.

- *Hypertensive encephalopathy*: Sudden marked elevation of blood pressure leading to neurological manifestations and loss of consciousness due to brain edema. Treatment: Sodium nitroprusside to control blood pressure rapidly.
- *Drugs of choice*: Again, remember that HCTZ is the drug of choice to start in any patient with HTN, except for the following particular scenarios:

  1. HTN plus DM: ACEI or ARB to delay progression of diabetic nephropathy.
  2. HTN plus severe COPD or asthma: Calcium channel blocker.

  3. HTN in African Americans: Diuretics or calcium channel blockers.
  4. HTN in elderly: Diuretics or calcium channel blockers.
  5. HTN in pregnancy: Alpha methyl dopa or Hydralazine.
  6. HTN 2ry to Hyperaldosteronism: Spironolactone.

Congestive Heart Failure (CHF)

- *Mechanism*: Failure of the heart to pump out enough blood.
- *Starling's law*: Force of contraction is directly proportional to length of muscle fiber, until a certain limit, at which muscles undergo dilatation and failure.
- *Types*:

  1. Systolic: Low EF. Caused by myocardial infarction, alcohol and illicit drugs.
  2. Diastolic: Normal EF and decreased ventricular compliance. Caused by long-standing hypertension and is characterized by S4.
  3. High output CHF, e.g., Thyrotoxicosis.
  4. Low output CHF: Most cases of CHF fall in this category.

- *Clinical picture*: Refer to Table 1.9.
- *Diagnosis*:

  1. Clinical picture.
  2. *CXR: Butterfly shaped pulmonary venous congestion* on chest X ray + *Kerley A and B* lines. Refer to Fig. 1.29.
  3. EF <50% on echocardiogram.

TABLE 1.9 Congestive heart failure.

	Left ventricular failure	Right ventricular failure
Symptoms	• Dyspnea • Orthopnea • Paroxysmal Nocturnal Dyspnea (P.N.D.) • Frothy blood tinged sputum	• Lower extremities edema • Right hypochondrial pain due to liver congestion
Signs	• Bilateral basal crackles • Pulsus alternans • S3 gallop	• Jugular venous distension • Hepatomegaly • +ve Hepatojugular reflux • Pitting edema of lower extremities • Pulsus paradoxus • S3 gallop

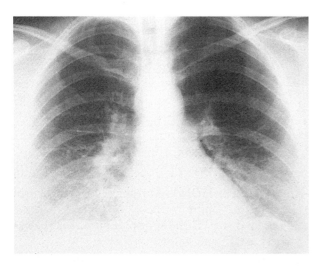

FIG. 1.29 Pulmonary edema and Kerley B lines in CHF

4. Elevated serum B-Type Natriuretic Peptide (BNP) *above 400 pg*, due to stretch of ventricles.

- *Treatment*: Heart failure is treated by 4 classes of medications, as follows:

1. Diuretics

- Low cardiac output leads to decreased renal blood flow, which leads to stimulation of the renin angiotensin aldosterone system, and ultimately salt and water retention.
- Examples: *Furosemide, Hydrochlorothiazide.*
- Spironolactone is a *K-sparing anti-aldosterone* diuretic that is beneficial in *severe* CHF, and has been proven to *reduce morbidity and mortality.*

2. Vasodilators

- *Venodilation leads to decreased pre-load*, while *arteriodilation leads to decreased after-load.*

Angiotensin Converting Enzyme Inhibitors (ACEI)

- *Mechanism*:

  1. Prevent conversion of angiotensin I to angiotensin II. This leads to inhibition of aldosterone formation, and decreases preload and afterload.
  2. ACEI has also been proven to *decrease remodeling of the myocardium* and to *delay progression of diabetic nephropathy.*

- *Side effects*:

  1. Hypotension.
  2. Hyperkalemia and elevated creatinine.

3. Dry cough: Due to accumulation of *bradykinins* in the lungs. If this occurs, you can switch the patient to *angiotensin receptor blockers (ARBs)*.
4. Angioedema: More common in *African Americans.*

- *Contraindications: Bilateral renal artery stenosis. ACEI is the drug of choice to treat HTN in patients with unilateral RAS.*
- *Examples of ACEI: Enalapril, Lisinopril, Captopril.*
- *Examples of ARBs: Losartan, Irbesartan.*

Smooth Muscle Relaxants

- *Hydralazine and nitrates* used in combination have been proven to be beneficial for *african american* patients with CHF.

3. Inotropics

Digoxin

- *Mechanism: Inhibits Na-K ATPase*, which leads to increased intracellular Na and Ca. This leads to increase myocardial contractility.
- *Indications*:

  1. *Left sided systolic dysfunction (not right and not diastolic).*
  2. Arrhythmia: Decreases conduction velocity in A-V node.

- *Bioavailability of oral digoxin*: 50–75%.
- *Side effects*: Bradycardia and Gynecomastia.
- *Elimination*: Excreted in the urine.
- *Toxicity*: Hypokalemia, nausea and vomiting, *yellow vision* and haloes.
- Toxicity risk is increased in the presence of *hypokalemia, hypomagnesemia, hypercalcemia, diuretics or quinidine.*
- *Treatment of toxicity: Potassium* and *digoxin binding* fragments (*Digibind*).
- *Digitoxin*: Has longer half life and more affinity, and is excreted in *bile*.
- *Note*: Digoxin and digitoxin have been proven to decrease the frequency and duration of hospitalization secondary to CHF; however *they do not decrease mortality.*

Phosphodiestrase Inhibitors

- *Mechanism*:

  1. Inhibit phosphodiestrase enzyme, which in turn leads to increased cAMP. cAMP activates Ca channels by phosphorylation, leading to Ca influx.
  2. Inodilators: These drugs act as vasodilators and inotropics.

- *Examples*: *Amrinone, Milrinone.*

4. Beta blockers

- *Mechanism*:

  1. Negative inotropic and negative chronotropic action, leading to decreased myocardial oxygen consumption.
  2. Block the renin-angiotensin aldosterone system.

- They have been proven in many studies to significantly *decrease morbidity and mortality secondary to CHF and coronary artery disease (CAD)*.
- *Side effects*: Bradycardia, Hypotension, sexual dysfunction and fatigue.
- *Contraindications*:

  1. Vasospastic (Prinzmetal) angina: Allows unopposed vasoconstrictor alpha action.
  2. Diabetes mellitus (Relative contraindication): Masks the signs of hypoglycemia. Besides, can cause fasting hypoglycemia by inhibiting glycogenolysis.
  3. Severe asthma and COPD (Relative contraindication): Might worsen the bronchospasm.

- *Precautions*: Sudden stoppage leads to rebound tachycardia and arrhythmia.
- *Examples: Carvedilol, Metoprolol.*

Atherosclerosis

- *Introduction*: Disease of the *large* and *mid-sized* arteries.
- *Predisposing factors*: Smoking, old age and DM.
- *Complications*: Myocardial infarction (MI), Cerebrovascular accidents (CVA).
- *Pathology*: Starts with *fatty streaks* and *foam cell* formation (Where macrophages phagocytose oxidized LDL), then a *plaque* is formed. The end point is interfering with blood flow to an organ and causing an infarct, which is either:

  1. Red: Made of *blood,* e.g.. *Lungs, GI.*
  2. Pale: As in *MI* and *CVA.*

Myocardial Infarction

- *Clinical picture*: Crushing substernal chest pain radiating to left shoulder, along with diaphoresis, nausea and dizziness.
- *Risk factors*: Male >55, Female >65, smoking, dyslipidemia, family history. So you can tell that *age* is the most important risk factor.

- *Diagnosis*:

  1. Elevated troponin-I and CK-MB, and *LDH1>LDH2 flip ratio*.
  2. EKG shows changes in the ST segments or T waves.

- *Markers*: Myoglobin is the first to rise *(After 1 h)*, and troponin is the last to disappear (*Rises after 3 h and lasts for 10 days*).
- *Treatment*:

  1. First step: MONA: *M*orphine, *O*xygen, *N*itroglycerin, *A*spirin.
  2. Second step: Heparin drip, aspirin, beta-blockers, ACEI and statins.
  3. If patient is *unstable* or has *ST elevation MI (STEMI)*, urgent heart catheterization is done. If heart catheterization is more than *90 min* away, thrombolytic therapy is indicated, e.g., Tissue plasminogen activator (tPA).
  4. Glycoprotein IIb/IIIa inhibitors are indicated in Non-ST elevation MI (NSTEMI) and after stent placement, as *they inhibit platelet aggregation and fibrinogen production*.

- *Pathologically*: Coagulative necrosis in the myocardium starts within hours:

  1. Day 1: Neutrophils migration occurs.
  2. Week 1: Granulation tissue formation.
  3. Week 3 after the MI: Myocardial scar is complete.

- *Angina*: Chest pain that occurs to myocardial ischemia and has 3 types:

  1. Stable angina: Due to uncomplicated atheroma.
  2. Unstable angina: Due to a complicated plaque, i.e., rupture.
  3. Prinzemetal angina: Due to *coronary vasospasm.* Shows *ST elevations*, and *beta blockers are contraindicated, as allows full uninhibited alpha action on blood vessels.*

- *Complications*:

  1. Arrhythmia and heart failure.
  2. Rupture of interventricular septum or papillary muscles: Rupture of papillary muscles and/or chordae tendineae of mitral valve is the most common, and its presents in the USMLE with an MI followed by the appearance of new mitral regurgitation murmur and sudden onset pulmonary edema. *Note that papillary muscles attach posteriorly and are supplied by right coronary artery.*
  3. Ventricular aneurysm: Suspected by *persistent ST elevation* after resolution of MI. A thrombus can form inside the aneurysm and embolization can ensue.

4. Dressler syndrome: Pericarditis that might occur few weeks after resolution of the MI, and is treated with steroids.

- *Notes*:

  1. Chest pain that starts days after the MI indicates pericarditis or re-infarction.
  2. MI is the most common complication after carotid endartrectomy.
  3. Most common cause of death in MI is *arrhythmia*.
  4. Cessation of smoking for 5 years decreases risk of MI by *50%*.
  5. Indications for bypass surgery: Left main coronary artery involvement, or 3+ vessel disease. Anything else could be treated with stenting.

Pericarditis

- *Causes*: Multiple, but mostly *viral*.
- *Clinical picture*: Chest pain, *worse on lying flat and relieved by sitting up or leaning forwards*.
- *On exam: Friction rub*.
- *EKG*: *Diffuse PR depressions and ST elevations* with normal troponins. Refer to Fig. 1.30.
- *Treatment*: Non-steroidal anti-inflammatory medications (NSAIDs).

Pericardial Effusion and Tamponade

- *Mechanism*: If *any amount of fluid* collects *rapidly* between the visceral and parietal layers, tamponade occurs.
- *Clinical picture*:

  1. *Hypotension*.
  2. *Distant heart sounds*.
  3. *Inspiratory drop of blood pressure aka Pulsus paradoxus*.
  4. *Inspiratory filling of jugular veins aka Kaus-maull's sign*.

- *Diagnosis*:

  1. Echocardiogram confirms and evaluates degree of effusion.
  2. CXR: *Flask shaped heart*.

- *Treatment*: Urgent pericardiocentesis.
- *Notes*:

  1. *Malignant effusions are hemorrhagic,* and *uremic effusions are serous*.
  2. *During pericardiocentesis, internal mammary artery is at risk of injury*.
  3. *In tamponade, the left atrial pressure is equal to right atrial pressure and is equal to right ventricular end diastolic pressure. LAP = RAP = RVEDP.*

Rheumatic Fever

- *Mechanism*: Post-group *A beta-hemolytic streptococcal* infection, due to cross sensitivity between streptococcal antigen and cardiac tissue.
- *Clinical picture*: Unique *CCASE* that you can never forget once you see a patient with *fever plus 2 or more of Jones criteria*:

  1. Chorea: Known as Sydenham chorea.
  2. Carditis: Valve lesions, *mitral* being most common.
  3. Arthritis: Migratory and fleeting.
  4. Subcutaneous nodules.
  5. Erythema marginatum on the trunk and proximal extremities.

- *Diagnosis*: High ESR and Anti-streptolysin O titers (ASLO).
- *Complication*: Most common is *mitral stenosis*.
- *Pathology*:

  1. *Aschoff bodies: Central fibrinoid necrosis surrounded by fibrosis*.
  2. *Antischkow cells*.

- *Treatment*: Penicillin. If allergic to PCN, give erythromycin.

Endocarditis

- *Causes*:

  1. Streptococcus viridans: *Most common cause.* Responsible for subacute cases.
  2. *Staphylococcus aureus*: Has rapid onset, more aggressive and common in IV drug users.

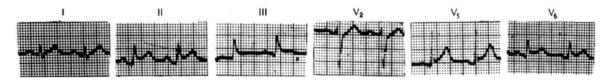

FIG. 1.30 EKG changes in pericarditis

3. Abacterial: also known as marantic endocarditis, e.g., renal failure, cancer.

- *Valves involved*:

  1. Just like rheumatic fever, the most common is *mitral valve*.
  2. Tricuspid valve is more common to be involved in IV drug users.

- *Clinical picture*:

  1. *Fever* and sepsis in a patient with a *new murmur*.
  2. Osler nodes: Tender nodular lesions on fingers.
  3. Janeway lesions: Erythematous lesions on palms.
  4. Roth spots: White spots in the retina.
  5. Splinter hemorrhage: Linear hemorrhage under the nails.

- *Diagnosis*:

  1. Positive blood cultures: *First thing to order when you suspect this disease*.
  2. *Trans-esophageal* echocardiogram: To diagnose valvular vegetations.

- *Treatment*: Broad spectrum antibiotics for 4-6 weeks, e.g., PCN + aminoglycoside. Treatment aims at sterilizing the vegetations, and decreasing risk of septic emboli.
- *Note: Antibiotic prophylaxis before procedures aims at decreasing the risk of endocarditis. Amoxicillin (2 g) is given orally to any patient with heart murmur at least 1 h before most procedures. Clindamycin or azithromycin are given in case of a penicillin allergy.*

Hypertrophic Obstructive Cardiomyopathy (HOCM)

- *Mechanism*: Familial disease (AD) characterized by *disproportionate thickening* of the interventricular septum leading to subaortic stenosis, hence also known as Idiopathic Hypertrophic Subaortic Stenosis (IHSS).
- *Clinical picture*:

  1. Syncope or sudden death on exertion, so always think of this in USMLE for a young patient who suddenly collapsed during exercise.
  2. Aortic stenosis murmur, which is decreased by anything that increases the venous return, e.g., Squatting, laying supine, hand grip etc....

- Complications: Fatal arrhythmia, e.g., *Ventricular fibrillation*
- *On exam: Pulsus bisferious.*

- *Diagnosis*: Echocardiogram.
- *Treatment*: Beta blockers and vasodilators. An implantable cardioverter defibrillator (AICD) is also indicated for any patient with HOCM.
- *Contraindication*: Inotropic agents, e.g., Digoxin.
- *What to advise your HOCM patient*: All family members should be evaluated for HOCM.

Coarctation of the Aorta

- *Types*:

  1. *Preductal*: Proximal to the origin of the left subclavian artery origin; usually associated with patent ductus arteriosus.
  2. *Postductal*: More common, and is distal to the origin of the left subclavian artery origin. Clinically there is higher flow and pressure into the upper half of the body, and lower flow into the lower half, and blood takes a detour through the intercostal arteries to be able to reach the superior epigastric. This leads to dilated intercostal arteries and *rib notching mainly posteriorly, which is pathognomonic for this disease.*

- *Clinical picture*:

  1. Significant difference between blood pressure in the *upper and lower* extremities.
  2. Systolic murmur over the left 3rd interscapular area, along with machinery murmur over the collaterals.
  3. A common finding in coarctation of aorta is bicuspid aortic valve, and you can easily hear the *systolic ejection click on the apex.*

- *Diagnosis: Aortography is diagnostic.* Rib notching on chest X-ray can be seen.
- *Treatment*: Surgical correction.
- *Note: Think about coarctation in any case presenting with Turner syndrome.*

Aortic Dissection

- *Clinical picture*:

  1. *Chest pain radiating to the back* mainly in-between the scapulae.
  2. Significant difference between the blood pressure readings of *left and right* upper extremities.

- *Diagnosis*:

  1. CXR: *Wide mediastinum is suggestive of dissection.*

2. Diagnosis is confirmed by:
   - Gold standard: *Aortography.*
   - Emergency situations: *Trans-esophageal Echocardiogram.*
   - Non-emergency situations: *MRI.*
   - Practically: Spiral CT of the chest.

- *Treatment*:
  1. Dissection of ascending aorta: *Urgent surgical repair.*
  2. Dissection of descending aorta: Medically, by lowering blood pressure using beta-blockers as drug of choice. Avoid inotropic agents and vasodilators (e.g.: Nitroprusside) without initial beta blockade, as this will worsen the dissection.

Aortic Aneurysm

- *Introduction*: Aortic arch aneurysm can compress on the trachea if it was huge and the pulsations could be felt at the sternal notch, however most aortic aneurysms are below the level of renal arteries, and are secondary to atherosclerosis and HTN. Abdominal Aortic Aneurysm (AAA) is discussed below.
- *Clinical picture*: Abdominal pain radiating to the back.
- *On exam*: Pulsatile abdominal mass.
- *Diagnosis*: Aortography or ultrasound of the abdomen.
- *Treatment*: Abdominal aortic aneurysm is treated surgically only if they exceed *5 cm* in diameter (or *6 cm in thoracic ones*). If smaller, you only need to control risk factors and follow up by ultrasound every 6 months.
- *Note*: True aneurysms are formed of intima, media and adventitia, while false ones are formed only of adventitia.

Arrhythmias
Sinus Tachycardia

- *Definition*: Regular, HR >100, caused by exercise, fever or anxiety.
- *Treatment*: treat the cause.

Supraventricular Tachycardia (SVT)

- *Definition*: Regular, HR>100, caused by exercise, fever or anxiety.
- *EKG*: Deformed P waves and short PR intervals. Refer to Fig. 1.31.
- *Treatment*: IV Adenosine and treat the cause.

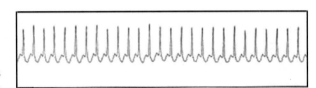

FIG. 1.31 Supraventricular tachycardia

Ventricular Tachycardia

- *Definition*: Regular, A-V dissociation present, caused by fluid shifts and ischemic heart disease.
- *EKG*: Wide complex tachycardia. Refer to Fig. 1.32.
- *Signs*: Cannon neck vein waves.
- *Treatment*: DC cardioversion is the first step, followed by epinephrine, amiodarone and lidocaine.
- *Note*: Torsades de Pointe is a multifocal V. tach.- treated as above plus *magnesium sulfate* and overdrive pacing.

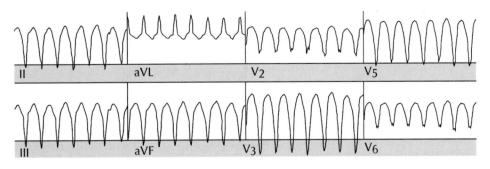

FIG. 1.32 Ventricular tachycardia

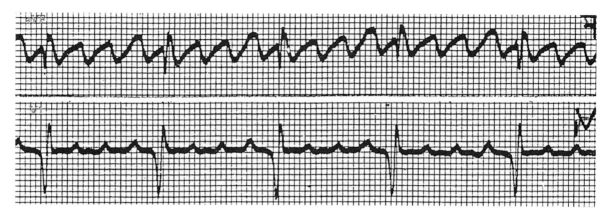

FIG. 1.33 Atrial flutter

Atrial Flutter

- *Definition*: Regular, HR>100 (Atrial rate = 300–400).
- *EKG*: *Saw-tooth* appearance. Refer to Fig. 1.33.
- *Signs*: Neck vein pulsations > Radial pulsations.
- *Treatment*: Rate control, e.g., Digoxin, Beta blockers or CCB, and anticoagulation with warfarin for an INR target of 2–3.

Atrial Fibrillation

- *Definition*: Irregularly irregular, HR>100.
- *Causes*: Ischemic heart disease, thyrotoxicosis, pulmonary embolism or in most cases without any cause (Lone A. Fib.).
- *Signs: Absent neck (a) waves*, and *pulsus deficit of more than 10/min*.
- *EKG: Irregularly irregular, absent P waves*. Refer to Fig. 1.34.
- *Complication*: Left atrial thrombus, which might embolize and cause CVA.
- *Treatment*: Rate control, e.g., Digoxin, Beta blockers or CCB, and anticoagulation with warfarin for an INR target of 2–3. DC cardioversion is done only if the patient is hemodynamically unstable.

Extrasystole

- *Definition*: Regularly irregular, HR variable.
- *Signs: Pulsus deficit <10/min* and normal neck vein waves.
- *Treatment*: No need to treat unless they are ventricular or multifocal, then beta blockers or CCB are warranted.

Wolff Parkinson White (WPW) Syndrome

- *Mechanism*: Premature atrial or ventricular contraction leading to re-entrant tachycardia that follows an accessory pathway (Wolff Parkinson White bundle).
- *Clinical picture: Recurrent dizziness episodes mostly in young adults.*
- *EKG*: Short P-R and slurred upstroke (*J wave*) before QRS complex.
- *Treatment*: Radiofrequency ablation of the accessory tract.

Heart Block

- *1st degree*: PR interval of more than *0.21 seconds* without any dropped beats.
- *2nd degree*: Divided into 2 different types:

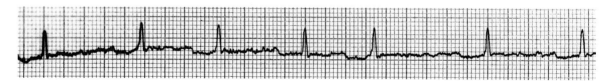

FIG. 1.34 Atrial fibrillation

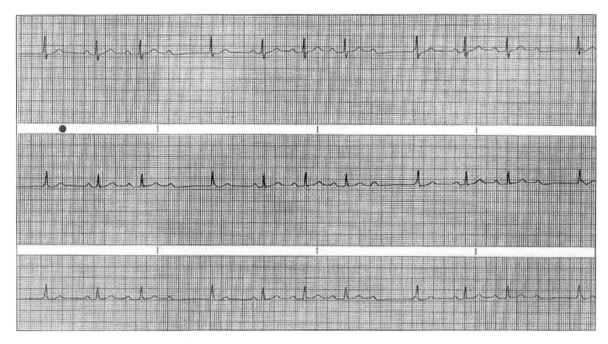

FIG. 1.35 Second degree AV block (Mobitz I)

1. Mobitz I (Wenckbach): Increasingly prolonged PR followed by a dropped QRS. Refer to Fig. 1.35.
2. Mobitz II: Dropped QRS without any preceding PR prolongation. Refer to Fig. 1.36.

• *3rd degree*: Complete AV dissociation with *cannon neck vein (a) waves*. Refer to Fig. 1.37.

• *Treatment*:

1. 1st degree: Adjust medications and watch closely
2. 2nd and 3rd degrees: Atropine and pacemaker placement. *Remember: Pacing is also needed in Torsades de Pointe and Left bundle branch block.*

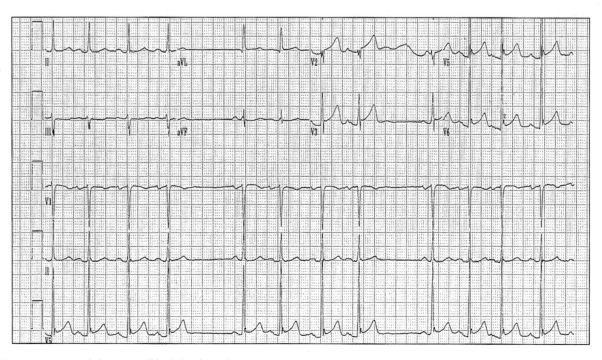

FIG. 1.36 Second degree AV block (Mobitz II)

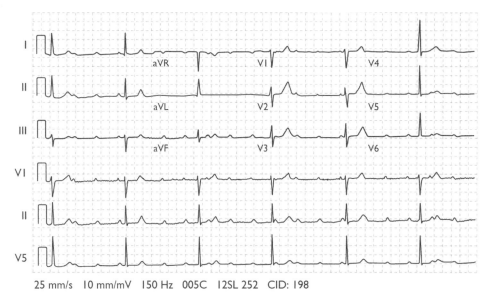

25 mm/s 10 mm/mV 150 Hz 005C 12SL 252 CID: 198

FIG. 1.37 Third degree AV block

Ventricular Fibrillation

- *Definition*: Emergency, caused by electrolyte imbalance or ischemic heart disease.
- *EKG*: Broad bizarre irregular fine waves. Refer to Fig. 1.38.
- *Treatment*: Similar to V. tach.

Pulseless Electrical Activity (PEA)

- *Definition*: Formerly known as Electro-mechanical Dissociation (EMD).
- *Causes*: Pneumothorax or cardiac tamponade.
- *Diagnosis*: Normal electrical activity on the monitor with absent pulses on exam.
- *Treatment*: IV fluids, epinephrine and atropine. DC cardioversion is contraindicated.

Hypothermic Arrhythmia

- *EKG*: *Osbourne (J) waves* and ventricular fibrillation.
- *Note*: Other complications of hypothermia include rhabdomyolysis and pontine myelinolysis.

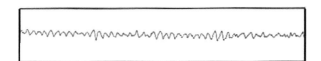

FIG. 1.38 Ventricular fibrillation

Asystole

- Known as *Flat line*, caused by hypotension or electrolyte imbalance or ischemic heart disease. Treatment: Similar to PEA.

Shock

- *Definition*: Systolic blood pressure *below 90*, or mean arterial pressure *below 60*.
- *Pathophysiology*:

  1. *Compensated stage*: Contraction of pre-capillary sphincters to maintain circulation.
  2. *Cell distress stage*: Anaerobic metabolism due to opening of A-V shunts.
  3. *Decompensated stage*: Contraction of post-capillary sphincters and relaxation of pre-capillary ones, leading to capillary sludge and DIC.

- *Types*: Refer to Table 1.10 for defining parameters obtained through Swan-Ganz catheter placed through the internal jugular vein into the pulmonary artery.
- *Treatment*:

  1. *Hypovolemic*, e.g., Dehydration, bleeding: Aggressive hydration ± vasopressors and treat the cause.
  2. *Distributive*, e.g., Septic: Aggressive hydration and antibiotics ± vasopressors (*Septic shock has 2 phases: Warm shock with cutaneous vasodilatation, followed by Cold shock with diffuse vasoconstriction*).

TABLE 1.10 Types and Swan-Ganz parameters of all 4 types of shock. PCWP: Pulmonary capillary wedge pressure. SVR: Systemic vascular resistance. CO: Cardiac output.

Type	PCWP	SVR	CO
Hypovolemic	Low	High or normal	Low
Distributive	High or normal	Low	High initially then low
Cardiogenic	High or normal	High or normal	Very low
Obstructive	High or normal	High or normal	Low

3. *Cardiogenic,* e.g., MI: Dobutamine infusion and treat cause. Do not give too much fluids in this type of shock.
4. *Obstructive,* e.g., Pulmonary embolism, pneumothorax: Treat the cause + Hydration ± vasopressors.

3. LDL below 160 mg/dl if no risk factors, below 130 if up to 2 risk factors, and below 70 if 3 or more risk factors and/or CAD.
4. HDL above 40 mg/dl in males, and above 50 in females.

- Refer to Table 1.11 for details on medications.

Dyslipidemia

Goal:
1. Total cholesterol below 200 mg/dl.
2. Triglycerides below 150 mg/dl.

Neurology

Cerebral Cortex (refer to Fig. 1.39)

Frontal Lobe

- *Areas 4, 6*: Injury causes *contralateral spastic paresis.*

TABLE 1.11 Cholesterol lowering medications.

Class	Examples	Mechanism	Indications	Side effects
Statins	Atorvastatin Simvastatin	Inhibit HMG-coA reductase enzyme, which normally converts HMG-coA to mevalonic acid	• High total cholesterol • High LDL	• Elevated liver enzymes • Myositis: patient presents with muscle aches and elevated serum creatine phosphokinase CPK
Fibrates	Clofibrate Gemfibrozil	• Stimulate lipoprotein lipase enzyme • Stimulate cholesterol excretion in bile and stools	• High TG • Type III dyslipidemia	• Cholesterol gall stones • Malignancy; especially due to Clofibrate
Bile acid sequestrants	Cholestyramine Colestipol	Inhibit enterohepatic circulation, so the liver uptakes LDL and cholesterol from circulation to synthesize bile	• Type II dyslipidemia • Itching in obstructive jaundice	• Deficiency of fat soluble vitamins: A, D, E and K • Folic acid deficiency
Niacin	Niacin	Inhibit triglyceride lipolysis in adipose tissue	• Low HDL • Type IIb dyslipidemia	• Flushing and pruritis: prevented by taking an aspirin half hour before each dose • Hyperuricemia • Hyperglycemia
Probucol	Probucol	Inhibit oxidation of cholesterol and LDL, thus prevent foam cell formation	• Atherosclerosis • Type II dyslipidemia	*Probucol prolongs* Q-T interval

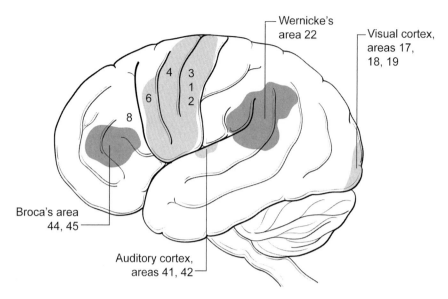

FIG. 1.39 Brain areas

- *Area 8*: Injury causes *ipsilateral eye deviation*.
- *Areas 44, 45 (Inferior temporal gyrus)*: Injury causes expressive (a.k.a. *Broca's*) aphasia, in which the patient understands but cannot articulate.
- *Areas 9, 10, 11, 12*: Injury causes *sphincter and gait disturbances*.

Temporal Lobe

- *Areas 41, 42*: Injury causes *sensorineural hearing loss*.
- *Area 22 (Superior temporal gyrus)*: Injury causes receptive (a.k.a. *Wernicke's*) aphasia, in which the patient cannot understand language or symbols. The patient *can articulate, but does not make any sense*. That is why it is known as *Fluent aphasia*.
- *Anterior temporal lobe*: Injury causes *Kluver-Bucy syndrome*, which presents with *hypersexuality* and *hyperphagia*.
- *Inferomedial occipitotemporal cortex*: Injury causes *prosopagnosia*, where the patient cannot recognize faces.

Parietal Lobe

- *Sensory cortex areas 3, 1, 2*: Injury causes *contralateral hemihyperesthesia*.
- *Superior parietal areas 5, 7*: Injury causes *contralateral sensory neglect*.
- *Inferior parietal area*: Injury causes *Gerstmann syndrome*, which is full of *(Dys)*, i.e., *Dys*lexia, *Dys*graphia, *Dys*calculia.

Occipital Lobe

- *Unilateral injury*: Causes *contralateral hemianopsia*.
- *Bilateral injury*: Causes *complete blindness*.

Alzheimer's Disease

- *Introduction*: *Most common cause of dementia in the elderly*, with multi-infarct dementia ranking second.
- *Mechanism*: Decreased *Choline Acetyltransferase (CAT)* enzyme responsible for *acetylcholine synthesis, and loss of cholinergic neurons in the forebrain*.
- *Genetics*: Abnormality in chromosomes 1, 14 and 21 has been suggested, also the presence of at least one copy of E4 gene on chromosome 19.
- *Clinical picture*: Gradual steady dementia. Multi-infarct dementia is *stepwise*. In both cases, *recent memory is the first thing to be affected*, followed by *language* (Patient cannot find the words), and finally *spatial ability* (Deals with figures and perception of dimensions of objects).
- *CT head*: *Ventricular dilatation and cortical atrophy*.
- *Pathology*: *Amyloid plaques, Hirano bodies and Neurofibrillary tangles*. Also, degeneration of *the nucleus of Meynert*.
- *Treatment: Cholinestrase inhibitors*, e.g., Donepezil.
- *Notes*:

  1. *Pick's disease*: Another cause of dementia that affects the *frontal and temporal* lobes, and is well know for the intracytoplasmic inclusion bodies known as *Pick bodies*.

2. *Normal pressure hydrocephalus*: Another cause of dementia with the unique triad: *Dementia, wide based ataxia and urinary incontinence.*

Glioblastoma Multiforme

- *Introduction*: *Most common primary brain tumor.*
- *Pathologically*: *Grade IV astrocytoma* with poor prognosis. *Pseudopalisading* of cancer cells around a central area of hemorrhage and necrosis is seen on histology.
- *Clinical picture*: High intracranial pressure, i.e., Early morning headache, vomiting and blurry vision due to papilloedema.
- *Diagnosis*: CT or MRI of the brain shows a mass with necrotic center surrounded by edema. Also known as *Butterfly glioma*. Refer to Fig. 1.40.
- *Notes*:

  1. Brain tumors in adults are mainly *supratentorial*, with *metastatic tumors* being the most common brain tumor.
  2. Brain tumors in children are mainly *infratentorial*, with *astrocytoma* being the most common tumor.
  3. Metastatic brain tumors show a *ring enhancement* on the CT scan.

Pseudotumor Cerebri

- *Mechanism*: Elevated intracranial pressure without a space occupying lesion.

- *Age group*: *Adolescent overweight females.*
- *Causes*: Vitamin A toxicity, tetracyclines, steroid withdrawal and OCPs.
- *Clinical picture*: Early morning headache, vomiting and blurry vision due to papilloedema.
- *Diagnosis*: Diagnosis of exclusion, CT brain and LP are normal.
- *Complication*: Long-standing untreated cases can lead to permanent blindness.
- *Treatment*:

  1. Treat the cause.
  2. Steroids and acetazolamide: To decrease intracranial pressure.
  3. Resistant cases: Shunt operation.

Cavernous Sinus Thrombosis

- *Causes*: Progression of infection from the sinuses or the orbit.
- *Clinical picture*: Conjunctival congestion, with proptosis, fever, chills and ophthalmoplegia.
- *Treatment*: Antibiotics. Surgical drainage is reserved for resistant cases.
- *Note*: Always look for other clues in any patient with "Pink eye."

Meningitis

- *Definition*: Infection of the meninges, whether by bacteria or viruses.

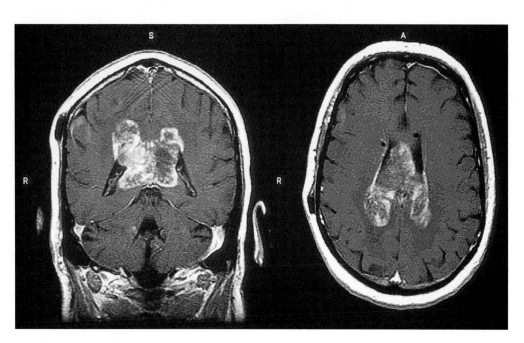

FIG. 1.40 Glioblastoma multiforme

- *Cause*: Most common organisms differ with age and condition:

  1. *Newborn group*: *Group B streptococcus*.
  2. *Children*: *Streptococcus pneumoniae*.
  3. *Adults*: *Neisseria meningitidis*.
  4. *Elderly*: *Streptococcus pneumoniae*.
  5. *HIV patients*: *Cryptococcus neoformans*, a form of yeast with *extracapsular halo*, found in *pigeon's droppings*, diagnosed by *india ink* staining and cultured on *Sabouraud agar*.

- *Clinical picture*:

  1. Fever, headache, photophobia, and *neck stiffness*.
  2. On exam: Stiff neck, positive *Kerning's* and *Brudzinski's* signs.

- *Diagnosis*: Lumbar puncture. *Agglutination test to detect soluble antigens in CSF is the most sensitive and specific test to diagnose meningitis.*
  1. CSF in bacterial meningitis would show *high protein content*, *high pressure*, *high WBC count*, and *low glucose* level.
  2. CSF in viral meningitis would show only *high protein content*, *high pressure* and *high lymphocyte* count with normal glucose level. *TB meningitis' CSF will show the exact thing like viral's CSF except that the glucose level will be very low.*

- *Complications*:

  1. Adrenal hemorrhage a.k.a. *Waterhouse Friedrichson syndrome*, which could be seen as *Shell-like calcifications* on the X-ray.
  2. Encephalitis: Shown on EEG as *Sharp triphasic complexes*. Herpes encephalitis is unique in causing olfactory hallucinations and showing mononuclear pleocytosis and RBCs in the CSF.
  3. Fulminant meningococcemia: High fever, sepsis and *purpura fulminans*.

- *Treatment*:

  1. Drug of choice is *3rd generation cephalosporin* + Vancomycin.
  2. Treatment of Cryptococcus neoformans: Amphotericin B + Flucytosine.

- *Prophylaxis for close contacts*: Drug of choice is *Rifampicin*.
- *Notes*:

  1. TB meningitis causes injury of cranial nerves *III, VI, VII* and *VIII* only.
  2. If you face a case in the exam with meningitis, along with extremely elevated amylase level with no clear abdominal source, think of *acute viral parotitis as the culprit*.

Meningiomas

- *Introduction*: Arise from the *arachnoid villi* of meninges: 90% of them are benign, and 90% are supratentorial.
- *Clinical picture*: Asymptomatic, or present with a focal deficit.
- *Diagnosis*: CT or MRI of the brain. Confirmation of diagnosis by biopsy.
- *Treatment*: Surgical only if symptomatic.
- *Pathological clue*: Suspect meningioma on the exam if a case is presented with intracranial hypertension along with *psammoma bodies*.
- *Notes*:

  1. *Oligodendrogliomas arise from frontal lobes; slow growing tumors and very commonly show calcifications.*
  2. *Psammoma bodies could be seen in (PMS): Papillary carcinoma of thyroid, Meningioma, Serous ovarian cyst.*

Hydrocephalus

- *Communicating*: Obstruction is in the *subarachnoid space*.
- *Non-communicating*: Obstruction is before the CSF reaches the subarachnoid space. There is an anatomical obstruction as follows:

  1. *Congenital aqueductal stenosis*: *X-linked* hydrocephalus causing dilatation of *lateral* and *third* ventricles. Refer to Fig. 1.41.

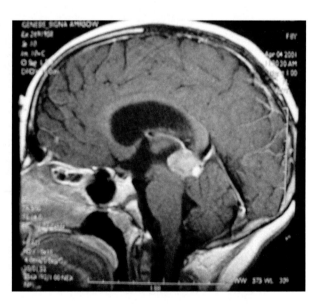

FIG. 1.41 Hydrocephalus secondary to obstruction of aqueduct of Sylvius by a tumor

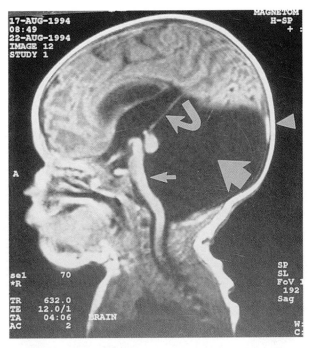

FIG. 1.42 Hydrocephalus (Dandy Walker)

2. *Dandy-Walker deformity*: Obstruction in the foramina of *Luschka and Magendie*, which leads to dilatation of the *4th ventricle*, along with an *atrophied cerebellum* and *occipital meningocele*. Refer to Fig. 1.42.

• *Remember*: If a hydrocephalus question mentions:

1. Dilated *third and lateral* ventricles: Obstruction is at the *aqueduct*.
2. Dilated *4th ventricle* and normal 3rd and lateral: *ventricles Dandy-Walker*.

• *Normal pressure hydrocephalus*: Occurs due to *failure of the arachnoid villi to absorb the CSF*. Patients are usually elderly with a slow progression of symptoms or just had a recent traumatic brain injury and intracranial hemorrhage. They present with a triad of *D*ementia, *U*rinary incontinence and *A*taxia.

• *Treatment of hydrocephalus*: *Surgical placement of a shunt*.

Arnold-Chiari Malformation

• *Mechanism*: Elongation of the *cerebellum* and *medulla oblongata* through the foramen magnum. Cranial nerves compressed are *IX, X and XI*.

• *Clinical picture*: *Stridor, dysphagia, vocal cord paralysis* and *hydrocephalus. Arnold with big head who cannot talk, breathe or eat.*

• *Treatment*: Surgical decompression and placement of a shunt.

Cerebrovascular Accident (CVA) (refer to Fig. 1.43)

• *Introduction*: Also known as *stroke*; this could be ischemic or hemorrhagic.

• *Risk factors*:

1. Ischemic stroke is common in patients with *arrhythmia*, e.g, Atrial fibrillation.
2. Hemorrhagic stroke is common in patients with head injury, e.g., Falls.
3. Amyloid deposition in intracranial vessels of the elderly could be a risk factor.

• *Clinical picture*:

1. *Middle Cerebral Artery (MCA)* stroke: *Slurred speech*, contralateral *hemiplegia* and *hemihypoesthesia*. Common with internal capsule (Lacunar) stroke. *Note that MCA is the mother artery of lenticulostriate artery.*
2. *Anterior Cerebral Artery (ACA) stroke*: Contralateral hemiplegia and hemihypoesthesia, *more pronounced in the lower extremity*.
3. *Posterior Cerebral Artery (PCA) stroke*: Contralateral homonymous hemianopia with macular sparing.
4. *Vertebrobasilar stroke*: Vertigo, vertical nystagmus and incoordination signals suggestive of cerebellar injury, e.g., Ataxia, dysmetria (e.g., Finger to nose test), and *intention tremors*.

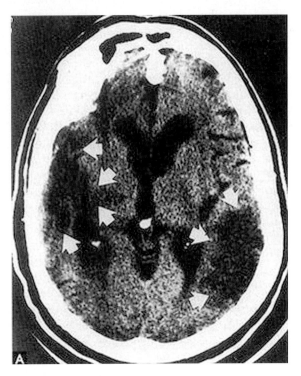

FIG. 1.43 Bilateral ischemic CVA

5. *Right parietal lobe infarction*: (Neglect syndrome) Patients have *sensory neglect to left side of the body but move it normally*; they also have *visual field defects*.
6. *Left parietal lobe infarction*: Patients have *speech and language abnormalities*.

- *Diagnosis*: *CT of the head* is diagnostic, but most ischemic cases won't develop changes until after 48 h.
- *What to order*:

  1. *Repeat CT head in 24–48 h*.
  2. *Carotid Doppler*.
  3. *Echocardiogram* and *EKG*.

- *Treatment*: Never drop the blood pressure too quickly; it is usually high to maintain cerebral perfusion; *Cushing reflex is hypertension and bradycardia*.

  1. Ischemic cases: Thrombolytic therapy with tPA if patient presented within the *first 3 h* after onset of CVA. Other options include *antiplatelet* agents, e.g., aspirin, dipyridamole, Clopidogrel.
  2. Hemorrhagic cases: Treated conservatively unless hemorrhage is severe (e.g., *causing midline shift*), then surgical drainage is necessary.

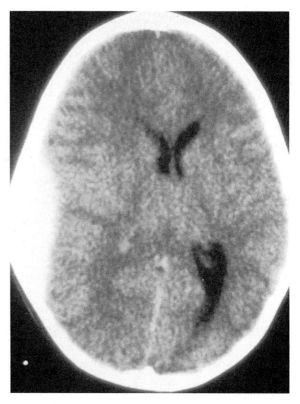

FIG. 1.44 Epidural hematoma

Intracranial Hemorrhage

- *Clinical picture*: Patient has trauma followed by headache, photophobia, nausea and vomiting.
- *Epidural*: *Convex-shaped*. Bleeding is from *middle meningeal artery*, which runs between the *2 roots of auriculotemporal nerve*. Refer to Fig. 1.44.
- *Subdural*: *Crescent-shaped* and is the *most common* traumatic intracranial injury. Bleeding is from *bridging superior cerebral veins*. Refer to Fig. 1.45.
- *Subarachnoid*: Patient has the *worst headache of his life* and fundus exam might show *retinal hemorrhage*. Most common cause is trauma followed by rupture of an aneursym, mostly in *communicating arteries*. Diagnosis: Lumbar puncture is the test of choice. CT head can also be used but it is less sensitive; refer to fig. 1.46.
- *Notes*:

  1. Anterior communicating artery connects the *anterior cerebral arteries* with each other. Injury (e.g., rupture of aneurysm): *Subarachnoid hemorrhage* and *bitemporal lower quadrantanopia*. The most common location of Berry aneurysms is the *at the bifurcation* of the anterior communicating artery.
  2. Posterior communicating artery connects the *middle cerebral with posterior cerebral* arteries. Injury:

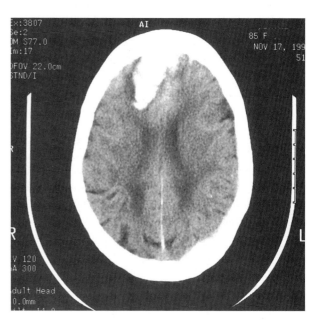

FIG. 1.45 Subdural hematoma

Subarachnoid hemorrhage and *injury of third cranial nerve. Suspect in a patient presenting with the worst headache of his life plus ptosis and diplopia.*

- *Note*: Any intracranial process causing midline shift, e.g., hemorrhage or mass, is managed using

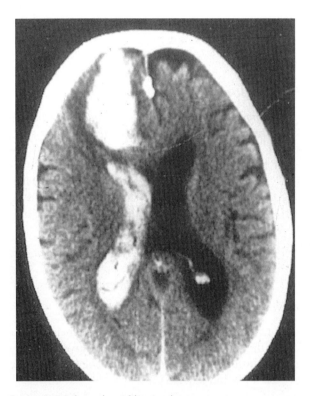

FIG. 1.46 Subarachnoid hemorrhage

dexamethasone, diamox, mannitol and inducing a *hyperventilation* state if the patient is on mechanical ventilation.

Concussion

- *Mechanism*: Temporary loss of consciousness *due to failure of neurological signaling.*
- *Causes*: Mechanical brain injury, e.g., Car accident.
- *Phases*:

  1. Concussion: Immediate but temporary loss of consciousness.
  2. Lucid interval: Full consciousness is regained, but a hematoma is building up.
  3. Compression: Due to the compressive effect of the hematoma.

- *Complication*: *Recent memory loss*; regained gradually over up to 6 months.
- *Diagnosis*: Clinical. *All radiology work up is normal.*
- *Treatment*: Conservative. Resolves spontaneously.

Spina Bifida

- *Mechanism*: *Defect in the vertebral column that allows contents of spinal canal to herniate outside the body*; common in the *lumbosacral* spine area.
- *Prevention*: *Folic acid supplementation during pregnancy.*

- *Screening*: Ultrasound (US) in the first trimester shows *Lemon sign.*
- *Treatment*: Surgical.
- *Notes*:

  1. Hypertrichiosis in the lower lumbar area could be a sign of *spina bifida occulta.*
  2. If the same defect occurs in the back of the skull, it is called *Encephalocele.*

Craniopharyngioma

- *Introduction: Most common cause of hypopituitarism in children.*
- *Mechanism: Remnant of Rathke's pouch, resulting in an anterior pituitary tumor.*
- *Clinical picture*:

  1. *Headache, nausea, vomiting* and *bitemporal hemianopia.*
  2. Growth hormone, ADH and gonadotrophin deficiency.

- *Treatment*: Excision of the tumor.

Cerebellar Lesions

Cerebellar Anterior Vermis Syndrome

- Common in *alcoholics.*
- Clinical picture: *Lower extremity incoordination.*

Cerebellar Posterior Vermis Syndrome

- Common in *children*; a classic cause is *medulloblastoma.*
- Clinical picture: *Truncal and upper extremity incoordination.*

Cerebellar Tumors

- Most *m*idline tumors are *M*edulloblastoma.
- Most lateral ones are Astrocytoma.
- The most common brain tumors in children are *posterior fossa tumors*, mainly *infratentorial*, with *Astrocytoma being the most common.*
- Clinical picture: *Incoordination, ataxia, nystagmus* and *high intracranial pressure.*
- Treatment: Surgical resection and possibly radiation and chemotherapy.

Hypothalamus Lesions

- As a rule, the *posterior part of hypothalamus regulates the sympathetic system*, while the anterior part regulates the parasympathetic.
- Supraoptic nucleus regulates *ADH* secretion.

- Paraventricular nucleus regulates *oxytocin* secretion.
- Anterior nucleus regulates the process of *cooling*.
- Posterior nucleus regulates the process of *heating*.
- Lateral nucleus regulates the process of *hunger*.
- Medial nucleus regulates the process of *satiety*.
- Septate nucleus regulates *sexual urges and emotions*.
- A common question on the exam is about the hypothalamic structure that is injured in alcoholism and Wernicke's encephalopathy. The answer is the *mammillary bodies* and they have an unforgettable clinical picture:

  1. *Encephalopathy, ataxia* and *nystagmus*: Due to *Thiamine (B1) deficiency*.
  2. Korsakoff's confabulations: Patients can also develop *anterograde amnesia* and start *fabricating stories*. This is caused by injury to the *hippocampus*.

- To sum up, here are the injury sites in alcoholism:

  1. *Wernicke's encephalopathy* (Due to vitamin B1 deficiency): *Mammillary bodies of hypothalamus; Mediodorsal nucleus of thalamus*.
  2. *Korsakoff's syndrome*: *Hippocampus*.

Basal Ganglia Lesions
Parkinson's Disease

- *Mechanism*: Depletion of dopamine-producing neurons in the *substantia nigra*, interfering with the transmission of movement signals to the striatum.
- *Causes*: Combination of genetic and environmental factors. However, it could result from use of illegal drugs contaminated with *MPTP* (1-methyl-4-phenyl-1,2,3, 6-tetrahydropyridine), or *Metoclopramide*.
- *Clinical picture*: *(5R)* main symptoms:

  1. *R*igidity, mostly cogwheel.
  2. *R*esting tremors.
  3. Hypo*r*eflexia or A*r*eflexia.
  4. B*r*adykinesia.
  5. Othe*r*s: Shuffling gait, mask face and Micrographia.

- *Microscopy*: Lewy bodies, and *degeneration of substantia nigra*.
- *Treatment*:

  1. Levodopa (L-dopa) plus carbidopa: It is the mainstay of treatment. L-dopa is preferred over dopamine as it is lipophilic and can easily cross the blood-brain barrier. *Carbidopa is added as it decreases the peripheral effects and metabolism of L-dopa*.

2. Other drugs that can be used are newer dopamine agonists, anticholinergics (*to decrease tremors*) and MAO-B inhibitors.

Huntington's Chorea

- *Mechanism*: Atrophy of the caudate nucleus and degeneration of its cholinergic and GABAergic neurons.
- *Genetics*: Inherited as an *autosomal dominant* disease on *chromosome 4*.
- *Clinical picture*: Dementia, hypotonia and *choreoathetoid movements* due to *hyperactive N-Methyl D-Aspartate (NMDA)* and *glutamate*.
- *Diagnosis*: Brain CT or MRI shows:

  1. *Atrophy of frontal and temporal gyri and caudate nucleus*.
  2. Dilated anterior horns of lateral ventricles.

- *Notes*:

  1. Chorea is sudden purposeless movements, while athetosis is slow, distal writhing movements.
  2. Huntington's patients usually have *low substance P levels* in the CNS.
  3. If you see a case with chorea in the exam, look for these clues:

     - If the patient has *rheumatic fever* picture: *Sydenham's chorea*.
     - If the patient is *pregnant and in her 2nd trimester*: *Chorea gravidarum*.
     - If the patient has a *strong family history*: *Huntington's chorea*.

Tardive Dyskinesia

- *Definition*: Movement disorder in patients using *antipsychotics* or *metoclopramide* for an extended period of time.
- *Clinical picture*: Repetitive chorea-like movements of the face, tongue and neck.

Hemiballismus

- *Mechanism*: Vascular lesion injuring the *subthalamic nuclei*.
- *Clinical picture*: Sudden, aggressive flinging movements on the contralateral arm, *i.e., Similar to swinging a baseball bat*.

Midbrain Lesions
Parinaud Syndrome (Dorsal)

- Most common cause is a pinealoma. Lesions may be located in various locations:

1. Superior colliculi: Causes *paralysis of upward, downward and convergent gaze.*
2. Aqueduct of Sylvius: Causes *non-communicating hydrocephalus.*

Benedikt Syndrome (Paramedian)

- Ipsilateral oculomotor nerve palsy.
- Contralateral medial leminiscus injury.
- Contralateral cerebellar ataxia.

Weber's Syndrome (Medial)

- Ipsilateral oculomotor nerve palsy.
- Contralateral corticospinal tract injury.
- Contralateral paralysis of face, tongue and palate.
- Patients classically present with their uvula directed *towards the unaffected side* plus symptoms of posterior cerebral artery injury.

Pontine Lesions

Inferior Pontine Syndrome

- Two distinct syndromes secondary to vascular compromise:

1. *Medial*: Due to injury of *basilar artery*, affecting the corticospinal tract, medial leminiscus and abducens nerve (VI).
2. *Lateral*: Due to injury of the *anterior inferior cerebellar artery*, causing an ipsilateral facial nerve lesion, and ipsilateral sensorineural hearing loss.

Medial Longitudinal Fasciculus Syndrome (MLF)

- Also known as *internuclear ophthalmoplegia.*
- Pathognomonic sign of *multiple sclerosis.*
- Injures the nerve fibers *between the abducens and oculomotor nerve.*
- Patients have a palsy of the *medial rectus muscle* along with *nystagmus.*

Pontine Hemorrhage

- Due to an injury of *basilar* or *cerebellar* arteries.
- Clinical picture: *Unilateral facial* and *contralateral body* paralysis.
- *Pinpoint pupils are observed if bleeding is severe. This is a common case in USMLE, so remember that pontine hemorrhage causes pinpoint pupils.*

Medullary Lesions

Medial Medullary Syndrome

- Due to injury of the *anterior spinal artery*. Affected areas include:

1. *Corticospinal pyramid*: Causing contralateral spastic paresis.
2. *Medial leminiscus*: Causing contralateral loss of touch and proprioception.
3. *Hypoglossal nucleus*: Causing ipsilateral flaccid paralysis of the tongue. The tongue veers *towards the affected side.*

Wallenburg Syndrome (Lateral)

- Due to an injury of the *posterior inferior cerebellar* artery. Affected areas include:

1. *Nuclei of cranial nerves IX, X and XI*: Causing dysphagia, dysarthria, dysphonia and loss of the gag and cough reflexes.
2. *Sympathetic chain*: Causing ipsilateral Horner's syndrome.
3. *Trigeminothalamic tract*: Causing ipsilateral loss of pain and temperature sensations from *the face.*
4. *Lateral spinothalamic tract*: Causing contralateral loss of pain and temperature sensations from *the body.*
5. *Vestibular nuclei*: Causing vertigo and nystagmus.
6. *Cerebellar peduncles*: Causing ipsilateral cerebellar ataxia.

Tracts and Injuries

Dorsal Column

- *Composition*: Gracile fibers from lower limbs and cuneate fibers from upper limbs.
- *Function*: Transmits *fine touch* and *proprioception* from the limbs.
- *Course*: Fibers ascend in the dorsal column and *decussate in the medulla* forming the *medial leminiscus,* and end in *Brodmann areas 1, 2 and 3.*
- *Injury*:

1. Below decussation: Loss of fine touch and proprioception from the same side of the body.
2. Above decussation: Loss of fine touch and proprioception from the contralateral side of the body.

Lateral Spinothalamic Tract

- *Function*: Transmits *pain and temperature* sensations from the body.
- *Receptors*: *Fast A* and *slow C* fibers.
- *Course*: Fibers run in the *Lissauer tract* then decussate in the *anterior white commisure* at the same level they enter the cord. Fibers ascend in the *lateral funiculus* and end in *Brodmann's area 1, 2, and 3*.
- *Injury*: *Contralateral loss of pain and temperature sensations*.

Anterior Spinothalamic Tract

- *Function*: Transmits *deep touch* and *pressure* sensations from the body.
- *Injury*: *Contralateral loss of deep touch and pressure sensations*.

Lateral Corticospinal Tract

- *Function*: Transmits voluntary motor signals.
- *Course*: Fibers arise from the cerebral cortex and *decussate in the medulla*.
- *Injury*: *Spastic paresis*.
- *Note*: This tract is characterized by *delayed myelination. Myelination is not completed until 2 years of age*.

Hypothalamospinal Tract

- *Course*: Runs from the *hypothalamus* to the *intermediolateral column* of the spinal cord.
- *Injury: Ipsilateral Horner's syndrome*.
- *Spinocerebellar tract*: Transmits *proprioception from the muscles and joints*.
- *Ventral trigeminothalamic tract*: Transmits *pain and temperature from the face*.
- *Dorsal trigeminothalamic tract*: Transmits *touch and pressure from the face*.

Spinal Cord Lesions (Refer to Fig. 1.47)
Introduction

- Upper motor neuron lesions (UMNL) cause *hypertonia* and *hyperreflexia*.
- Lower motor neuron lesions (LMNL) cause *hypotonia, hyporeflexia* and *fasciculations*.
- Spinal cord injury *above C3* may cause *quadriplegia*.
- Systemic steroids given in the *first 10 hours* after spinal cord injury help minimize damage.
- Spinal cord tumors include astrocytomas, meningiomas, and metastatic cancers.

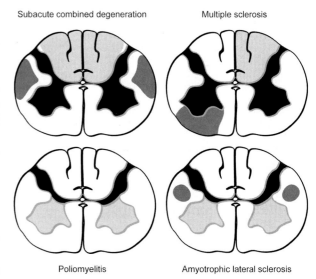

Subacute combined degeneration   Multiple sclerosis

Poliomyelitis   Amyotrophic lateral sclerosis

FIG. 1.47 Transverse section of spinal cord showing spinal tract lesions

- Note: *Dumbbell-shaped spinal cord tumors are common in Neurofibromatosis type 2. They are Schwannomas and they show Antoni bodies on histology.*

Multiple Sclerosis (MS)

- *Introduction*: *Demyelinating disease* affecting the brain and spinal cord. It is most common in *females 20–40 years* of age.
- *Clinical picture*: Suspect MS in a young woman presenting with *nonspecific limb weakness* and *visual deficits due to optic neuritis or internuclear ophthalmoplegia*.
- *Diagnosis*:

  1. *MRI* of brain which shows *periventricular white matter plaques*. Refer to Fig. 1.48.
  2. CSF: *High IgG level*.

- *Treatment: Systemic corticosteroids*.
- *Prophylaxis: Beta-interferon*.

Poliomyelitis

- *Cause*: Polio virus, transmitted *feco-orally* and replicates in the *oropharynx*.
- *Mechanism*: LMNL, due to injury of the *anterior grey horn*.
- *Clinical picture*: *Hypotonia, hyporeflexia, muscle wasting* and *fasciculation*.
- *Diagnosis*:

  1. Isolation of polio virus from oropharynx or stools.
  2. CSF shows *lymphocytosis* and elevated protein count.

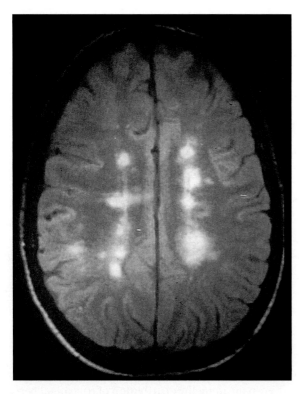

FIG. 1.48 Periventricular plaques of MS

Amyotrophic Lateral Sclerosis (ALS)

- *Mechanism*: Also known as *Lou Gehrig disease*. Due to combined UMNL and LMNL. Affects the *anterior grey horn* and the *corticospinal tracts*.
- *Clinical picture*: *Asymmetrical* limb weakness and combination of signs of UMNL (Hypertonia, hyperreflexia, Babinski sign) and LMNL (Hypotonia, hyporeflexia, fasciculation).

Tabes Dorsalis

- *Mechanism*: *Dorsal column damage* due to *untreated syphilis*.
- *Clinical picture*:

  1. Loss of propioception and vibration sensations along with *electric like pains in the upper and lower extremities*.
  2. *Ataxia* and positive *Romberg sign* (Inability of the patient to maintain an upright posture with his eyes closed without swaying or falling over).

- *Note*: Tabetic crisis patients present with *abdominal pain* and *bladder dysfunction*.

Brown Sequard Syndrome

- *Mechanism*: *Hemisection of the spinal cord*.
- *Clinical picture*:

1. *Ipsilateral: Flaccid paralysis and Horner's syndrome*.
2. *Contralateral: Loss of pain and temperature sensations*.

Anterior Spinal Artery Occlusion

- *Introduction*: Common in Abdominal aortic aneurysm surgeries.
- *Clinical picture*:

1. Flaccid paralysis and loss of pain and temperature *bilaterally below the lesion*.
2. *Bilateral Horner's* syndrome.

Subacute Combined Degeneration (SCD)

- *Mechanism*: Affects the dorsal and lateral columns, secondary to *vitamin B12 deficiency*.
- *Clinical picture*: *Ataxia, loss of propioception and loss of vibration sense* in a *stocking/glove distribution*.
- *Note*: Presents in the USMLE as a patient with lower extremity neurological manifestations along with *high Mean corpuscular volume (MCV) and mean corpuscular hemoglobin (MCH)* (Suggesting B12 def.)

Syringomyelia

- *Mechanism: Central cavitation of the cord* which injures the *anterior grey horns*, and the *anterior white commisure*.
- *Clinical picture*: Bilateral hand and arms weakness, along with *loss of pain and temperature sensation in both hands*.

Guillain Barre Syndrome

- *Mechanism: Ascending LMNL* that affects *facial muscles in 50% of cases*. Most common pathogen associated with this syndrome is *Campylobacter jejuni*.
- *Clinical picture*: Recent flu like illness, followed by *lower limb weakness, progressing proximally*.
- *Diagnosis*: CSF: *Abnormally high protein count with normal cell count*.
- *Treatment: Plasmapharesis*.

Cranial Nerves

I: Olfactory nerve

- Originates from the *olfactory bulb* and ascends through the *cribriform plate of the ethmoid bone*. Terminates in the olfactory cortex of the uncus (*area 34*).

- Lesion: Ipsilateral anosmia.
- Lesion in the uncus: Olfactory hallucinations.

II: Optic nerve

- Embryologically derived from the *diencephalon,* and is made of the axons of ganglion cells.
- Pupillary light reflex begins with light stimulating the retina → Optic nerve → Pretectum → Edinger-Westphal nucleus → Ciliary ganglion → Pupils. Refer to Figs. 1.49 and 1.50.
- Pupil *constricts with light* and *dilates in dark.* This process is mediated by the *ciliospinal center of Budge.*
- *Argyl Robertson pupil:* Pupil that *accommodates to near vision* but *cannot react to light.* Common in patients with *syphilis.*
- *Papilledema:* Occurs with *high intracranial pressure* and patients present with *blind spots* and a *normal visual acuity.* Refer to Fig. 1.51.
- Uncal herniation causes *bilateral dilated fixed pupils.*

III: Oculomotor nerve

- Motor nerve to eye muscles.
- Supplies all the oculomotor muscles except:

  1. *Superior oblique* muscle: Innervated by cranial nerve IV. (*SO4*)
  2. *Lateral rectus* muscle: Innervated by cranial nerve VI. (*LR6*).

- Refer to Fig. 1.52 for actions of the oculomotor muscles.

IV: Trochlear nerve

- Action: Innervates the *superior oblique* muscle.
- Injury: Weak downward gaze and vertical diplopia.

V: Trigeminal nerve

- Motor: Supplies the *muscles of mastication.*
- Sensory: Supplies *face, mouth* and *supratentorial dura.*
- Trigeminal nerve has three divisions:

  1. *Ophthlamic (V1):* Passes through *superior orbital fissure.*
  2. *Maxillary (V2):* Passes through *foramen rotandum.*
  3. *Mandibular (V3):* Passes through *foramen ovale.*

- Injury: Hemianesthesia of the face along with weak mastication. *Patient's jaw will deviate towards the paralyzed side due to unopposed action of lateral pterygoid muscle on the healthy side.*
- *Trigeminal neuralgia* (Tic douloureux): Sharp stabbing pain along the distribution of trigeminal nerve. Treatment: *Carbamazepine.*

VI: Abducens nerve

- Action: Innervates the *lateral rectus* muscle.
- Injury: *Convergent strabismus* and *horizontal diplopia.*

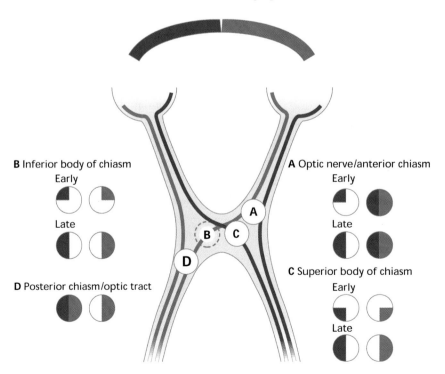

B Inferior body of chiasm
Early
Late

A Optic nerve/anterior chiasm
Early
Late

C Superior body of chiasm
Early
Late

D Posterior chiasm/optic tract

Fɪɢ. 1.49 Visual pathway injuries 1

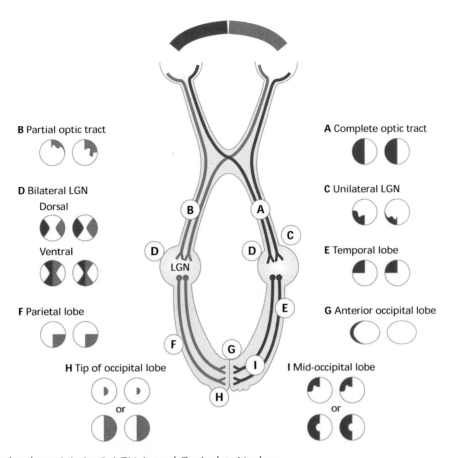

Fig. 1.50 Visual pathway injuries 2, LGN: Lateral Geniculate Nucleus

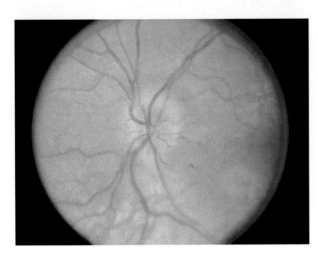

Fig. 1.51 Papilledema

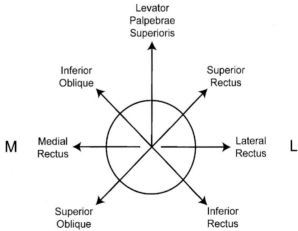

Fig. 1.52 Diagram showing actions of oculomotor muscles, M: Medial, L: Lateral

VII: Facial nerve

- Motor: Innervates *muscles of facial expression.*
- Taste: *Anterior two thirds of the tongue.*
- Relays in the superior olivary nucleus; hence also supplies the *lacrimal* and *submandibular salivary glands.*

- Clinical picture of injury:

  1. Facial droop and loss of the nasolabial fold on the affected side.
  2. Inability to *show teeth, blow cheeks, raise eyebrows* or *close eyes tightly.*

- Division of facial nerve to upper face receive bilateral corticobulbar fibers, while the division to the lower face receive only contralateral corticobulbar fibers, so:

1. *UMNL*: Weakness of the *contralateral lower face* (Forehead spared).
2. *LMNL* (Bell's palsy): Weakness of the *ipsilateral upper and lower face* (Forehead affected).

VIII: Vestibulocochlear nerve

- Action: *Vestibular portion regulates balance* and the *cochlear controls hearing*.
- Pathways:

  1. Hair cells in the inner ear relay signals to the *vestibular ganglion and nuclei*.
  2. Bipolar cells of cochlea relay signals to the *superior olivary nucleus, medial geniculate body* (MGB), and finally to the *auditory cortex (Areas 41, 42)* in the *temporo-lateral sulcus*.

- Injury to the vestibular branch: *Vertigo and nystagmus*.
- Injury to the cochlear branch: *Tinnitus and senorineural hearing loss*.
- Horizontal nystagmus may be either:

  1. *Vestibular*: Fast phase is in the same direction.
  2. *Post-rotatory*: Fast phase is in the opposite direction.
  3. *Caloric*: Eyes deviate *toward the warm water* and away from cold water in the ear canal.

Deafness

- *Conductive hearing loss*: Caused by obstruction in the auditory canals, e.g., Cholesteatoma in middle ear or atresia of the auditory canal.
- *Sensorineural hearing loss*: Caused by injury to the auditory neurological pathway, e.g., Congenital rubella infection during the 8th week of pregnancy.
- *Weber test*: Place a tuning fork on the forehead. Vibration is louder in the ear with conductive hearing loss, and is diminished in the one with sensorineural hearing loss.
- *Rinne test*: Moving a tuning fork from the mastoid process to in front of the external auditory meatus. The sound is louder on the mastoid in conductive cases, and is louder in front of the ear in *normal* and *sensorineural hearing loss* cases.
- *Acoustic neuroma*: *Schwann cell tumor* arising from the *vestibulocochlear nerve at the cerebellopontine angle*. May compress cranial nerves *V* and *VII*. The tumor is *benign* and patients present with *worsening hearing loss* and *tinnitus*. Diagnosed by *MRI* and treated *surgically*.

IX: Glossopharyngeal nerve

- Functions:

  1. Sensory: *Taste and sensory to the posterior one third of the tongue*.
  2. Innervates the *parotid* glands.
  3. Carries input from the carotid sinus (baroreceptor) and the carotid body (chemoreceptor).

- Injury:

  1. Loss of taste and sensation from posterior one third of the tongue.
  2. Loss of gag reflex.
  3. Carotid hypersensitivity causing *syncope*.

- Glossopharyngeal neuralgia is a condition similar to trigeminal neuralgia.

X: Vagus nerve

- *The main parasympathetic supply to the human body*.
- Injury: Paralysis of the *soft palate, pharynx* and *larynx*. Could be fatal.
- Clinical picture: *Dysphagia, hoarsness* of voice and loss of cough and gag reflexes. The *uvula deviates towards the paralyzed side*.

XI: Accessory nerve

- Innervates the *sternocleidomastoid* and *trapezius* muscles.
- Injury:

  1. Shoulder drop: Due to a paralyzed *trapezius*.
  2. Neck looking toward the side of the lesion: *Due to the unopposed action of the contralateral sternocleidomastoid*.

XII: Hypoglossal nerve

- Innervates all the tongue muscles *except the palatoglossus, which is innervated by vagus nerve*.
- Injury: Tongue deviates toward the paralyzed side *due to unopposed action of the contralateral genioglossus muscle*.

Seizures

- *Types*:

  1. Seizures can present in different forms, e.g., Grand mal, Absence, Myoclonic, status epilepticus or febrile convulsions.
  2. Seizures are either *partial* affecting a localized part of the body, or *generalized* affecting the whole body at the same time.

3. Seizures could also be simple or complex. The only and main difference is that complex seizures, unlike simple ones, are associated with *altered or loss of consciousness*.

- *Clinical picture*:

1. *Grand mal seizures*: Starts with generalized increased muscle tone (*Tonic phase*), followed by generalized convulsions (*Clonic phase*) during which loss of control over bowel and bladder, and tongue biting might occur. The last stage is *postictal phase*, during which the patient is lethargic and confused.
2. *Absence seizures*: Patient presents with *episodes of staring spells*, during which he/she continuously performs repeated movement, e.g., smacking lips, mumbling. EEG: *3-Hz spike and wave pattern on EEG*.
3. *Temporal lobe seizures*: Preceded by olfactory hallucinations *due to uncus stimulation*.
4. *Benign Rolandic epilepsy: Manifests as muscle twitching and is common in school age children.*

- Seizures are followed by *postictal state (confusion)*, and sometimes *transient paralysis (Todd's paralysis)*.
- *Diagnosis: EEG. MRI of the brain is also needed to rule out organic causes.*
- *Most common cause of seizures in children: Infection (Febrile seizures).*
- *Most common cause of seizures in adults: Head trauma.*
- *Most common cause of seizures in elderly*: Cerebrovascular accident.
- *Treatment*:

1. Grand mal seizures: Phenytoin (*Side effects: Megaloblastic anemia, Gingival hyperplasia*), or carbamazepine (*Side effects: Bone marrow depression and hepatotoxicity*).
2. Absence seizures: Ethosuximide (*Side effect: Steven's Johnson syndrome*) or valproic acid.
3. Myoclonic seizures: Clonazepam.
4. Febrile seizures: Phenobarbitone (*Side effect: Morbilliform rash*).
5. Status epilepticus: *Diazepam first*, then Fosphenytoin.

Muscular Disorders
Myasthenia Gravis

- *Mechanism: Antibodies against acetylcholine or its receptors in the muscles*, linked to *HLA-DR3*. Some cases are associated with a *thymus tumor*.
- *Clinical picture: Muscle weakness and diplopia, worse later in the day.*

- *Diagnosis: Edrophonium test (Tensilon test)* and *EMG* are diagnostic.
- *Treatment*: Cholinestrase inhibitors, e.g. pyridostigmine, neostigmine.
- *Note*: Eaton Lambert syndrome is a paraneoplastic syndrome that occurs due to *antibodies against calcium channels*. It stands as the mirror image of myasthenia gravis as patients have similar symptoms, but both the symptoms and the EMG – unlike M.Gravis- get better by exertion.

Werdnig-Hoffmann Disease

- *Introduction*: Lower motor neuron lesion (LMNL).
- *Clinical picture*:

1. Generalized *symmetrical* hypotonia, hyporeflexia, hypothesia.
2. *Tongue fasciculations.*

- *Note*: Polio also causes LMNL, but unlike Werdnig-Hoffmann, polio is *asymmetrical* and *there is no sensory loss.*

Disc Prolapse

- *Cause*: Herniation of the nucleus pulposus due to trauma or degeneration of annulus fibrosus.
- *Clinical picture*:

1. Radicular back pain shooting down the affected extremity, e.g., Neck pain radiating down one arm, or low back pain radiating down one leg.
2. Posterior prolapse of the disc causes spinal stenosis or cauda equina syndrome. The latter is an emergency that presents with tingling and numbness below level of lesion, saddle hypoesthesia and bowel/bladder incontinence.

- *On exam*: Positive straight leg raising test. The test is done with the patient laying in supine position; raise each leg separately from the table; test is positive if the patient develops *radicular pain* (explained above) upon leg raising. (*Remember, radicular pain, not lower back pain or pain in the back of the thigh*).
- *Diagnosis*: MRI of the spine.
- *Treatment*:

1. NSAIDs and physical therapy: *Best next step*.
2. Surgery, e.g., Discectomy or laminectomy: Last resort unless there are signs of severe compression, e.g., weakness and muscle atrophy.

Carpal Tunnel Syndrome

- *Mechanism*: Median nerve compression under the flexor retinaculum.

- *Causes*: Pregnancy, RA or occupational, e.g., Computer work, drilling.
- *Clinical picture*: Hand weakness and numbness, more at *night, exacerbated by flexion of the wrist* and *alleviated by dangling the hand in a dependant position.*
- *On exam*:

  1. Atrophy of thenar muscles.
  2. *Tinel sign*: Tapping of peroneus longus tendon reproduce symptoms.
  3. *Phalen test*: Dorsal sides of both wrists are approximated to achieve at least a 90° wrist flexion; this reproduces the symptoms.

- *Diagnosis*: Clinically, however, confirmation is via *nerve conduction studies.*
- *Treatment*: *Wrist splints.* Surgery is the last resort.

Migraine

- *Clinical picture: Unilateral throbbing headache* associated with *photosensitivity* and nausea, more common in *females*, and usually preceded with an aura of *light flashes.*
- *Physiology*: Serotonin levels are *elevated during the aura*, and they drop as headache worsens.
- *Prophylaxis (Chronic cases)*: *Beta blockers,* e.g., Propranolol or *Methysergide*; however the latter carries the risk of causing *retroperitoneal fibrosis.*
- *Treatment (Acute): Sumatriptan (5HT-1D agonist)* or *Ergotamine.*
- *Note*: Cluster headache occurs in clusters, each lasting few days at a time. Patients have headache behind a red inflamed eye, lacrimation and rhinorrhea. Treatment: 100% O_2.

Nerve Injuries

Injury of Upper Trunk of Brachial Plexus

- Aka Erb's palsy or *waiter's tip deformity.*
- Patient arm is *adducted, extended, pronated,* and *medially rotated.*

Injury of Lower Trunk of Brachial Plexus

- A.k.a. Klumpke paralysis.
- Patient presents with *loss of motor power and sensation over the medial three and half fingers of the injured hand.*

Radial Nerve Injury

- Common in *midshaft humerus fractures.*
- *Motor*: Patient presents with *inability to extend his wrist and fingers,* hence *wrist drop ensues.*

- *Sensory*: Loss of sensation over the *dorsum of the hand.*

Ulnar Nerve Injury

- Commonly due to *compression at the elbow or wrist.*
- *Motor*: Paralysis of *interossei* and *medial 2 lumbricals,* causing *claw hand deformity.*
- *Sensory*: Loss of sensation along the *medial third of the hand.*
- *Note*: Palmar interossei *ad*duct fingers *PAD,* while dorsal ones *ab*duct fingers *DAB.*

Median Nerve Injury

- Common in *wrist injury,* as it lies *deep to flexor retinaculum.*
- *Motor*: Paralysis of *opponens pollicis* and *flexor digitorum superficialis* causing *wasting of thenar eminence,* and *pointing index*; which does not flex when making a fist. This deformity is known as *Ape hand.*
- *Sensory*: Loss of sensation over *the lateral two thirds of the palm.*
- *Note*: Flexor digitorum superficialis controls the PIP joints, while flexor digitorum profundus controls the DIP joints.

Axillary Nerve Injury

- Commonly injured in fractures of the *surgical neck of the humerus and anterior displacement of humeral head.*
- Two muscles suffer paralysis:

  1. Deltoid: Leading to adduction of the arm.
  2. Teres minor: Leading to medial rotation of the arm.

Common Peroneal Nerve Injury

- Common in *upper fibular fractures.*
- Clinical picture:

  1. *Decreased sensation over lateral leg and foot.*
  2. *Impaired dorsiflexion and eversion of the foot.*

Keywords for Nerve Injuries

- *Loss of knee reflex*: Femoral nerve injury.
- *Waddling gait*: Superior gluteal nerve injury.
- *Loss of plantar flexion of the foot*: Tibial nerve injury (L4-S3).
- *Loss of dorsiflexion (Foot drop)*: Common peroneal nerve injury (L4-S2).

Ophthalmology

- *Macular degeneration*: Most common cause of blindness in the elderly. Patient presents with gradual painless loss of vision. Treatment: Laser photocoagulation.
- *Central retinal artery occlusion (CRA)*: Patients present with sudden unilateral painless blindness. Retinal exam: Cherry rod fovea. Treatment: Thrombolytics.
- *Central retinal vein occlusion (CRV)*: Presents in the same way as CRA occlusion. Retinal exam: Retinal hemorrhage and exudates. Treatment: Laser photocoagulation.
- *Ischemic optic neuropathy*: Occurs due to involvement of *posterior ciliary artery*. Common in cases of giant cell arteritis.
- *Hollen Horst plaques*: Retinal plaques that occur mostly due to *embolization*.
- *Chemical burns*: Emergency, *alkaline is more dangerous than acidic*. Treatment: Irrigation with water or saline is the first thing to do.
- *Superficial corneal foreign bodies*: Removed by irrigation or by a sterile cotton swab in the office after applying topical anesthetic eye drops. Next step after removal is eye patch application, antibiotic eye drops and ophthalmology evaluation. *Intraocular foreign body is a contraindication to MRI and to any superficial manipulation of the eye.*
- *Open angle glaucoma*: Patient presents with gradual loss of peripheral vision with an end result of complete blindness.
- *Closed angle glaucoma*: *Ophthalmological emergency*. Patient presents with sudden severe eye pain, halos around light, nausea and vomiting. Urgent treatment: *Topical Pilocarpine, Topical Timolol and systemic Acetazolamide.*
- *Treatment of glaucoma*: Achieved by 2 mechanisms as described below:

  1. *Decrease aqueous humor synthesis.*
     - Diuretics: Mainly carbonic anhydrase inhibitors, e.g., Acetazolamide.
     - Beta-blockers, e.g., Timolol.

  2. Increase aqueous humor excretion.

     - Cholinergic agonists: Stimulate contraction of ciliary muscle and increased outflow of aqueous humor through trabecular meshwork, e.g., Pilocarpine.
     - Alpha-agonists, e.g., Epinephrine.
     - Prostaglandins, e.g., Latanoprost.

E.N.T.

- *Otitis externa*: Usually caused by *Pseudomonas aeuroginosa*, and patient presents with painful ear and tenderness on movement of the ear pinna. Treatment: *Antibiotic ear drops.*
- *Otitis media*: Usually caused by Strept. Pneumoniae. Complication: Repeated infections lead to hearing loss. Treatment: Amoxicillin.
- *Inner ear infections*: e.g., *Viral labyrinthitis, Vestibular neuritis*. Patients present with vertigo, nausea, vomiting and horizontal nystagmus. Treatment: Meclizine. *Vertical nystagmus indicate a central process, e.g., Vertebrobasilar CVA.*
- *Sinusitis*: Usually caused by *S. Pneumoniae*, and patient presents *with facial pressure* and *postnasal drip*. On exam: Oropharyngeal cobblestoning and opacification of sinuses on *transillumination*. Treatment: *Amoxicillin.*
- *Nasal meatuses*: Nasolacrimal duct opens into inferior meatus, Sphenoid sinus opens into sphenoethmoidal recess, Posterior ethmoid sinus opens into the superior meatus, where all other sinuses open into the middle meatus.
- *Meniere's disease*: Due to *endolymphatic hydrops*. Patient presents with recurrent episodes of ear fullness, deafness and vertigo. Treatment: Diuretics.

Important Notes and Keywords

- *Negri bodies* in the Purkinje cells of the cerebellum is pathognomonic of *rabies*.
- *Hirano rods* and *neurofibrillary tangles* are pathognomonic of *Alzheimer's disease*.
- Degeneration of the *basal nucleus of Meynert* is pathognomonic of *Alzheimer's disease*.
- *Lewy bodies* and *absence of melanin* from substantia nigra is pathognomonic of *Parkinson's disease*.
- Brain stem is the origin of cranial nerves III to XII.

  1. Midbrain: III–IV.
  2. Pons: V–VIII.
  3. Medulla: IX–XII.

- *Reflexes*:

  1. Biceps reflex: Mediated by *C5 and C6*.
  2. Triceps reflex: Mediated by *C7 and C8*.
  3. Knee reflex: Mediated by *L2, L3 and L4*.
  4. Ankle reflex: Mediated by *S1*.
  5. Babinski reflex: Dorsiflexion of big toe and fanning of the toes on stimulation of lateral sole of the foot. It is a sign of an *upper motor neuron lesion*.

- Causes of bilateral facial nerve paralysis: Bilateral Bell's palsy, e.g., Lyme disease, Sarcoidosis and Guillian Barre syndrome.
- Spongiform encephalopathy (Mad cow disease): Caused by Crutzfeld Jacob (CJ) virus, and patient presents with altered mental status, seizures and myoclonus. Remember the mycoclonus very well.

Respiratory System

Important Definitions

- *TV*: Amount of air that enters the lung on normal inspiration; it is equal to *500 cc*.
- *IRV*: Amount of air that enters the lung on forced inspiration.
- *ERV*: Amount of air left in the lung after normal expiration.
- *RV*: Amount of air left in the lung after forced expiration.
- *Note: Residual volume cannot be measured by spirometry and the only way to measure it is by doing complete pulmonary function tests (PFTs).*
- FRC is reduced in any disease with low lung volume, e.g., Lung collapse or fibrosis.
- FRC is increased in any disease with large lung volume, e.g., Emphysema.
- Refer to Fig. 1.53 for important equations and definitions.

Pulmonary Function Tests (PFTs)

- *Key*: The secret number here is *80%*; anything below 80% is abnormal.
- *Obstructive lung diseases,* e.g., COPD: Low FVC and *very low* FEV1 result in a *FEV1/FVC ratio of less than 80%*; however *TLC is above 80%*.
- *Restrictive lung diseases,* e.g., Interstitial lung disease: Low FVC and *equally low* FEV1, so the *ratio is more than 80%*; however *TLC is below 80%*.
- *Mixed (Obstructive and Restrictive)*: FEV1/FVC <80% and TLC <80%.

Dead Space

- *Anatomical dead space*: Around *150 mL* and is measured by the *Fowler method.*
- *Physiological dead space*: Measured by *Bohr method.*

Respiratory Muscles

- *Passive inspiration: Diaphragm.*
- *Forced inspiration: External intercostals* and *accessory muscles.*
- *Passive expiration: Passive.*
- *Forced expiration: Internal intercostals* and *abdominal muscles.*

Compliance

- *Definition: Lung distensibility,* which is *inversly proportional to lung elasticity.*
- *Note*: At functional residual capacity level, the force of lung collapse and chest wall expansion are equal in power and opposite in direction.

Bronchio-Alveolar-Pulmonary System

- Maximum resistance to airflow occurs at the level of *medium sized bronchi.*
- There is a *fourth power inverse proportion* between radius of airway and airflow resistance.
- Surfactant a.k.a. *Diplamitoyl-phosphatidylcholine* is formed by *type II pneumocytes,* and is completely formed by the *35th week of gestation.* It lines the alveoli to keep them open. This is achieved by

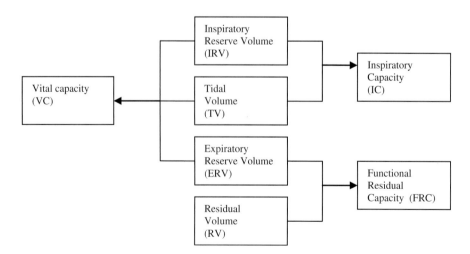

FIG. 1.53 Lung volumes and capacities. Total lung capacity (TLC) = IRV + TV + ERV + RV

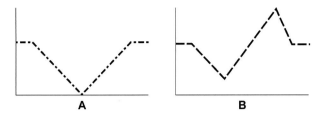

FIG. 1.54 **A** Intrapleural pressure changes during respiratory cycle. **B** Alveolar pressure changes during respiratory cycle

decreasing surface tension and increasing compliance of the alveoli.

- Large alveoli are stable. It is the small sized ones that easily collapse, especially in absence of surfactant.
- During the respiratory cycle, alveolar pressure and intrapleural pressure measured by a ballon catheter in esophagus change as shown in Fig. 1.54.
- Ventilation and perfusion are highest in the lung bases and least in the apices.
- Ventilation/Perfusion ratio (V/Q): *At apex = 1–3, at base = 0.6–0.8.*
- *If V/Q ratio is equal to zero, that indicates complete airway obstruction, while extremely elevated V/Q ratios indicate circulation obstruction resulting in perfusion defect.*

Breathing and Gases

- *Respiratory centers*: Medullary reticular formation contains the major respiratory centers as follows:

  1. Dorsal group: Controls *inspiration.*
  2. Ventral group: Controls *expiration.*
  3. Apneustic and Pneumotaxic centers in pons: *Inhibit inspiration.*

- *Gases*:

  1. Diffusion limited: *Oxygen* and Carbon monoxide (CO).
  2. Perfusion limited: *Carbon dioxide (CO₂),* NO₂ and Oxygen.

- *Chemoreceptors*:

  1. Central: In medulla, and is stimulated by *high CO₂* and *high H.*
  2. Peripheral: In carotid and aortic *bodies.* Stimulated by *low oxygen, high CO₂* and *high H.* So when they ask you in the USMLE about how breathing is stimulated in a patient with low oxygen but normal CO₂, the answer is obviously peripheral receptors.

- *Notes*:

  1. Hypoxia causes vasodilatation everywhere in the body *except the lungs, where it causes vasoconstriction.*
  2. CO₂ is transported in the blood mainly in the form of *bicarbonate* and to a lesser extent bound to hemoglobin.
  3. Pulmonary venous congestion leads to rapid shallow breathing due to stimulation of *J receptors.*
  4. Hering Bruer reflex: Inhibition of inspiration due to stretch of lung tissue.

Asthma

- *Mechanism*: Inflammatory process of the airways characterized by *reversible bronchospasm,* and increased airway secretions.
- *Clinical picture: Shortness of breath, wheezing* and *chronic cough.*
- *Diagnosis*: PFTs and *Methacholine challenge test.*
- *Treatment*:

  1. *Inhaled steroids* is the mainstay of treatment: Steroids *suppress the hyperreactivity of airways to various stimuli.* Side effects: *Oral thrush,* which is prevented by *washing the mouth after inhalation.*
  2. Exercise induced asthma: *Albuterol* before exercise.
  3. Allergy induced asthma: *Mast cell stabilizer* inhaler, e.g., Nedocromil.
  4. Others:

     - *Beta2 agonist bronchodilators*: Short acting, e.g., Albuterol, or long acting, e.g., Salmeterol.
     - *Anticholinergic inhalers,* e.g., Ipratropium: They cause bronchodilation and suppression of the respiratory airways' secretions.
     - *Theophylline*: Bronchodilator. *Side effects: Arrhythmia and seizures.*
     - *Leukotreine inhibitors,* e.g., Montelukast: *Last resort in severe asthma.*

- *Notes*:

  1. Atopic (Extrinsic allergic) asthma is mediated by antigen antibody complexes on mast cells, and the release of interleukins and O₂ radicals by eosinophils and T lymphocytes.
  2. Sputum of asthmatic patients shows *Charcot Laden crystals*; a breakdown product of *eosinophils.*

Chronic Obstructive Pulmonary Disease (COPD)

- *Mechanism*: combination of *chronic bronchitis* and *emphysema*, leading to *expiratory* airway obstruction.
- *Chronic bronchitis*: Expectorant cough for at least *3 successive months/year,* for at least *2 successive years.*
- *Emphysema*: Dilatation of the airspaces *distal to terminal bronchioles*, mostly *centroacinar (Pancinar only in alpha-1 anti-trypsin deficiency).*
- *Clinical picture*:

    1. *Blue bloaters*: Patients with predominant *bronchitis* have *cough* as their main symptom, plus cyanosis and edema.
    2. *Pink puffer*: Patients with predominant *emphysema* have *dyspnea* as their main symptom, plus continous puffing with expiration.

- *Diagnosis*:

    1. *PFTs*: Show obstructive picture (*FEV1/FVC <80*).
    2. *Chest X-ray*: *Hyperinflated lungs and flattened diaphragm.* Refer to Fig. 1.55.

- *Complications*: Multiple, the most significant is *Cor-pulmonale*, which is right ventricular failure. Refer to CHF for more details.
- *Treatment*: *Oxygen* is the mainstay of treatment of COPD, and is the only factor that reduces morbidity and mortality. Practically, treatment is the same as asthma.
- *Notes*:

    1. In emphysema, there is low alpha-1 globulin levels.
    2. Patients with alpha-1 antitrypsin deficiency also have recurrent hepatitis. So keep your eyes open in the USMLE for this patient who was born with emphysema and is presenting with elevated transaminases.

Respiratory Failure

- *Definition*: Decline in the respiratory function leading to $PO_2 <60$, and $PCO_2 >50$.
- *Types and causes*:

    1. *Type I*: Hypoxic normocapnic (Low O_2, normal CO_2): Caused by emphysema, pneumonia and pulmonary edema.
    2. *Type II*: Hypoxic Hypercapnic (Low O_2, High CO_2): Caused by asthma and COPD.

- *Clinical picture*:

    1. Hypoxia: Cyanosis and tachycardia.
    2. Hypercapnia: Headache, full bounding pulse and lethargy (*CO_2 narcosis*).

- *Treatment*:

    1. Type I: O_2 with *high* concentrations.
    2. Type II: O_2 with *low* concentrations to maintain the respiratory center's stimulation. *This is one case where high oxygen flow can be fatal.*

Pneumothorax

- *Types*: Air in the pleural sac, which could be:

    1. *Closed,* e.g., due to ruptured blebs or bullae.
    2. *Open*: Air enters and leaves the pleura without trapping.
    3. *Tension pneumothorax*: Air enters and only partially leaves the pleural sac due to *check valve* mechanism. Refer to Fig. 1.56.

- *Causes*:

    1. *Primary*: Suspect in *tall, thin, middle aged smoker.*
    2. *Secondary*: To COPD or cystic fibrosis.

- *Clinical picture*:

    1. *Sudden* respiratory distress.
    2. Chest pain on inspiration due to severe pleurisy.

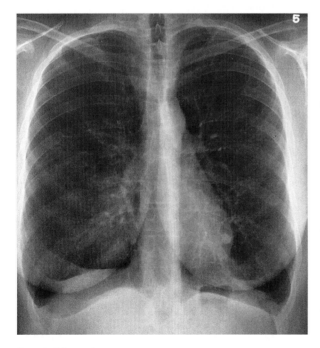

Fig. 1.55 Emphysema

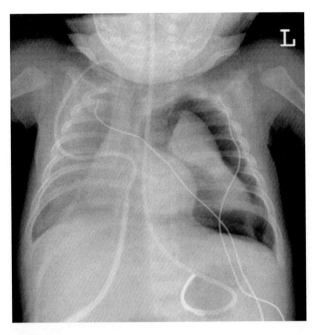

FIG. 1.56 Left tension pneumothorax

3. Hemodynamic instability in severe cases due to compression on the heart.

- *On exam*:

  1. *Hyperresonance on chest percussion* on affected side.
  2. Limited air entry on auscultation of affected lung.

- *Diagnosis*: CXR shows *hyperinflation and shift of mediastinum to the opposite side.*
- *Treatment*: *Chest tube insertion*; however, if not immediately available and patient is unstable, insert a wide bore needle into the 2nd intercostal space in the mid-clavicular line to allow the trapped air out, till the chest tube is inserted.
- *Pleurodesis* (Sealing of both pleural layers together) is considered in:

  1. First pneumothorax episode in secondary cases.
  2. Second episode in primary cases.

Lung Cancer

- *Introduction*:

  1. Second most common malignancy in men after prostate cancer, and the third in women after breast and colon cancers; however, *it is the number 1 cause of death from cancer in both genders.*
  2. *Most common cause of pleural effusion.*
  3. Smoking increases the lung cancer risk by *10 times more than normal.*

- *Types*: Refer to Table 1.12.
- *Clinical picture*: Cough, hemoptysis, weight loss and pleural effusion or sometimes completely asymptomatic.
- *Diagnosis*: *Biopsy*; peripheral ones by *CT guided biopsy*, and central ones by *bronchoscopic guided biopsy or mediastinoscopy.*
- *What else to order*: *Bone scan, CT of abdomen and pelvis, and CT of the head to rule out metastases.*
- *Treatment* : Surgery (only if the tumor has not metastasized yet), radiation and chemotherapy for all types, *except for small cell cancer, where surgery is not an option.*
- *Remember*: Central tumors are (SS) *S*quamous and *S*mall cell. The rest are peripheral.
- *Notes*:

TABLE 1.12 Types of lung cancer.

Type	Location	Para-neoplasia	Miscellaneous
Adenocarcinoma	Peripheral	None	• Most common lung cancer • Early metastases
Squamous cell carcinoma	Central	Hypercalcemia: due to release of PTH related peptide	• 2nd most common lung cancer • Causes lung cavitations • Squamous cells are eosinophilic with hyperchromatic nuclei
Small cell carcinoma	Central	• ACTH: Cushing syndrome • ADH: Syndrome of inappropriate ADH. (SIADH) • Muscle weakness: Eaton Lambert, due to antibodies against calcium channels antibodies • Sensory neuropathy: Due to anti-neuronal antibodies (ANNA-1)	• Eaton Lambert is just like Myasthenia Gravis , except: 1. Activity makes symptoms better 2. Activity makes EMG waves stronger • Small cells are basophilic and lymphocyte sized
Large cell carcinoma	Peripheral	Gynecomastia	

1. Any type of lung cancer infiltrating the sympathetic chain will cause *Horner's syndrome,* and is called *Pancoast tumor.* Horner's syndrome presentation:

   - *Ptosis*: Due to paralysis of *superior tarsal muscle.*
   - *Miosis*: Due to paralysis of *dilator pupillae muscle.*
   - *Anhydrosis.*

2. Bronchopulmonary segment is formed histologically of a bronchus with its supplying artery and vein, plus the lung segment that they all supply.
3. Mesothelioma is a pleural based malignancy that occurs due to exposure to asbestos for long duration, at least *10 years.*
4. Bronchial adenoma is a benign tumor arising from bronchial mucosa. Patient presents with recurrent hemoptysis and carcinoid syndrome (Diarrhea, Flushing, Bronchospasm, right heart valve lesions mainly the tricuspid valve, high urinary 5-HIAA).

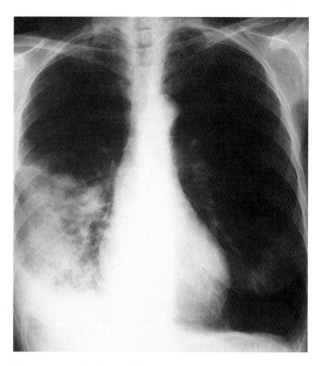

Fɪɢ. 1.57 Right lower lobe pneumonia

Pneumonia

- *Definition*: *Infection* and *consolidation* of the pulmonary tissue.
- *Cause*: *Community acquired,* unless the patient has been in a hospital or a nursing home for more than *72 h* before symptoms start; that's when it is called *nosocomial pneumonia.* Refer to Fig. 1.57.
- *Types*: Lobar pneumonia is the most common form and is caused by *Streptococcus pneumoniae*; however pneumonia could be interstitial or bronchopneumonia.
- *Phases*:

   1. Congestion.
   2. Red hepatization (2–4 days): *Mediated by neutrophils.*
   3. Grey hepatization (4–8 days): *Characterized by high fibrin content.*
   4. Resolution: After 8–10 days from the initial phase.

- *Clinical picture*: Cough and expectoration, fever and shortness of breath.
- *On exam*: The area with pneumonia is *dull to percussion, has high Tactile Vocal Fremitus (TVF), Rales and crackles, bronchial sounds* and *egophony* (if the patient says "e", you hear it as "a" on auscultation).
- *Diagnosis*: Chest X-ray and sputum culture.
- *Treatment*: Any pathogen can cause pneumonia, but be sure to remember that community acquired

pneumonia is best treated by Quinolones, e.g., Levofloxacin or a combination of Macrolide, e.g., Azithormycin, and 3rd generation cephalosporin.

- *Notes*:

1. *Atypical pneumonia*:

   - If the chest X-ray looks worse than how the patient clinically presents, think of atypical pneumonia, *especially if the patient also has diarrhea or change in mental status*; most common causes are:

      1. *Legionella: Diagnosed by Direct immunofluorescence and culture on charcoal agar. Typical sources are shower heads and air conditioners.*
      2. *Mycoplasma: Diagnosed by high mycoplasma IgM titers.*

   - Treatment of atypical pneumonia: Macrolides, e.g., *Erythromycin.*

2. *Aspiration pneumonia*: Caused by *anaerobes* and is more common in the right lung, due to the large right main bronchus that is more in line with the trachea. Suspect aspiration in patients with *gastrostomy feeding tubes, alcoholics* and *after coma or seizure.*
3. *Key facts*:

   - *Staphylococcus aureus*: Causes *lung cavitation* and *hemoptysis. Also the most common*

cause of pneumonia following an influenza infection. Methicillin Resistant S. aureus (MRSA) is treated with Vancomycin.
- Klebsiella: Causes apical (Friedlander) pneumonia and red current jelly sputum.
- H. Influenza is one common cause of pneumonia in patients with COPD.

Bronchiectasis

- Mechanism: Combination of airway obstruction and infection, leading to abnormal persistent dilatation of the bronchi.
- Most common sites: Bases of the lungs.
- Clinical picture: Cough and expectoration, more on stooping forwards. Also hemoptysis due to mucosal ulceration.
- On exam:

  1. Lung bases: Dull to percussion with high TVF.
  2. Lung apices: Resonant to percussion with low TVF: due to compensatory emphysema.

- Diagnosis: CXR or CT chest shows honeycomb appearance.
- Treatment: Postural drainage and antibiotics.

Pulmonary Embolism (CPE)

- Source: Most common source is DVT in the lower extremities, which could be explained by Virchow's triad: Flow stasis, endothelial damage and hypercoagulable state.
- Clinical picture: Sudden dyspnea, hyperventilation and pleuritic chest pain in a patient with normal CXR. Presents in the USMLE as a hospitalized or immobile patient who suddenly develops unexplained respiratory distress few days after surgery.
- Diagnosis:

  1. Gold standard for diagnosis: Pulmonary angiography.
  2. Practically, we use V/Q scan (test of choice) which will show ventilation/perfusion mismatch.
  3. If the CXR is not clear, V/Q will not be accurate, so a CT chest is done.
  4. Patients with PE have normal chest X ray.
  5. Right ventricular strain on EKG.

- Treatment: Heparin is the first step, followed by warfarin for 3–6 months (Target INR = 2–3).
- Fat pulmonary embolism: Occurs after long bone fractures; patients have dyspnea and skin petechiae. Treatment is mainly supportive.

Pleural Diseases
Pleurisy

- Causes: Any nearby infection or irritation, e.g., Pneumonia, Pneumothorax.
- Clinical picture: Stitching chest pain increased with deep inspiration and cough.
- On exam: Pleural rub.
- Treatment: Treat the cause + NSAIDs.

Pleural Effusion

- Causes: Transudative, e.g., CHF, Exudative, e.g., Pneumonia, Chylous, e.g., Thoracic duct obstruction, or hemorrhagic, e.g., Malignancy.
- Clinical picture: Dyspnea and pleuritic chest pain (Increased with inspiration).
- On exam: Decreased everything, i.e., Decreased chest movement on inspiration, Decreased Tactile Vocal Fremitus (TVF), Dullness on percussion and Decreased air entry on auscultation.
- Diagnosis: Chest X-ray shows leveling of fluid filling the costophrenic angle. Large effusion pushes the mediastium towards the opposite lung. Refer to Fig. 1.58.
- Treatment:

  1. Thoracocentesis is diagnostic and therapeutic. Fluid is sent for analysis to diagnose its nature, e.g., Exudate, transudate, etc....
  2. If fluid reaccumulated after thoracocentesis, chest tube should be inserted.
  3. If fluid reaccumulated after removal of chest tube, pleurodesis should be done (Sealing of the pleural layers).

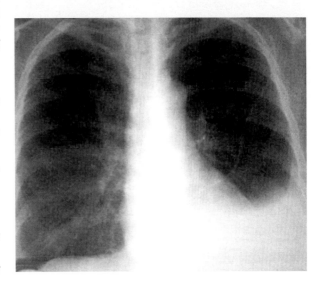

FIG. 1.58 Left pleural effusion

- *Notes*:

  1. Malignant effusions are *bloody* and they re-accumulate rapidly and pleurodesis is indicated.
  2. Empyema is accumulation of pus in the pleural cavity. Treatment: *Antibiotics and intercostal tube drainage.* If fails: Open drainage and removal of the pleura (Decortication).
  3. Lung collapse and lung fibrosis are 2 other diseases with "*Decreased everything*" on exam, but the mediastinal shift here is *towards the opacified lung, not towards the opposite side.*

Interstitial Lung Disease (ILD)

- *Mechanism*: Infiltration of the lung tissue with inflammatory cells leading to restrictive lung disease.
- *Causes*: Silicosis, asbestosis, Sarcoidosis, drugs (e.g., Amiodarone).
- *Clinical picture (5C)*: Cough, Cyanosis, Clubbing, Crackles and Core-pulmonale.
- *CXR*: Diffuse *reticulonodular infiltrate*. Refer to Fig. 1.59.
- *Diagnosis: open lung biopsy.*
- *Treatment*: Steroids.
- *Notes on some ILDs*:

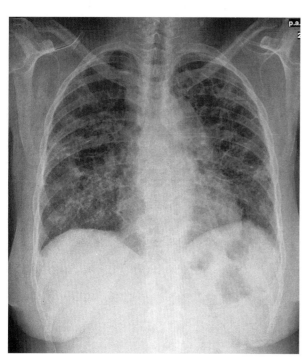

FIG. 1.59 Ground glass appearance of Interstitial lung disease

1. *Idiopathic pulmonary fibrosis (IPF)* is a rapidly progressive ILD with bad prognosis. Most patients end up on steroids and O2 at all times.
2. *Eosinophilic granuloma*: a.k.a. Langerhan cell granulomatosis (Formerly Histiocytosis X) is more common in *male smokers*. *Diagnosis*: Langerhan cells on lung biopsy or bronchioalveolar lavage. *Complication*: Pneumothorax. *Hand Schuller Christian disease*: Eosinophilic granuloma + Lytic bone lesions + Diabetes inspidus + exophthalmia.
3. *Aspergillosis*: Immune complex mediated ILD. *Brownish* sputum with *branching hyphae* under microscope.

Silicosis and Asbestosis

- *Silica*: Exposure occurs in *glass and sand industry*. Clinical picture: *Upper* lung zones injury and *hilar egg shell calcifications*.
- *Asbestos*: Exposure occurs in *brakes and shipyard industry*. Clinical picture: *Lower* lung zones injury and *pleural calcifications*. Unique feature: *Ferruginous bodies* in lungs (Asbestos + Hemosiderin) with *clubbed ends*. Complications: *Mesothelioma* and bronchogenic carcinoma.

Sarcoidosis

- *Mechanism*: *Non-caseating granuloma*, more common in *African Americans. Remember that granuloma is a type IV hypersensitivity reaction.*
- *Clinical picture*:

  1. Uveitis, lacrimal and parotid glands swelling.
  2. CVS: Cardiomyopathy.
  3. CNS: Bilateral facial nerve palsy.
  4. Lungs: Hilar lymphadenopathy and restrictive lung disease.
  5. Metabolic:

     - Hypercalcemia: Due to secretion of activated vitamin D by macrophages.
     - Diabetes insipidus: Due to posterior pituitary dysfunction.

- *Diagnosis*:

  1. High serum angiotensin converting enzyme level (ACE).
  2. Transbronchial biopsy showing non-caseating granuloma is diagnostic. Microscopy shows *Schumann* and *Asteroid* bodies.

- *Treatment*: Self resolving; however severe and non-resolving cases are treated with systemic steroids.

- *Notes*:

  1. In sarcoidosis, there is *low albumin* and *high gamma globulin* levels.
  2. Mucocutaneous forms of sarcoidosis are treated with *chloroquine*.

Tuberculosis (TB)

- *Causes*: Mycobacterium Tuberculosis (Acid fast bacillus) is the most common cause; however, in immunocompromised patients Atypical Mycobacteria are involved, e.g., M. Avium, M. Marinum, M. Kansasi.
- *Primary complex*: *Ghon's focus* in the upper lung lobe.
- *Pathology*: Mycobacterium Tuberculosis live *inside macrophages*, after inhibiting the *phagosome-lysosome fusion process*.
- *Clinical picture*:

  1. *2 nights, 2 losses*: Night fever, night sweats, loss of weight and loss of appetite. Mediated by *interleukins*.
  2. Cough and expectoration.
  3. Hemoptysis: Due to erosion of a blood vessel, or oozing from friable granulation tissue.

- *Diagnosis*:

  1. Isolation of the organism on a culture is the diagnostic test of choice. Sample obtained from the sputum or gastric aspirate.
  2. CXR: Apical infiltrate or cavitation.
  3. Tuberculin test: Purified Protein Derivative (PPD) is injected intradermally in the forearm, and the induration (*not erythema*) is measured in 48–72 h. *Note: PPD test becomes positive 3–10 weeks after infection, and not immediately afterwards.*

- *PPD interpretation*:

  1. Induration less than 10 mm in immunocompetent person: Normal.
  2. Induration more than 10 mm in immunocompetent person: Next step is to obtain a CXR:

     - Normal CXR (Latent TB): INH therapy for 9 months.
     - Abnormal CXR: TB treatment.

  3. Induration less than 5 mm in immunocompromised patient: Normal.
  4. Induration more than 5 mm in immunocompromised patient: Next step is to obtain a CXR:

     - Normal CXR (Latent TB): INH therapy for 12 months.
     - Abnormal CXR: TB treatment.

- *Treatment*: 6 months treatment course: 2 months of INH, Rifampin, Pyrazinamide and *Ethambutol (or Streptomycin)*, followed by 4 months course of INH and Rifampin.
- *Side effects of therapy*:

  1. INH: Hepatotoxicity and peripheral neuritis (*Vitamin B6 during therapy is necessary*).
  2. Rifampin: Orange discoloration of body fluids and hepatotoxicity.
  3. Pyrazinamide: Hepatitis and gout.
  4. Ethambutol: Optic neuritis.

Sleep Apnea

- *Definition*: Cessation of breathing during sleep.
- *Types and Causes*:

  1. Central: Respiratory center depression, e.g., Alcohol, BDZ.
  2. Obstructive: Narrow airway, e.g., Large tongue, large palate, big neck.
  3. *Pickwickian syndrome (Obesity hypoventilation syndrome)*: Obstructive sleep apnea + Obesity + CO_2 retention.

- *Clinical picture*:

  1. Loud snoring during sleep.
  2. Episodes of apnea during sleep followed by waking up gasping for air.
  3. Daytime sleepiness and fatigue.

- *Diagnosis*: Sleep study (Polysomnography) showing at least *10* apnea episodes/hour, each episode lasting at least *10* seconds.
- *Complications*: Pulmonary hypertension (>20), Cor pulmonale and sudden death.
- *Treatment*:

  1. Continous Positive Airway Pressure (*CPAP*) during sleep, and *weight loss*.
  2. Avoidance of alcohol and BDZ before bedtime.
  3. For resistant cases: Uvulo-Palato-Pharyngo-Plasty (UPPP).

Solitary Lung Nodule

- *Definition*: Any nodule that is *less than 5 cm* in diameter, discovered accidentally on a CXR or CT without any related symptoms.
- *Characteristics*:

  1. Benign: Central, round, regular border, uniform calcification.
  2. Malignant: Peripheral, irregular shape, speculated, irregular calcification.

- *Management*:

  1. High risk patient (Old, smoker, Family history of cancer): Biopsy.
  2. Low risk patient (Young, Non smoker, No family history): Repeat CXR every 3 months for 2 years:

     - If any change in characteristics mentioned above: Biopsy.
     - If stable: Follow up on symptoms.

Cough

- *Introduction*: Cough is a protective reflex in cases of infection and in post-operative patients.
- *Most common cause of cough*: Smoking.
- *Causes of chronic cough*: Chronic sinusitis, GERD and Asthma.
- *Antitussives*: Decrease cough by 2 mechanisms:

  1. Peripheral: Anesthesize peripheral receptors. Best is *Benzonatate*.
  2. Central: Increase threshold of cough center. Best is *Dextromethorphan*.

- *Note*: One of the complications of lack of cough, deep breaths and using incentive spirometry in post-operative patients is *atelectasis. Suspect atelectasis in a patient developing fever 1–2 days after surgery.*

Drug-Induced Pulmonary Diseases

- *Interstitial lung diseases*: Amiodarone, Nitrofurantoin.
- *Cough*: ACE inhibitors (Treatment: Switch to ARB).
- *Bronchospasm*: Aspirin and non-selective beta blockers.
- *Pulmonary eosinophilia*: Gold, penicillamine.

Infectious Diseases

Human Immunodeficiency Virus (HIV)

- *Introduction*:

  1. *Enveloped DS RNA* virus with multiple functional enzymes including reverse transcriptase, protease, and integrase.
  2. The outer shell is formed of capsid protein, gp41 and gp120 capsid proteins, and *p24 (Early marker)*.
  3. Reverse transcriptase (*RNA dependant DNA polymerase*) converts the virus's RNA to DNA.

- *HIV genome*: Has Long Terminal Repeat sequences (*LTRs*) which include:

  1. Sticky ends: Recognized by integrase.
  2. Promotor/Enhancer region: DNA transcription.
  3. gag (Group antigens): Code for viral antigenic proteins.
  4. pol (Protease, integrase and reverse transcriptase): *Protease is the agent that makes HIV contagious.*
  5. tat (Transactivator): Activates transcription.
  6. env (Envelope proteins).

- *Transmission*: Infection is mainly through blood or sexual intercourse*; more in females and those who engage in anal intercourse.*
- *Pathology*: HIV targets the following cells:

  1. T lymphocytes: Mainly *CD4. If CD4 count drops below 200, the patient requires treatment, even if he does not have any obvious infection.*
  2. B lymphocytes: Can trigger other immunological disease.
  3. Monocytes and macrophages: Act as *reservoir* for the virus. Can also transport it to the CNS, causing aseptic meningitis and neuropathy.

- *Clinical picture*:

  1. Initial viremia followed by a latent period of *5–10 years.*
  2. AIDS related complex (ARC): Weight loss, fever, and night sweats.

- *Diagnosis*: Positive Enzyme-Linked Immunosorbent Assay (ELISA) test is the first step. If positive, confirm diagnosis by doing *Western Blot* test.
- *Follow up*: Best done through the viral RNA load, and CD4 count. *They are used for prognostic purposes, early detection of progression of HIV to AIDS, and to assess response to treatment.*
- *Complications*:

  1. Kaposi sarcoma (*Purple skin nodules*): By *Human Herpes Virus-8 (HHV-8). Kaposi sarcoma occurs due to vascular proliferation and hemosiderin deposition.*
  2. Oral hairy leukoplakia: By *Epstein-Barr virus (EBV)*. Can be seen on the lateral borders of the tongue.
  3. Chorioretinitis: By *Cytomegalovirus (CMV)*.
  4. Esophagitis: By *Candida albicans*.
  5. Diarrhea: By *Cryptosporidium parvum*. Treatment: *Azithromycin*.
  6. Meningitis: By *Cryptococcus neoformans*.
  7. Seizures: By *Toxoplasma Gondii, which causes diffuse intracranial calcifications*, and *contrast enhancing mass*. Treatment: *Sulfadiazine +*

Pyrimethamine. Drug of choice to treat toxoplasmosis during pregnancy is *Spiramycin*.

8. Leukemia: *Human T-cell Leukemia Virus-1 (HTLV-1) causes hairy cell leukemia, while HTLV-2 causes T cell leukemia.*

9. Pneumonia:

   - *Pneumocystis Jiroveci (Formerly P. Carinii "PCP")*. Suspect when CD4 count is less than 200. *Diagnosis*: Bronchoalveolar lavage or lung biopsy. *Culture*: Does not grow in vitro, but stains with methenamine silver. *Treatment*: SMX/TMP and/or pentamidine.

   - *Mycobacterium-Avium-Complex (MAC)*: Acid fast bacillus. Suspect when CD4 count is less than 50. *Clinical picture*: Pneumonia. *Diagnosis*: Lung biopsy. *Treatment*: Clarithromycin, ethambutol and rifabutin.

- *Treatment of HIV*:

  1. *Reverse transcriptase inhibitors:*
     - Zidovudine (AZT): Inhibits HIV *replication*. Side effects: Severe *headache. Note: Given to pregnant HIV patients to decrease risk of fetal transmission.*
     - Didanosine (ddi), Zalcitabine and Lamivudine: All cause *pancreatitis* and *peripheral neuropathy*.

  2. *HIV protease inhibitors*, e.g., Indinavir and Ritonavir. Side effects:

     - Elevated liver transaminases.
     - *Indinavir causes nephrolithiasis.*

- *Note*:

  1. Prophylaxis against HIV after a contaminated needle stick injury is a *1 month course of LIZ (Lamivudine, Indinavir, Zidovudine)*. The main factor deciding the probability of transmission is *the depth of the injury*.

  2. Risk of materno-fetal transmission of HIV is significantly reduced by treating the mother during pregnancy with *zidovudine*.

Rabies

- *Introduction*: *Rhabdovirus* which replicates *locally in a wound,* and may travel up neuronal axons into the CNS to cause encephalitis.
- *Source*: Multiple; most famous are dogs, cats, bats and raccoons.
- *Pathology*: Brain tissue shows virions, a.k.a. *Negri bodies*.
- *Clinical picture*: Fever, headache and *hydrophobia* due to pharyngeal muscles spasm. This may

lead to *foaming of the mouth*, a classic symptom of rabies.

- *Treatment: Immunoglobulins and active immunization*, using five injections of a killed virus vaccine.
- *Note*: Washing the wound with soap and water dissolves the lipid envelope of the virus, which leads to prolongation of its incubation period.

Clostridium Tetani

- *Introduction*: *Spore forming, Gram positive anaerobic* bacillus with *terminal spores (C. Tetani has Terminal spores)*.
- *Mechanism*: *Tetanospasmin* toxin cause tetany by inhibiting the release of GABA from cerebellum, and glycine from Renshaw cells of spinal cord.
- *Clinical picture*:

  1. Muscle spasms and lockjaw.
  2. Risus sardonicus: Fixed smile due to muscle spasm. (Sign of advanced disease).

- *Prevention*: Vaccination, and tetanus toxoid is given every 10 years.
- *After exposure*, e.g., Patient injured his foot by stepping on a rusty nail.

  1. If last toxoid dose was within the last 5 years: No toxoid needed.
  2. If last toxoid dose was more than 5 years ago: Give a new dose of toxoid.
  3. If patient has never been immunized: Give tetanus toxoid and immunoglobulin.

- *Treatment of tetanus*:

  1. Airway protection, and clean wound.
  2. Medications: Vaccine + Immunoglobulin + Muscle relaxants.

Clostridium Difficile

- *Introduction*: *Spore forming, Gram positive anaerobic* bacillus.
- *Mechanism*: Exotoxins. Toxin A causes diarrhea. Toxin B is cytotoxic.
- *Clinical picture*: *Pseudo-membranous colitis*. Usually follows the use of broad spectrum antibiotics, e.g., Ampicillin, Clindamycin. Patient presents with severe watery malodorous diarrhea and abdominal pain.
- *Diagnosis*: Detecting C. Diff. toxins in the stools.
- *Treatment*: Oral metronidazole or Vancomycin. They have to be given orally as they act *locally* inside the intestine.

Listeria Monocytogenes

- *Introduction*: Non-spore forming, Gram positive bacillus, with unique features:

    1. *Facultative intracellular* organism.
    2. The only Gram positive organism capable of releasing *endotoxins*.
    3. *End over end motility,* a.k.a. *tumbling*.

- *Clinical picture*: Meningitis and sepsis. Third most common cause of meningitis in neonates (After Strept. Agalactiae, and *E. coli*). It also causes meningitis in immunocompromised patients, e.g., HIV.
- *Treatment*: *Ampicillin + Sulbactam* or *SMX/TMP*.

Salmonella

- *Introduction*: A motile *H₂S releasing* bacterium, with *Vi antigen*.
- *Source*: Food or water contaminated with animal feces. A famous source is *undercooked eggs. S. typhi is carried only by humans in the gall bladder and not carried by animals.*
- *S. typhi*: A facultative intracellular organism, causing *typhoid (Enteric) fever*, where patient presents with:

    1. *Step-ladder fever.*
    2. *Rosy spots on the abdomen.*
    3. RLQ abdominal pain: Often confused with appendicitis.
    4. Treatment: *Ciprofloxacin* or *Ceftriaxone*.

- *S. cholera-suis*: Causes bacteremia which targets lungs, liver or even the brain.
- *S. enteritidis*: Causes mucous or watery diarrhea. Treatment: Self resolving. *Antibiotics will prolong bacterial shedding.*

Rickettsia

- *Introduction*: Gram negative, *intracellular* organism with *ATP/ADP translocator*.
- *Characteristics*: Same antigens as Proteus mirabilis (OX-2, OX-19, OX-K), which can be distinguished and diagnosed by *Weil-Felix test*.
- *Clinical picture*:

    1. *Rocky Mountain spotted fever*: Caused by *Rickettsia rickettsii*, transmitted by ticks (*Dermacentor*). Clinical picture: Fever, and petechial rash that *starts in the palms and soles and creeps towards the trunk*.
    2. *Epidemic typhus*: Caused by *Rickettsia prowazekii*, transmitted by *ticks*. Clinical picture: Fever,

and rash that involves the whole body *except palms and soles*.
    3. *Endemic typhus*: Caused by *Rickettsia typhi*, transmitted by *rats*. Clinical picture: Fever, and *rash that starts on the fifth day of fever*.
    4. *Q fever*: Caused by *Coxiella burnetti*, transmitted through contact with animals and animal products. Clinical picture: Fever and pneumonia, due to inhalation of *endospores. It is the only rickettsia that doesn't cause rash.*
    5. *Bartonella henselae*: Causes *Cat Scratch disease*. Clinical picture: Cat scratch, followed by fever, rash and *swollen tender pustular lymphadenopathy*. Complication: *Bacillary angiomatosis*, which is proliferation of blood vessels, common in AIDS patients.
    6. *Ehrlichia canis*: From dog *licks*, causing fever and rash. Peripheral smear shows *numerous morulae inside the monocytes.*

- *Diagnosis*: Complement Fixation Test (CFT).
- *Treatment: Doxycycline plus chloramphenicol*. Drug of choice for cat scratch disease is azithromycin.

Bacillus Cereus

- *Introduction: Spore forming, Gram positive* bacillus.
- *Mechanism*: Heat stable or labile toxin in *undercooked rice*.
- *Clinical picture: Diarrhea, mostly after ingestion of undercooked rice.*
- *Treatment*: Self resolving without treatment.

Cryptococcus Neoformans

- *Introduction: Polysaccharide encapsulated yeast.*
- *Transmission: Pigeon droppings.*
- *Clinical picture*: Meningitis in immunocompromised patients, e.g., AIDS.
- *Diagnosis*:

    1. *India ink* staining of CSF shows a *halo around the yeast cells.*
    2. Culture: Grows on *Sabouraud's agar*.

- *Treatment*: Combination of *Amphotericin B and flucytosine.*
- *Notes*:

    1. Amphotericin B: Causes phlebitis, nephrotoxicity and febrile reaction. Prevention: Give aspirin or acetaminophen before Amphotericin treatment.
    2. Flucytosine: Causes bone marrow depression and GI upset.

Coccidiodes Immitis

- *Introduction*: Thick walled spherules, causing Cocci-diodomycosis (*San Joaquin valley fever*).
- *Location*: Common in the *southwestern United States* (*Desert areas*).
- *Clinical picture*: Atypical pneumonia and *erythema nodosum* (Tender red nodules on tibia).
- *Diagnosis*: Positive complement fixation test (CFT).
- *Treatment*: Fluconazole or itraconazole. Amphotericin B is used in severe cases.
- *Note*: So, when you see a patient in the USMLE who has been to a desert area in the southwestern US recently, and now has pneumonia and bumps on his legs, you know what to think!

Entamoeba Histolytica

- *Introduction*: A parasite that moves by means of *pseudopodia*, and it exists in 2 forms:

  1. *Mature cyst*: Infective form.
  2. *Trophozite*: Pathogenic form.

- *Clinical picture*: Severe watery diarrhea, *with blood and mucus*.
- *Complication*: Liver abscesses; mainly involving the *right lobe*.
- *Diagnosis*: Stool culture shows *trophozites with intracytoplasmic RBCs*.
- *Treatment*: *Metronidazole*.
- *Note*: Homosexual men are frequent carriers.

Giardia Lamblia

- *Introduction*: A parasite that also exists in 2 forms:

  1. *Mature cyst*: Infective form.
  2. *Trophozite*: Pathogenic form. It is *pear shaped*, with *2 nuclei* and *4 pairs of flagella*.

- *Clinical picture*: Watery malodorous diarrhea, and abdominal distention and bloating. So, when you see a patient in the USMLE who just traveled outside the US recently, and now has abdominal pain, and watery, *non-bloody diarrhea*, you know what to think!
- *Diagnosis*: Stool analysis shows cysts and/or trophozites.
- *Treatment*: *Metronidazole*.
- *Note*: *Well water* and *day care centers* are notorious sources of Giardia lamblia.

Plasmodium

- *Introduction*: Parasite causing *malaria*, transmitted by the *female anopheles*.

- *Clinical picture and causative organism*:

  1. *Tertian*: Attacks of fever and sweats every 48 hours: *Plasmodium vivax* and *Plasmodium ovale*.
  2. *Quartan*: Attacks of fever and sweats every 72 hours: *Plasmodium malariae*.
  3. *Malignant malaria* with variable attack periods: *Plasmodium falciparum*.

- *Prophylaxis*: *Chloroquine*. If chloroquine resistant, give *Mefloquine*.
- *Treatment*:

  1. *P. vivax, P. ovale* and *P. malariae*: Chloroquine for blood forms, and primaquine for tissue forms.
  2. *P. falciparum*: Chloroquine. If chloroquine resistant, give quinine, mefloquine or artemether.

- *Notes*:

  1. *Plasmodia vivax* and *P. ovale* reproduce in the liver to form *hypnozites*. These stages can causes multiple relapses (*Relapsing malaria*).
  2. African-Americans resist infection by *P. vivax*, because they do not have *Duffy A* and *Duffy B* antigens on their RBCs.
  3. Sickle cell patients are resistant to infection by *P. falciparum*, due to *HbS*.
  4. Anti-malarial medications induce hemolysis in patients with *G6PD deficiency*.

Miscellaneous

- *Sporothrix schenkii*: Cigar shaped budding yeast. *Transmission*: Contact with rose thorns (a.k.a. *Rose gardener's disease*). *Clinical picture*: Subcutaneous nodules and ulcers. *Treatment*: Potassium iodide (KI) or itraconazole for cutaneous forms, and Amphotericin B for extracutaneous forms.
- *Aspergillus*: Inhalation causes hypersensitivity reactions *type I and III*, which leads to bronchospasm. May form aspergilloma in lungs. Also releases *aflatoxins* which have been linked to *liver cancer*. Shows *branching hyphae* under microscope (Candida shows *pseudo-hyphae*). *Note*: Aspergillus is the nightmare of any bone marrow transplant unit.
- *Chromoblastomycosis*: Causes cauliflower-like masses with copper colored sclerotic bodies and *B*road *B*ased *B*udding (BBB) on microscopy. Treatment: *Itraconazole*.
- *Histoplasmosis and blastomycosis*: Transmitted through birds' feces and may cause pneumonia.
- *Actinomycosis*: Causes formation of yellow sulfur granules. Treatment: *Penicillin*

- *Shigella*: A pathogen transmitted by contaminated hands and water. Releases *Verotoxin*, which causes *bloody diarrhea; rich in WBC count*.
- *Campylobacter jejuni*: Causes *bloody loose diarrhea*. Treatment: *Erythromycin*. Association: *Guillian-Barre syndrome*.
- *Yersinia enterocolitica*: Causes *appendicitis-like pain*, mucosal ulceration and diarrhea. Mechanism: Release of enterotoxins and direct intestinal cells invasion.
- *Trypanosoma cruzi*: Transmitted by *Reduviid (Kissing) bug*, and causes skin chagoma (Nodule or papule), a.k.a. *Romana sign*. Late stages might develop *Chagas disease* (Toxic megacolon, cardiomypoathy and achalasia). *Treatment: Nifurtimox*.

Miscellaneous

- *Normal labs in the elderly*: Low PO2, Low FEV1, Low Hb, Low GFR and elevated alkaline phosphatase. They also high level of *vitamin A* due to decreased liver clearance.
- *Tumor markers*:

1. *Carcinoembryonic Antigen (CEA): Colorectal cancer.*
2. *CA 19-9: Pancreatic cancer.*
3. *CA 125: Ovarian cancer.*
4. *Alpha Fetoprotein (AFP): Hepatocellular cancer and teratoma.*
5. *Prostatic Specific Antigen (PSA): Prostate cancer.*
6. *Human Chorionic Gonadotrophin (HCG): Choriocarcinoma, Vesicular mole and seminoma.*
7. *S-100: Melanoma.*

- *Metastases*:

1. Most common tumor to send metastases: *Breast cancer.*
2. Most common organ to receive metastases: *Adrenal medulla.*

TABLE 1.13 Vitamins and minerals.

Vitamin	Properties	Deficiency
Vitamin A	• Fat soluble • Retinoic acid is used in cases of acne. • Isotretinoin is a teratogenic form	• Night blindness. *Bitot spots*. Dry skin and hair. • Toxicity: Increased intracranial pressure and joint pains
Vitamin D	• Fat soluble • D2 is consumed in milk • D3 is formed under the skin by UV stimulation • Active form is 1,25 dihydroxycholecalciferol • It increases calcium and phosphate absorption from intestine	• Fatigue, muscle and bone weakness, and fractures • Toxicity: hypercalcemia manifested by altered mental status, polyuria and constipation. Common in hyperparathyroidism and sarcoidosis
Vitamin E	• Fat soluble • Antioxidant function: protects RBCs from hemolysis	• Fragile RBCs and higher risk of hemolysis
Vitamin K	• Fat soluble • Synthesized by intestinal flora • It forms gamma-carboxy-glutamate, upon which some clotting factors depend for activation; namely *factors II, VII, IX and X, and proteins C and S*	• Causes: 1. Vitamin K antagonists, e.g., warfarin 2. Destruction of intestinal flora by long term use of antibiotics. • Coagulopathy with high bleeding tendency • Patients have *high PT and APTT*
Vitamin B1 (Thiamine)	• Water soluble • Thiamine pyrophosphate is a co-factor for 2 reactions: 1. Oxidative decarboxylation of keto acids 2. Transketolase of HMP shunt.	• 2 important deficiency syndromes: 1. *Beri Beri*: Polyneuropathy and CHF. 2. *Wernicke-Korsakoff syndrome*: Triad of *encephalopathy, nystagmus* and *ataxia*. Korsakoff is manifested by *anterograde amnesia* and *confabulations*.
Vitamin B2 (Riboflavin)	• Water soluble • It is a co-factor in oxidation and reduction reactions forming FAD and FMN	• Angular stomatitis • Cheilitis • Corneal vascularization

TABLE 1.13 (continued).

Vitamin	Properties	Deficiency

Vitamin B3 (Niacin)	• Water soluble
	
	• It is a co-factor in oxidation and reduction reactions forming NAD and NADP
	• It inhibits lipolysis, so used in type II hyperlipidemia to *increase HDL* and decrease LDL and VLDL
	• Side effects: *Facial flushing and pruritis*
		• Pellagra triad:
		
		  1. *Diarrhea*
		  2. *Dermatitis*
		  3. *Dementia*
		
		• Dermatitis of pellagra is mainly on the face and neck arranged in a *necklace like* distribution.

Vitamin B5 (Pantothenic acid)	• Water soluble • It is the provider of co-A	• Rash and diarrhea

Vitamin B6 (Pyridoxine)	• Water soluble
	• Forms pyridoxal phosphate, which is essential for transamination and decarboxylation reactions
		• Peripheral neuropathy
		• Hyper-excitability and seizures
		• Causes:
		
		  1. *INH*
		  2. OCPs

Vitamin B12 (Cobalamin)	Water soluble
	• Stores in the liver last for at least 5 years
	• Absorbed in the ileum, and presence of intrinsic factor is essential for absorption
	• Co-factor for homocysteine and methylmalonyl co-A reactions
		• Macrocytic hyperchromic anemia
		• Subacute combined degeneration SCD
		• *Causes*:
		  1. Vegetarians
		  2. Malabsorption
		  3. Infestation e.g.: Diphyllobothrium latum
		  4. Lack of intrinsic factor = Pernicious anemia
		  5. Lack of ileum

Vitamin C (Ascorbic acid)	• Water soluble
	• It is needed for 2 important processes:
	
	  1. Intestinal iron absorption by keeping it in the ferrous state
	  2. Collagen synthesis by hydroxylation of proline and lysine
		• Caused by decreased intake, most pronounced in people not eating vegetables
		• *Vegetarians → Vit. B12 def. Meat eaters → Vit. C def.*
		• *Scurvy*, manifested by:
		
		  1. Gingival hypertrophy
		  2. Easy bruising and bleeding
		  3. Poor healing

Folic acid	• Pteridine + Glutamic acid + PABA → Folic acid • Dihydrofolate reductase converts folic acid to FH4. This reaction is inhibited by methotrexate • FH4 reacts with homocysteine to form methionine. This reaction is regulated by B12 • Folic acid is essential for DNA and RNA synthesis	• *The most common vitamin deficiency in the U.S.* • Macrocytic hyperchromic anemia • Neural tube defects if supplementation is not adequate during pregnancy
Biotin	• Co-factor for many carboxylation reactions: Pyruvate → Oxaloacetate • It is a cofactor for fatty acid synthesis reactions: Acetyl co-A → Malonyl co-A	• Rash and diarrhea • Caused by ingestion of raw eggs, as the egg white contains *Avidin* which binds biotin; inhibiting its absorption
Fluorine	• Main source is drinking water	• Deficiency: Dental caries • Toxicity: Chalky white patches on teeth and osteosclerosis
Zinc	• Normal dietary intake is 6–16 mg/day, only 20% of which is absorbed	• Deficiency: Hair loss, paronychia, rash • Toxicity: Neurological manifestations
Selenium	• Serves as an anti-oxidant	• Deficiency: Cardiomyopathy • Toxicity: Hair loss, nail dystrophy
Copper	• A heavy metal	• Deficiency: *Menkes' syndrome*; patients have *kinky sparse hair.* • Toxicity: Hemolysis

3. Most common source of liver metastases: *Colon cancer*.
4. Most common sources of metastases to brain: *Breast, lungs and prostate cancers.*
5. Most common sources of metastases to bone: *Breast, prostate, thyroid and kidney cancers.*

- *Preventive medicine and screening*:

  1. Mammogram: Annually starting age 40.

  2. Pap smear: Annually after the onset of sexual activity till 3 successive normal smears are obtained, then it is done once every 3 years.
  3. Rectal exam and occult blood in stools: Annually starting age 40.
  4. Colonoscopy: Every 10 years starting age 50.
  5. PSA: Annually starting age 50.

- *Vitamins and minerals*: Refer to Table 1.13.

Chapter 2
Dermatology

Skin Lesions

- **Macule**: A circumscribed area of discolored skin, no elevations or vesicles.
- **Papule (<0.5 cm) or nodule (>0.5 cm)**: A circumscribed area of a skin elevation.
- **Plaque**: A disc-shaped, elevated lesion greater than 2 cm in diameter.
- **Vesicle**: A fluid-filled lesion, less than 0.5 cm in diameter.
- **Bulla**: A fluid-filled lesion, more than 0.5 cm in diameter.
- **Wheal**: A rapidly-formed skin elevation caused by edema of the dermis. Pathognomonic of *urticaria*.
- **Comedone**: A plug in the sebaceous gland orifice. Seen in acne vulgaris.
- **Burrow**: A grayish, irregular, linear elevation of the *horny layer* of the skin. Pathognomonic of *scabies*.
- **Ulcer**: Loss of skin layers *including the dermis*, healing with a scar.

A.W.A. Halim, *Passing the USMLE*, DOI: 10.1007/978-0-387-68984-5_2,
© Springer Science+Business Media, LLC 2009

- *Abrasion or excoriation*: Superficial loss of skin layers, *not involving the dermis*; *no scar* involved.
- *Scar*: Connective tissue that replaces lost tissue anywhere in the body.

Fungal Infections

Tinea Capitis (refer to Fig. 2.1)

- *Introduction*: Ringworm of the scalp.
- *Organisms*: Dermatophyte, Microsporum or Tricophyton.
- *Clinical picture*: Lesions are *itchy*, well circumscribed, and are usually multiple on the scalp. They are oval in shape, of variable sizes, and contain *hair stumps*.
- *Prognosis*: Lesions heal *without scar* formation.
- *Treatment*: *Oral antifungal*, such as terbinafine, itraconazole or griseofulvin for 4–6 weeks.
- *Notes*:

  1. *Kerion*: A subtype of tinea capitis infections. Clinical picture: Red, warm, tender swelling with pustular discharge, often confused with an abscess. Treatment: No incision and drainage is needed, antifungals usually suffice.
  2. *Favus*: A subtype of tinea capitis infections. Clinical picture: *Saucer-shaped*, crusty lesions in the scalp, known as *scatula*. Scatula is yellow in color with reddish margins. Unlike other tinea infections, this one heals *with a scar* and could cause alopecia.

Tinea Corporis (refer to Fig. 2.2)

- *Introduction*: Ringworm of the trunk.
- *Organisms*: All dermatophytes can cause this disease.

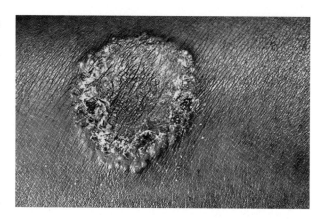

FIG. 2.2 Tinea corporis

- *Clinical picture*: Lesions are *itchy*, oval or rounded, with red elevated *circinate* margins and central clearing, hence also known as *Tinea Circinata*.
- *Treatment*: Topical antifungals. Oral antifungals are reserved for severe cases.

Tinea Cruris (Jock Itch)

- *Area involved*: Groin and buttocks.
- *Clinical picture*: Lesions are *itchy*, bilateral and symmetrical, reddish in color with raised *festooned* edges.
- *Treatment*: Topical antifungals. Oral antifungals are reserved for severe cases.

Tinea Pedis (refer to Fig. 2.3)

- *Introduction*: Athlete's foot.
- *Area involved*: Mostly in the *interdigital spaces*, but can occur anywhere in the foot.
- *Clinical picture*: *Itchy* erythematous *macerated* lesions.
- *Treatment*: Local antifungals. Oral antifungals are reserved for severe cases.

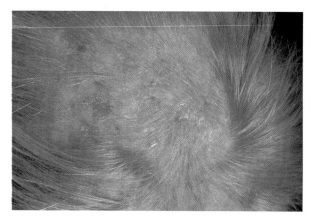

FIG. 2.1 Tinea capitis

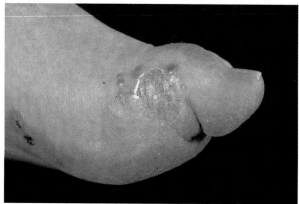

FIG. 2.3 Tinea pedis

Tinea Unguium (Onychomycosis)

- **Clinical picture**: Affects the *nails*, causing them to be *white* and *brittle*.
- **Treatment**: Oral *terbinafine*; *6 weeks for fingernails*, and *12 weeks for toenails*, plus local antifungals in severe cases.

Tinea (Pityriasis) Versicolor (refer to Fig. 2.4)

- **Organisms**: *Malassezia furfur*; a subtype of Pityrosporum orbiculare.
- **Area involved**: The trunk, usually the upper chest, neck and back.
- **Clinical picture**: Small, well-defined, scaling macules, of *various colors*. Some lesions are hypo-pigmented due to the *azelaic acid* produced by the fungus, which inhibits the melanocytes.
- **Diagnosis**: Examination of the lesions under Wood's light shows *yellow color*. KOH skin scraping shows the hyphae and yeast in *spaghetti and meatballs appearance*.
- **Treatment**: *Local with imidazole cream. Oral ketoconazole is reserved for severe cases.*

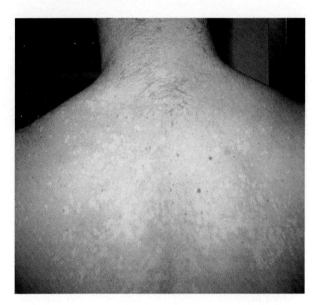

FIG. 2.4 Tinea versicolor

Candida Albicans

- **Introduction**: Candida albicans exists in two forms:

  1. **Yeast**: As flora.
  2. **Mycelia**: *Pathogenic form*.

- **Predisposing factors**: *Obesity*, *hyperhidrosis* and *DM*.
- **Diagnosis**: Presence of the pathognomonic *hyphae and pseudo-hyphae* under microscope. Refer to Fig. 2.5.
- **Treatment**: Mainly local, with nystatins or imidazole. Oral ketoconazole is reserved for severe and resistant cases.
- **Notes**:

  1. **Cutaneous candidiasis**: Common in skin folds, e.g.: diaper rash. Lesions are *red and moist with festooned edges*, and are surrounded by papules known as *Satellite lesions*. Refer to Fig. 2.6.
  2. **Oral candidiasis (Thrush)**: Common in patients using inhaled steroids. Lesions are multiple white plaques involving the tongue and esophagus. Refer to Fig. 2.7. Prevention: *Washing the mouth* after using steroid inhalers.
  3. **Genital candidiasis**: The *most common genital infection in females*. Clinical picture: *Whitish, milky vaginal discharge* and *curd-like patches*. Genital candidiasis are treated by a *single dose of oral fluconazole*.

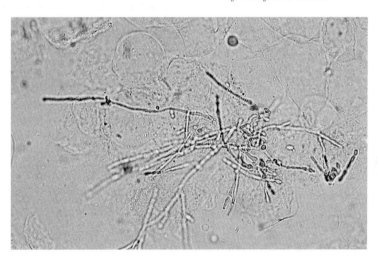

FIG. 2.5 Hyphae and spores of Candida Albicans

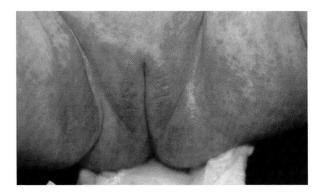

FIG. 2.6 Diaper candidiasis

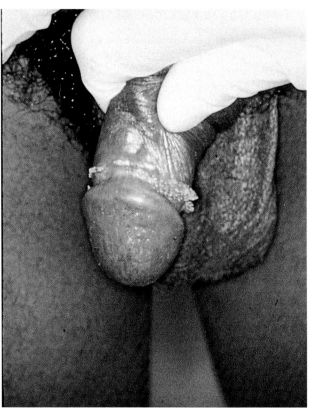

FIG. 2.8 Penile wart

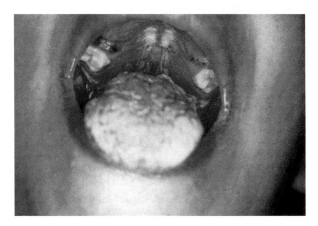

FIG. 2.7 Oral thrush

Notes

- Most fungal infections could be easily treated with a topical antifungal, e.g.: imidazole cream or ointment; except for two infections that require systemic therapy: *Tinea capitis* and *Tinea unguium.*
- Griseofulvin attacks only dermatophytes, and causes GI upset.
- Ketoconazole and terbinafine are *hepatotoxic.*

Viral Infections

Warts (refer to Fig. 2.8)

- *Introduction*: A common benign tumor from the *epidermal layer* of the skin.
- *Organism*: *Human papilloma virus (HPV).*
- *Clinical picture*: Starts as a *papule* and can occur at any part of the body. Commonly a *cauliflower-like lesion*; however it can occur in any shape or form.
- *Treatment*: *Cauterization*, either cryo, electrical or chemical using podophyllin resin in alcohol. *Topical imiquimod is an alternative treatment.*

- *Note*: Condyloma accuminata (venereal warts) are warts in the anogenital area.

Molluscum Contagiosum (refer to Fig. 2.9)

- *Organism*: *Pox virus.*
- *Area involved*: Mainly face and neck, but can also occur in the genital area.
- *Clinical picture*: Lesions are *pearly white, umbilicated papules.*
- *Diagnosis*: Identifying the *inclusion molluscum bodies* upon staining the contents of the lesion with *Wright* or *Geimsa* stains.
- *Treatment*: Lesions often regress spontaneously. Cauterization, either cryo, electrical or chemical using *ether* is reserved for non-resolving lesions.

Herpes Simplex (refer to Fig. 2.10)

- *Introduction*: Very common infection, mainly in children, age 2–5 years.
- *Organism*: Herpes simplex virus (*HSV*):

  1. *HSV type I targets the eyes and mouth.*
  2. *HSV type II targets the genitals.*

- **Clinical picture**: Red macule, which progresses into a pustule. The pustule ruptures leaving a *honey-colored crust*, which heals without scar formation.
- **Treatment**: Oral antibiotics, mainly penicillinase-resistant penicillins.
- **Notes**:

  1. Staphylococci release *exfoliatin* which can cause a bullous form of impetigo.
  2. If impetigo becomes deep enough to cause ulceration, it is called *ecthyma*.

Erythrasma

- **Clinical picture**: Red, scaly lesions found in skin folds, often confused with tinea.
- **Diagnosis**: Examination of the lesions under Wood's light shows red fluorescence. *Erythro = Red.*
- **Treatment**: Oral tetracycline.

Erysipelas

- **Area involved**: Face and lower limbs.
- **Organism**: *Group A streptococci.*
- **Clinical picture**: A superficial, well-demarcated, red, warm cellulitis.
- **Treatment**: Oral antibiotics, mainly *penicillin or cephalosporins*. In case of penicillin allergy, treat with *erythromycin*.

Erysipeloid

- **Organism**: *Erysipelothrix rhusiopathiae.*
- **Risk factor**: The patient is usually a *butcher* or a *fisherman* who uses sharp objects contaminated with animal flesh.
- **Clinical picture**: Lesion is a *small tender purplish area on the finger, where the injury with the sharp object has occurred.*
- **Treatment**: Penicillin.

Necrotizing Fasciitis

- **Introduction**: A deep infection of the fascia, usually polymicrobial. It is not well demarcated and could be very aggressive, to the point of fatality.
- **Clinical picture**: Affected area is red, warm, tender, swollen and might show bullae, discoloration and loss of sensation.
- **Treatment**: Broad-spectrum antibiotics and surgical debridement.

Folliculitis

- **Introduction**: Inflammation of the *superficial part of the hair follicle*.
- **Organisms**: *Staphylococcus aureus*, but *Pseudomonas aeruginosa* could also be blamed in some cases, e.g.: Hot tub folliculitis.
- **Predisposing factors**: Obesity, hyperhidrosis, DM.
- **Clinical picture**: Small, pustular lesions surrounding the hair follicles.
- **Treatment**: Oral antibiotics, mainly penicillinase-resistant penicillins. *Hot tub folliculitis is self resolving.*

Furunculosis

- **Introduction**: Inflammation of the *deep part of the hair follicle*.
- **Area involved**: Neck and buttocks.
- **Clinical picture**: Lesions are deep boils with pustular discharge.
- **Treatment**: Oral antibiotics and hot compresses. Incision and drainage is reserved for large, complicated lesions.
- **Note**: A collection of furuncles is known as a *carbuncle*.

Hidradenitis Suppurativa

- **Introduction**: Local inflammation of the *apocrine glands* in the axilla and groin.
- **Organism**: *Staphylococcus aureus*.
- **Clinical picture**: Reddish, painful nodules in the axilla or groin.
- **Treatment**: Oral antibiotics, *tetracycline* is best. Surgical drainage and debridement is also needed.

Paronychia (refer to Fig. 2.12)

- **Introduction**: Inflammation of the periungual tissue.

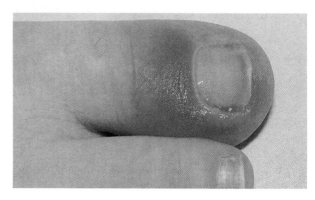

FIG. 2.12 Paronychia

- *Predisposing factors*: A hangnail or ingrown toenail.
- *Clinical picture*: The paronychial fold is erythematous, swollen and tender.
- *Treatment*: Hot compresses and penicillinase-resistant penicillin.

Lupus Vulgaris

- *Introduction*: The most common form of cutaneous TB lesions.
- *Area involved*: Face and neck.
- *Clinical picture*: Lesions are nodular plaques. Pressing the lupus vulgaris lesion with a glass slide reveals a characteristic brownish *apple jelly* color. This type of test is known as *diascopy*.
- *Treatment*: *TB treatment*.

Parasitic Infections

Scabies

- *Organism*: *Sarcoptes scabiei*.
- *Area involved*: Interdigital spaces; however, can occur anywhere.
- *Clinical picture*: Lesions start as *burrows* which are extremely itchy, especially at night. This leads to inflammation and even pustules in some severe cases.
- *Diagnosis*: Visualizing *burrows* and mites on an *oil mount* under microscopy.
- *Treatment*: Topical *permethrine* or *lindane*, and boiling clothes and bed sheets.
- *Notes*:

  1. *Scabies incognito* is one form of scabies that flares up with steroids.
  2. Children with scabies do not necessarily have burrows.

Pediculosis (Lice)

- *Pediculosis capitis*: Infects the scalp and looks just like dandruff, *except that the eggs cannot be easily pulled off the hairs*. Treatment: Topical *permethrin*.
- *Pediculosis corporis*: Infects the body. Treatment: Topical *lindane*.
- *Pediculosis pubis (a.k.a. Phthiriasis pubis)*: Infects the pubic area and inner thighs. The most common form of transmission is sexual contact. Treatment: Topical *lindane*. A common scenario on the USMLE would be finding Phthirus pubis in the eyelashes of a child upon examination, and the correct course

of action is to assume sexual abuse until proven otherwise.
- *Note*: Lindane is contraindicated in pregnancy and in children as it might cause CNS toxicity. The alternative treatment in both cases is permethrine.

Acne Vulgaris

- *Introduction*: Inflammation of the *pilosebaceous glands*; common in adolescents.
- *Area involved*: Face, chest and back.
- *Clinical picture*: Comedones which might progress to papules or even pustules.
- *Pathology*: The exact etiology of acne is not clear; however some theories suggest a link to hormonal imbalance, mainly increased androgens. Others link acne to infection with *Propionibacterium acne*.
- *Treatment*:

  1. Treatment of comedones: *Topical retinoids*.
  2. Treatment of papules or pustules: *Topical benzoyl peroxide plus topical antibiotics*, mainly clindamycin or erythromycin.
  3. In severe cases, *intralesional steroid injection* or *oral antibiotics*, such as tetracycline or erythromycin may be added.

Acne Rosacea

- *Introduction*: An inflammatory skin disease that is common in the *middle* part of the face and is common in the *middle* age group.
- *Clinical picture*: Erythema, telangiectasia and papules.
- *Complications*: Nose hypertrophy a.k.a. *rhinophyma*.
- *Treatment*: Oral tetracyclines and topical metronidazole.

Allergic Skin Diseases

Eczema

- *Introduction*: Allergic *type IV hypersensitivity* reaction of the skin to any factor:

  1. *Extrinsic* forms, i.e.: contact dermatitis, secondary to allergens or irritants like poison ivy, and the eczema ensues at least 4 or 5 days after contact, *never immediately afterwards*.
  2. *Intrinsic* forms of eczema are multiple and complicated, the most famous being atopic dermatitis, seborrheic dermatitis and pityriasis alba.

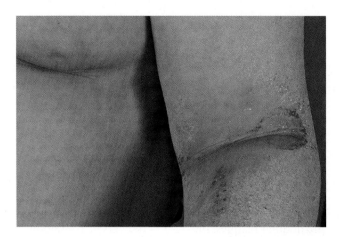

Fɪɢ. 2.13 Eczema

- **General clinical picture**: Lesions are always *itchy* and could form scales as they turn chronic.
- **Patch test**: Eczema is evaluated by testing different substances on the skin in diluted concentrations and noting their effect.
- **Treatment**: Topical corticosteroids, plus H1 blockers.
- **Atopic dermatitis**: refer to Fig. 2.13.

    1. A genetic dermatitis, and patients usually have other forms of allergy, such as asthma and allergic rhinitis.
    2. Lesions are erythematous and oozing, mainly on ante-*cubital* and *popliteal fossae* in children of 2 months up to 6 years of age.
    3. These lesions may form papules and develop *lichenification*.

- **Seborrheic dermatitis**: refer to Fig. 2.14.

    1. Occurs mainly, as the name suggests, in areas with sebaceous glands, e.g.: *Scalp and eyebrows*.
    2. Lesions are *yellowish, greasy* and *scaly*.
    3. Make sure to ask about risk factors for HIV in any young patient with these lesions.
    4. *Cradle cap* is seborrheic dermatitis that affects the scalp of newborns and can be treated with shampoos containing *selenium or zinc*.

- **Pityriasis alba**: A form of eczema that occurs mainly in children and is notorious, as the name suggests, for the *white patches* on the face, often confused with vitiligo.

Urticaria

- **Clinical picture**: A *wheal-shaped*, cutaneous *antigen-antibody reaction*, mainly in the *dermis*. The *wheals* are pale, elevated, rounded and surrounded by erythematous zone and are *intensely pruritic*. Refer to Fig. 2.15.

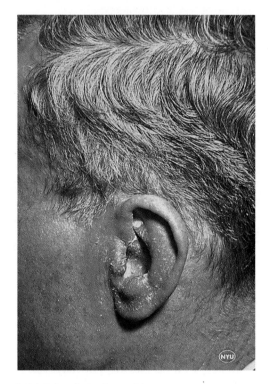

Fɪɢ. 2.14 Seborrheic dermatitis

- **Causes**: Factors to blame for urticaria are endless; any contact with or ingestion of a substance can lead susceptible patients to develop urticaria.
- **Treatment**: H1 blockers and avoidance of the cause, if known.
- **Note**: Angioedema is a fatal form of urticaria that involves the subcutaneous tissue. Patients become diffusely swollen very quickly, and death may result from laryngeal edema, so *look for stridor*. Treatment: *Epinephrine (life saving), steroids, H1 and H2 blockers*. In recurrent angioedema of unclear

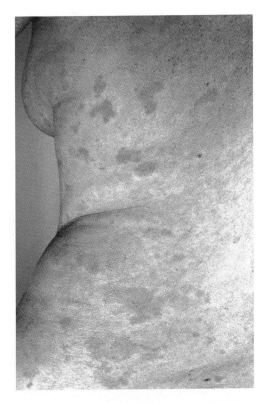

FIG. 2.15 Wheal reaction of Urticaria

cause, consider *hereditary angioedema* by checking for *C1 esterase inhibitor deficiency*.

Erythema Multiforme

* *Introduction*: A skin reaction to infections or drugs.
* *Clinical picture*:

1. *The minor form*: Characterized by *target-shaped* lesions known as or *iris*-lesions, which are skin lesions that look like a *bull's eye*. Just like

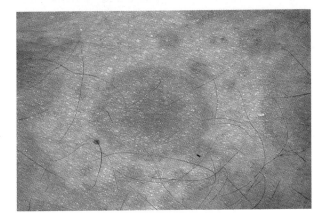

FIG. 2.16 Iris lesion of Erythema Multiforme

eczema, lesions start 4 or 5 days after the infection or ingestion of the drug. Refer to Fig. 2.16.
2. *The major form* (*Stevens's-Johnson syndrome*): Characterized by diffuse bullae, mainly around the mouth and eyes. In severe cases, renal failure and fatal pneumonitis may occur.

* **Skin biopsy**: *Necrotic keratinocytes* and *extensive lymphocytosis*.
* **Treatment**: Systemic corticosteroids, and avoidance of the cause if known.

Erythema Nodosum (refer to Fig. 2.17)

* *Pathogenesis*: Inflammation of the *dermis* and *subcutaneous fat*.
* *Causes*: Sarcoidosis, inflammatory bowel diseases, tuberculosis, streptococcal infections, malignancy and drugs, e.g. OCP. Of all these causes, *streptococcal infection* is the most common underlying cause.
* *Clinical picture*: Red, tender nodules that occur in the *pretibial region*.
* *Treatment*: Treat the cause plus NSAIDS.
* *Note*: Erythema nodosum in a case of sarcoidosis is a *good prognostic sign*.

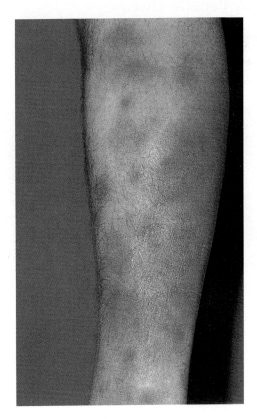

FIG. 2.17 Erythema nodosum

Toxic Epidermal Necrolysis

- *Introduction*: One of the most severe drug reactions.
- *Clinical picture*: Epidermis peels off in sheets, leaving painful erythematous lesions. This occurs even with gently touching the skin; a.k.a. *Nikolsky's sign*.
- *Treatment*: *Hospitalize the patient*, stop the offending medication and start systemic corticosteroids.
- *Note*: Toxic epidermal necrolysis is often confused in the clinical wards with *staphylococcal scalded skin syndrome*. They share similar symptoms, signs and Nikolsky's sign. *The latter, however, occurs mainly in newborns and is treated with penicillinase resistant penicillin.*

Medication-Induced Skin Diseases

- *Tetracycline*: Photosensitivity, pruritis and dermatitis.
- *Warfarin*: Skin necrosis through *depleting protein C* stores. This usually develops after about a week from starting the warfarin.
- *NSAIDs*: Toxic epidermal necrolysis, urticaria or Steven's Johnson syndrome.
- *OCPs*: Erythema nodosum and erythema multiforme.

Scaly Papular Diseases

Psoriasis (refer to Fig. 2.18)

- *Introduction*: A chronic skin disease which is only cosmetically disturbing and slightly itchy.

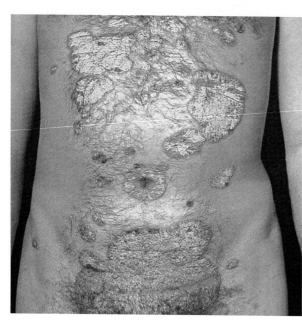

FIG. 2.18 Psoriasis

It is genetically determined, namely *HLA-B13* linked.

- *Pathology*: There are two important phenomena involved:

  1. *Parakeratosis*: Excessive proliferation of *stratum basale* and *spinosum*.
  2. *Acanthosis*: Retention of nuclei of superficial skin layers.

- *Area involved*: Extensor surfaces, mainly the knees and elbows.
- *Clinical picture*:

  1. Papular lesions, covered with the pathognomonic *silvery scales*.
  2. *Nail pitting*, and lifting of nail plate a.k.a *Onycholysis*.
  3. *Asymmetrical* arthritis that affects the *distal interphalengeal joints (DIP)*; it shows on X-ray as a *pencil in a cup*.
  4. *Koebner's phenomenon*: Development of lesions at sites of trauma or abrasion.
  5. *Auspitz sign*: Removal of scales reveals underlying *pin-point bleeding*.

- *Treatment*:

  1. Most lesions: Topical corticosteroids or topical vitamin D analogues.
  2. Pustular psoriasis: *Etretinate*.
  3. Resistant cases: Ultraviolet light or oral methotrexate.

Pityriasis Rosea (refer to Fig. 2.19)

- *Introduction*: An inflammatory, self-limited disease.
- *Clinical picture*:

  1. Starts with the pathognomonic *herald patch*, which is an oval, red patch on the trunk.
  2. Few days later, generalized patchy skin lesions follow, *sparing the extremities*. Lesions are well known for their *Christmas tree distribution* as they line themselves parallel to the ribs.

- *Prognosis*: The disease resolves spontaneously within 1–2 months.
- *Treatment*: Symptomatic.

Lichen Planus (refer to Fig. 2.20)

- *Introduction*: Papular, pruritic skin disease; more common in *females*.
- *Area involved*: Inner thighs and wrists.

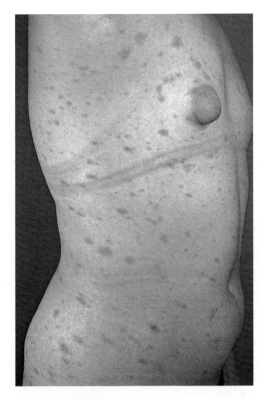

FIG. 2.19 Pityriasis rosea

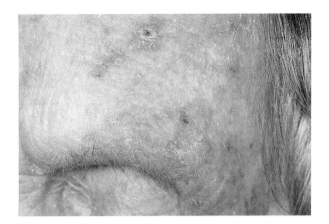

FIG. 2.21 Actinic keratosis

Actinic (Senile) Keratosis (refer to Fig. 2.21)

- *Introduction*: A pre-malignant skin lesion.
- *Clinical picture*: Patient is usually *elderly* presenting with discrete, scaly papular lesions only on *sun exposed areas*.
- *Prevention*: Sun screen before sun exposure.
- *Treatment*: Cryo-cauterization or 5-florouracil.
- *Note*: *All actinic keratosis lesions should be biopsied*, due to the potential of their transformation to *squamous cell carcinoma*.

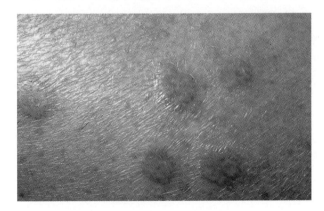

FIG. 2.20 Lichen planus

- *Clinical picture*: Lesions are *polygonal* papules with a *purplish* color, sometimes covered with white lines known as *Wickham's striae*.
- *Treatment*: Topical corticosteroids and H1 blockers.

Malignant Skin Diseases

Basal Cell Carcinoma (BCC) (refer to Table 2.1 and Fig. 2.22)

Squamous Cell Carcinoma (SCC) (refer to Table 2.1 and Fig. 2.23)

Melanoma (refer to Fig. 2.24)

- *Introduction*: Common in *fair skinned individuals*, due to sun exposure.
- *Pathology*: Lesions arise from the melanocytes of the *stratum basale*.
- *Risk factors*: Dysplastic nevi.

TABLE 2.1 Basal and squamous cell carcinomas of the skin.

	BCC	SCC
Layer	Epidermal basal cells	Epidermal keratinizing layer
Cause	Exposure to UV light	Transformation of premalignant lesions, e.g.: actinic keratosis, scars.
Macroscopic	Pearly translucent papule	Exophytic nodule with raised everted edges
Microscopic	Palisade pattern	Cell nest pattern, deep down to the dermis
Metastases	Locally malignant	Distant metastases
Treatment	Surgical excision	Surgical excision

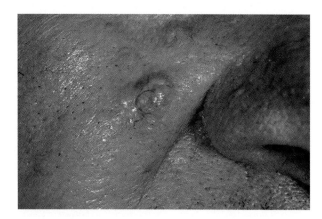

FIG. 2.22 Basal cell carcinoma

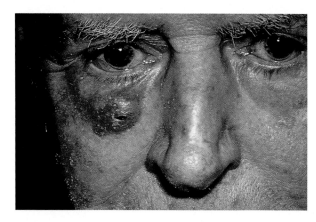

FIG. 2.23 Squamous cell carcinoma

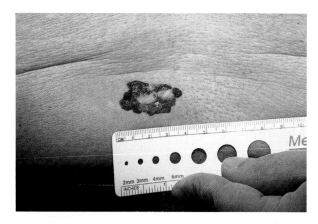

FIG. 2.24 Melanoma

- **Metastases**: *Distant metastases via blood*, especially to the *brain*.
- **Clinical picture**: Lesions are brownish in color, and are characterized by one or more of the following:

  1. A: *A*symmetrical.
  2. B: Irregular *B*order.

3. C: *C*olor changes.
4. D: *D*iameter of more than 6 mm.

- **Microscopically**: Lesions show melanocytes with malignant characteristics.
- **Prognosis**: The most important prognostic factor is *the depth of the lesions*.
- **Treatment**: Surgical excision, and chemotherapy with *interleukin-1*.
- **Note**: Melanoma of the *S*calp, *N*eck, *A*rm and *B*ack – *SNAB* – *carry worse prognosis*.

Miscellaneous

Vitiligo

- **Introduction**: Depigmentation disease of unknown etiology.
- **Clinical picture**: Lesions are white and macular and occur anywhere in the body. Vitiligo is not pruritic, which helps you differentiate it from other depigmenting skin diseases, e.g., Pityriasis alba.
- **Treatment**: Cosmetic, topical steroids and *ultraviolet A* light.
- **Note**: Vitiligo could be part of a polyglandular deficiency, so screen for other autoimmune diseases.

Pemphigus Vulgaris (refer to Fig. 2.25)

- **Introduction**: Autoimmune disease due to an *anti-epithelial antibody destroying the desmosomes*.
- **Pathology**: Desmosomes normally pull the epidermal cells together, so when they are destroyed, bullae develop. This phenomenon is called *Acantholysis*.
- **Clinical picture**: Bullous skin lesions.
- **Treatment**: Systemic corticosteroids.

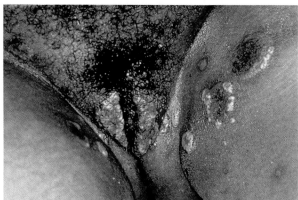

FIG. 2.25 Pemphigus vulgaris

- *Note*: Blistering of the skin could happen sometimes in healthy individuals after minor trauma; this is known as *Epidermolysis Bullosa*.

Acanthosis Nigricans

- *Clinical picture*: Hyperpigmented skin lesions that occur in skin folds, e.g.: axilla.
- *Note*: These lesions are indicative of:

  1. GI malignancy: Mainly *gastric*.
  2. Endocrine disorders: Mainly *insulin resistant DM*.

Lipoma

- *Introduction*: A benign tumor of the adipose tissue.
- *Clinical picture*: Patient presents with soft lobulated tumor.
- *On exam*: Two pathognomonic signs:

  1. *Dimpling of the skin* on displacing the tumor.
  2. *Slippery edge* on palpation: This is because the tumor is surrounded by *two capsules*.

- *Complications*:

  1. Intraluminal: Airway obstruction, intussusceptions.
  2. Others: Cosmetic, malignant transformation (rare).

- *Treatment*: *Enucleation*.

Keloid

- *Introduction*: Hypertrophied scar tissue, more common in *African-Americans*.
- *Clinical picture*: Patient presents with *skin growth at the site of a scar from previous trauma or surgery*.
- *Treatment*:

  1. Active (erythematous and pruritic): Topical steroids.
  2. Inactive (non-erythematous and non-pruritic): Excision.

Fibrosarcoma

- *Introduction*: A malignant tumor that arises from the muscles and tendons.
- *Clinical picture*: Well defined, un-capsulated smooth firm muscular swelling.

- *Diagnosis*: Muscle biopsy.
- *Next best step*: Chest X-ray to look for metastases.
- *Treatment*:

  1. Non-metastatic: Wide local excision of tumor, or amputation of the whole limb if bone is involved.
  2. Metastatic: Radiation therapy.

Desmoid Tumor

- *Introduction*: A fibrosarcoma of the rectus sheath of the abdomen, a.k.a. Paget disease of rectus sheath.
- *Clinical picture*: A tumor in the abdominal wall, *below the level of the umbilicus* that protrudes more with contraction of abdominal muscles.
- *Metastases*: Local infiltration only.
- *Treatment*: Wide local excision.

Dermoid Cyst

- *Introduction*: A cutaneous cyst that forms due to excessive epithelial growth.
- *Pathology*: Lined by *squamous epithelium,* filled with *sebaceous material*, and covered by a *fibrous capsule*.
- *Clinical picture*: Cystic, mobile, painless swelling, *usually at the site of a previous needle prick or injury*.
- *Complication*: Intracranial extension.
- *Treatment*: Excision after an X-ray to rule out intracranial extension.

Sebaceous Cyst

- *Introduction*: A *retention* cyst, due to *obstructed sebaceous gland's duct*.
- *Clinical picture*: Well defined cystic swelling, *usually on the face*, which opens up into the surface via a *punctum*.
- *Complications*: Infection or malignant transformation.
- *Treatment*: *Elliptical excision, which must include the punctum*.

Chapter 3
Obstetrics

Human Chorionic Gonadotrophin (HCG)

- **Definition**: A glycoprotein secreted by syncytiotrophoblast.
- **Production**: It starts at implantation (7 *days after fertilization*) and its levels double *every 2 days* till it peaks at around *10 weeks* gestational age (1,000,000 Units). After the peak, level decreases as the pregnancy progresses to full term.
- **Detection**: By urine analysis (Standard pregnancy test), or by measuring the beta subunit of HCG in serum (More sensitive and specific).

- **Uses of HCG**:
  1. Diagnosis of pregnancy: Appears in the urine 8 *days after fertilization*.
  2. Diagnosis and follow up of some ovarian and trophoblastic tumors.
  3. Evaluation of threatened abortion: If levels are doubling every 2 days, pregnancy is still intact. If no doubling, suspect missed abortion. Explained in detail later.

- **Functions of HCG**:

  1. Maintains corpus luteum until placental function is well established. (*10 weeks*).

A.W.A. Halim, *Passing the USMLE*, DOI: 10.1007/978-0-387-68984-5_3,
© Springer Science+Business Media, LLC 2009

2. Stimulates fetal testicular function in utero if the fetus is male.

- *Note*: Progesterone production during pregnancy:

  1. During the first 7 weeks: Corpus luteum.
  2. From 7 to 10 weeks: Corpus luteum *and* Placenta.
  3. 10 weeks onwards: Placenta.

Human Placental Lactogen (HPL)

- *Definition*: A polypeptide, which is very close in composition to *prolactin*.
- *Production*: It starts rising immediately after the missed period, and levels rise up to 7 Ug/ml by *36 weeks* gestational age.
- *Uses of HPL*: Good indicator of the functioning placental mass, so it is useful in some cases of high risk pregnancy, e.g., HTN or postmaturity; however, it is of little value in cases of large placenta, e.g., Diabetes mellitus or Erythroblastosis fetalis.
- *Functions of HPL*:

  1. Similar to growth hormone and prolactin: Stimulates growth of breasts.
  2. Inhibits glucose and protein metabolism by mother, sparing them for the fetus.

Feto-Placental Unit

- *Composition*: The co-operation of:

  1. Fetus: Through 16 Hydroxy-dehydroepiandrosterone-sulphate (DHEAS)
  2. Maternal placenta: Through her DHEAS

- *End result*: Estrogens, and it is a considered a good test of fetal well-being.
- *Normally*: (Estrone): E2 (Estradiol): E3 (Estriol) = 1:2:3. In pregnancy, the ratio of E1:E2:E3 is 1:2:30

Gametogenesis

- Refer to Figs. 3.1, 3.2 and 3.3
- *Spermiogenesis*: The process by which *spermatids* are converted to *mature sperm*.
- *The sperm's parts*:

  1. *Head*: Covered by an acrosomal cap and contains the genetic material.
  2. *Middle segment*: Composed of mitochondria.
  3. *Tail*: For movement.

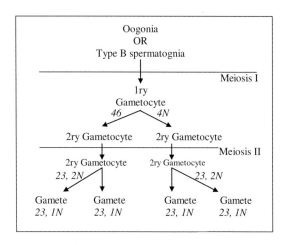

FIG. 3.1 Gametogenesis

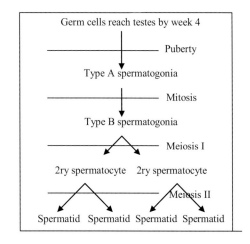

FIG. 3.2 Spermatogenesis

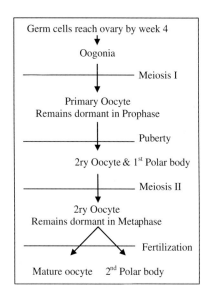

FIG. 3.3 Oogenesis

- Note: The acrosomal cap is derived from the *golgi apparatus*, and the tail is derived from the *centriole*.

Fertilization

- *Definition*: The union of male and female gametes to form the zygote.
- *Timing*: The *first 24 h after ovulation*.
- *Location*: Most common site is the lateral 1/3 of the Fallopian tube, namely the *ampulla*.
- *Steps*:

  1. Physiologically, after the sperm pierces the zona pellucida, zonal block occurs to prevent further penetrations and, similarly, when the sperm penetrates the vitelline membrane, vitelline block occurs. *Failure of the block systems results in multiple pregnancy*.
  2. Once the sperm comes into contact with the *zona pellucida* of the *secondary oocyte*, the sperm pronucleus forms and the mitochondria degenerates.
  3. This triggers oogenesis as mentioned earlier, and the female pronucleus is formed.
  4. Both pronuclei fuse to form the *zygote*.

Implantation

- The zygote (*Post fertilization day 2*) undergoes mitosis repeatedly to form the *blastula*, then a *morula* (*32 cell stage*, post fertilization *day 3*).
- The morula secretes fluid creating an internal cavity separating into two masses of cells. This structure is called the *blastocyst* (*day 5*). The inner cell mass is the *embryoblast*, and the outer is *trophoblast*.
- The zona pellucida then degenerates to allow the blastocyst to implant in the *posterior superior wall of the uterus* by post fertilization day 6 or 7.
- Afterwards, the trophoblast undergoes a differentiation process into syncytiotrophoblast and cytotrophoblast and forms villi.
- The invasion of the trophoblast into the endometrium is limited by the *fibrinoid (Nitabuch) layer*. Absence of this layer leads to pathological adherence of placenta.

Umbilical Cord

- *Composition*: Is around 50 cm long and has important components:

  1. Right and left umbilical arteries.
  2. Left umbilical vein: Carries oxygenated blood to the fetus.
  3. Connective tissue, e.g., Wharton jelly, allantoic duct, and amniotic epithelium.

- *Note*: The presence of a single umbilical artery in the cord (5%) is common in *pregnant patients with DM*, and is associated with *fetal cardiovascular anomalies* and *Edward's syndrome*.
- *Abnormalities of the cord after delivery*

  1. Patent urachal fistula: Presents with *urine* from the umbilicus.
  2. Vitelline fistula: Presents with *meconium* discharge from the umbilicus.
  3. Omphalocele: A *grey sack* surrounding the umbilicus.

Amniotic Fluid

- *Formation*: From fetal and maternal contributions:

  1. Fetal: *Urine* starting during the *10th week*.
  2. Maternal: *Transudation* from placental vasculature.

- *Maximum volume*: 1000 ml, and is normally reached by the *36th week* of gestation.
- *Composition*:

  1. Mainly water with some glucose and proteins.
  2. Sodium and bilirubin content of the fluid *decrease* throughout pregnancy.
  3. Creatinine and phospholipids content of the fluid *increase* throughout pregnancy.

- *Oligohydramnios*: Fluid <400 ml. Causes: Premature rupture of membranes (*most common cause*), renal agenesis (Potter syndrome), or posterior urethral folds.
- *Polyhydramnios*: Fluid >2000 ml. Causes: Esophageal atresia, anencephaly or maternal DM.
- *Amniotic band syndrome*: Bands in the amnion form in this syndrome. The fetus suffers *craniofacial anomalies*, *adhesions* and *amputations*.

Placenta

- *Composition*:

  1. Maternal: *Decidua basalis*.
  2. Fetal: *Chorion frondosum* or tertiary villi.

- *Surfaces*: The maternal surface has a *cobblestone* appearance and contains approximately *20 cotyledons*, while the fetal surface is *smooth and membranous*.

- *Parts*:

    1. In early pregnancy, the placenta is formed of:

        - Syncytiotrophoblast.
        - Cytotrophoblast.
        - Connective tissue.
        - Endothelium of fetal blood vessels.

    2. In late pregnancy, the placenta is formed only of the syncytiotrophoblast and *endothelium of fetal blood vessels*.

- *Pathological forms of placenta*:

    1. *Placenta Succentriata*: Accessory lobe, which may be retained and cause post-partum hemorrhage.
    2. *Placenta Circumvallata*: Chorionic plate is smaller than decidual plate, which may lead to abortion. The placenta will have a white decidual ring on its margin.
    3. *Placenta membranacea*: A large membranous placenta due to persistence of the *chorion leave*. May be associated with vasa previa, leading to antepartum hemorrhage.
    4. *Small placenta*: as in Pre-eclampsia, or *large placenta*: as in DM or Syphilis.
    5. *Pathological adherence (due to absent Nitabuch layer)*:

        - Placenta accreta: Implants deep down into muscle layer of uterus.
        - Placenta increta: Placenta penetrates through muscle layer.
        - Placenta percreta: Placenta completely perforates the uterus.

    6. *Abnormal cord attachments*: Central, marginal or velamentous (in membranes). The latter is associated with Placenta membranacea, and if the traversing vessels pass below the presenting part (vasa previa), antepartum hemorrhage of fetal origin could ensue and is a medical emergency.

- *Notes*:

    1. *The placenta lacks MHC antigens, so it does not elicit an immune response from the mother, preventing immunologic rejection.*
    2. *Dizygotic twins have 2 placentae, 2 chorions and 2 amnions.*

3. Monozygotic twins (in most cases) share a placenta, chorion, but have *2 amnions*.

Blood

- Refer to Table 3.1 for the differentiating points between fetal and maternal blood.

Amniocentesis

- *Definition*: Tapping of the amniotic fluid for diagnostic or therapeutic purposes.
- *Early amniocentesis (16–18 weeks)*:

    1. For diagnosis of chromosomal abnormalities.
    2. For diagnosis of neural tube defects by measuring Alpha-fetoprotein (AFP) in the amniotic fluid or the *m*aternal *s*erum, also known as (*MS*AFP):

        - High AFP (>2.5 mom): Anencephaly or Spina bifida
        - Low AFP (<0.4 mom):

            1. Down syndrome (Trisomy 21) (*Low AFP, Low estriol, High B-HCG*).
            2. Edward syndrome (Trisomy 18) (*Low AFP, Low estriol, Low B-HCG*).

- *Late amniocentesis (3rd trimester)*:

    1. For estimation of fetal lung maturity. Indicators of lung maturity include:

        - Lecithin/Sphingomyelin ratio > 2:1.
        - Phosphatidylglycerol content of 1% (last substance to appear in fluid).
        - Fluid creatinine level of 2 mg/dL or more.
        - Absence of bilirubin in the amniotic fluid.

    2. For amniography: A dye injection in the fluid for placental localization.

- *Therapeutic amniocentesis*: For polyhydramnios or inducing abortion.
- *Complications of amniocentesis*: Injury to internal organs or blood vessels, or premature rupture of membranes (PROM).

TABLE 3.1 Fetal and maternal blood.

Type of blood	Alkali denaturation test	Kleihauer Betke test	Nucleated RBC's	Hemoglobin
Fetal	Pink	Red	Positive	HbF
Maternal	Brown	Ghost cells	Negative	HbA

Diagnosis of Pregnancy

- **Symptoms**

  1. Amenorrhea, morning sickness, breast enlargement, and appetite changes, e.g., *Longing*.
  2. Quickening: Fetal movements could be felt starting at the *16th week in multiparous*, and the *18th week in nulliparous* women.

- **Signs**

  1. Breast enlargement and increased areolar pigmentation.
  2. Jaquemier sign: Vulva is soft and hyperpigmented.
  3. Chadwick sign: Vagina is soft, warm and hyperpigmented.
  4. Goodell sign: Cervix is enlarged, soft and hyperpigmented.
  5. Palmer sign: Early uterine contractions, which disappear throughout pregnancy.
  6. Hegar sign: Soft lower uterine segment (you can approximate one hand in the anterior fornix to another on the abdomen behind the uterus).
  7. Fetal heart sounds, uterine soufflé, and palpation of fetal body parts: In second and 3rd trimester.

- **Diagnosis**: B-HCG and ultrasound of the uterus.

Maternal Changes During Pregnancy

Genital Tract

- **Cervix, vagina and vulva**: Jacquemier, Chadwick and Goodell signs.
- **Uterus**: Weight increases from 50 g to almost 1 kg and it becomes ovoid in shape.

  1. At 12 weeks gestation: Fundus is at the level of *pubic symphysis*.
  2. At 24 weeks gestation: Fundus is at the level of *the umbilicus*.
  3. At 36 weeks gestation: Fundus is at the *xiphoid process*.

- The uterus performs fine contractions which can be felt by bimanual examination in early pregnancy (*Palmer sign*). These contractions decrease in frequency as the pregnancy progresses, and re-occur prior to labor (*Braxton Hick contractions*).
- The lower uterine segment becomes soft during pregnancy (*Hegar sign*), and it can be differentiated from the upper segment because it is thin with loose adherence of membranes and is passive (*Upper segment is thick and it can contract*).

- **Ovaries and Fallopian tubes**: Increased size and vascularity; also a pregnancy-induced luteoma may form in the ovaries, secreting androgens leading to maternal virilization.

Breast Glands

- **First few weeks**: Increased size and vascularity.
- **2nd month**: Increased pigmentation of primary areola and appearance of Montgomery tubercles.
- **3rd month**: Colostrum can be expressed.
- **6th month**: Increased pigmentation around the primary areola (*secondary areola*).

Cardiovascular and Pulmonary Systems

- Plasma volume increases by 50%, while RBCs count increases by 25%; thus, physiological hemodilution occurs. (A pregnant patient is anemic if Hb <11 g/dL).
- Increase in WBC count in mild degree is expected in pregnancy.
- Coagulation *factors I to X are increased*, while *factor XII is decreased*.
- ESR is increased during pregnancy, due to high levels of *fibrinogen*.
- Cardiac output is increased by 30%–40% (*Hyperdynamic circulation*).
- Blood pressure decreases during 2nd trimester due to *decreased peripheral resistance*.
- There is increased liability of formation of varicose veins, due to the vasodilatory effect of progesterone and compression of the gravid uterus.
- Pressure effect of the gravid uterus on the diaphragm throughout pregnancy causes:

  1. *Decreased: Total lung capacity (TLC), Residual Volume (RV) and Expiratory Reserve Volume (ERV)*
  2. *Increased: Tidal Volume (TV)*, and *mild respiratory alkalosis* (Increased pH)

Gastrointestinal System

- **Stomach**: *Decreased* gastric acid production; however, there is also *decreased* gastric emptying, so pregnant patients commonly complain of dyspepsia.
- **Morning sickness**: Disappears by the *16th to 18th week*.
- **Longing**: Due to vasodilatation of nasal blood vessels.
- **Hemorrhoids**: Due to progesterone effect.
- **Hepatic**: Increase in liver enzymes, and cholestasis leading to itching.

Urinary System

- *Increased*: GFR, renal blood flow, glucosuria, aminoaciduria and loss of water-soluble vitamins in urine.
- *Decreased*: Serum levels of urea and creatinine.

Endocrine System

- *Increased*:

  1. Size – *without proportionate increase in vascularity* – of pituitary gland, hence the risk for Sheehan syndrome. See endocrine section of IM.
  2. Serum prolactin levels.
  3. Thyroid binding globulin, hence an increase in bound thyroid hormones (physiological goiter). *Note: Free thyroxin levels are within normal limits.*

- *Decreased*: FSH and LH levels.

Skin

- Chloasma gravidarum: Butterfly pigmentation of the face, due to *placental and adrenal steroids*.
- Striae gravidarum on the abdomen and buttocks: Due to *rupture of elastic fibers*.
- Divarication of recti, especially in obese pregnant.
- Linea nigra in midline, spider angiomata and palmar erythema.

Metabolic Changes

- *Body weight*: Increased by an average of 12.5 kg (25–30 lbs), mainly in the second half of pregnancy.
- Pregnancy hormones have anti-insulin effect, so pregnancy is linked to impaired glucose tolerance and glucosuria.
- *Increased*: Serum cholesterol, fat-soluble vitamins, and immunoglobulins *A* and *M*.
- *Decreased*: Water-soluble vitamins.

Antenatal Care

- *Target*: Early diagnosis and treatment of any high risk pregnancy.
- *Inconsistent fundal height (fundus too high)*: *Most commonly due to incorrect dating of the pregnancy,* multiple gestation, or polyhydramnios.
- *Inconsistent fundal height (fundus too low)*: *Most commonly due to incorrect dating of the pregnancy,*

intrauterine growth retardation, fetal death, or oligohydramnios.

- *Test all pregnant women for rubella*: High levels of *IgM* against Rubella indicate an active infection. Fixed elevated levels of IgG denote *immunity*.
- *Vaccination*: *Only tetanus is indicated*. Live attenuated vaccines (e.g., MMR) are *contraindicated*. Other vaccines (e.g., Yellow fever, rabies) are given only if there is a strong indication.
- *Dietary daily supplementation during pregnancy*:

  1. Daily caloric requirements are 2200 Kcal/day.
  2. Calcium: 1 gm/day.
  3. Folic acid: 1 mg/day. Folic acid def. anemia puts the fetus at risk of *neural tube defects,* e.g., Anencephaly, spina bifida.
  4. Iron: 60 mg/day. During pregnancy, the mother needs an extra 800–1000 mg of iron compared to non-pregnant women. It is best to supplement an additional 30–60 mg of Fe daily, as only 10% of oral Fe is absorbed.

- *Urine analysis*: Urine should be checked as a routine test in antenatal care visits to rule out urinary tract infection. It is common for pregnant patients to develop asymptomatic bacteriuria leading to severe complications, so *treatment is warranted (even when asymptomatic)*.

Assessment of Fetal Wellbeing

- *Clinical picture*:

  1. Ten or more fetal movements in a 12-h period (starting 32 weeks onwards).
  2. Progressive weight gain and increase in abdominal girth.
  3. Progressive increase in fundal height.

- *Serology*: Serial measurements of HCG, HPL and Estriol (E3) levels.
- *Other tests*: Described below in detail.

Ultrasound

- To measure the gestational sac diameter (*to exclude Anembryonic pregnancy*), and to measure the crown-rump length.
- To measure body diameters; most importantly the *head circumference* (*used to estimate gestational age*), and Biparietal diameter (BPD).
- To assess fetal body growth in order to diagnose Intrauterine Fetal Growth Retardation (IUFGR), which has two types. Refer to Table 3.2.

TABLE 3.2 Intrauterine Fetal Growth Retardation (IUFGR).

	Type (I) IUFGR	Type (II) IUFGR
Cause	Fetal	Maternal
Onset	Early	Late
Type	Symmetrical	Asymmetrical
Prognosis	Bad	Excellent (catch up growth)

Cardiotocography (CTG)

- **Introduction**: Performed *after 32 weeks* gestation to assure maturity of fetus, and assess relation of fetal heart rate to uterine contractions.
- **CTG scoring**: *≥ 8 out of 10 is satisfactory*. If <8, it has to be repeated every 2 days.
- **Normal parameters**:

  1. Fetal heart rate is 120–160 bpm, with *beat to beat variability*.
  2. Accelerations (*Best sign of fetal well being*): Reflex fetal tachycardia in response to fetal movements.
  3. Decelerations: There are three types: Refer to Fig. 3.4
     - *Type 1 (Early)*: Bradycardia that occurs simultaneously *with* uterine contractions, *due to a vagal nervous reflex*.
     - *Type 2 (Late)*: Bradycardia that occurs *after* a uterine contraction, *due to transient cessation of placental blood flow with uterine contraction*, leading to transient fetal anaerobic metabolism.
     - *Variable deceleration*: Mechanical, *due to cord compression*, in which vein compression leads to reflex tachycardia, followed by artery compression leading to hypertension and bradycardia. *Amnioinfusion might be needed in some cases to overcome this problem.*

Non Stress Test

- **Reactive**: At least 2 accelerations (of at least 15 bpm) in a 20-min period.
- **Non reactive**: Less than 2 accelerations (of at least 15 bpm) in a 20-min period.

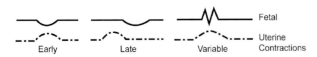

FIG. 3.4 Types of deceleration

Intrapartum Assessment of Fetal Wellbeing

- Monitoring of fetal heart rate.
- Meconium staining of amniotic fluid is a poor prognostic sign, but *not specific*.
- Fetal scalp pH measurement (Normal >7.25): If <7.2 think acidosis.

Abortion

- **Definition**: The termination of pregnancy *before 20 weeks gestation*.
- Causes:

  1. *Fetal* (e.g., Chromosomal or placental abnormalities). *This is the most common cause of 1st trimester abortions.*
  2. *Maternal*: General (e.g., Infections/hormonal), or structural (e.g., Patulous Os or hypoplastic uterus).

- **Clinical picture**: Amenorrhea, followed by abdominal pain and vaginal bleeding.
- **Notes**:

  1. Most common fetal genetic disease to cause abortion: *Trisomy 16*.
  2. Most common infection to cause abortion in early pregnancy: *Mycoplasma Hominis*.

- **Types of abortion**: Discussed below in detail.

Threatened Abortion

- **Definition**: Slight hemorrhage into the *choriodecidual space*. Stops spontaneously in most cases.
- **Pelvic exam**: *Closed cervix*.
- **Next best step**: *B-HCG measurement and monitoring* (Should double every 2 days. If no doubling, consider *missed abortion*).
- **Treatment**:

  1. Resuscitation and physical rest.
  2. Tocolytics (Anti-PG and B2 agonists) to relax the uterus: *Used in 2nd trimester abortion cases only*.
  3. 17-OH Progesterone: Used only if the cause is corpus luteum insufficiency.

Inevitable Abortion

- **Clinical picture**: The fundal level corresponds to the period of amenorrhea (correct height), but the pelvic exam reveals an *open cervix*, and products of conception protruding through the os.

- *Treatment*:

   1. Resuscitation.
   2. Evacuation of the uterine contents:

      - 1st Trimester: Suction or D&C (Dilatation and Curettage).
      - 2nd Trimester: Prostaglandins (PG) (*Best Choice*) or Oxytocin.

- *Note*: Incomplete abortion presents in the same manner as an inevitable abortion; however, in the latter case, the uterus has already expelled some of its contents, so the fundal height will be less than period of amenorrhea. In complete abortion, the uterus has already expelled all products of conception.

Septic Abortion

- *Definition*: Caused by superimposed infection complicating any type of abortion.
- *Most common organism*: *Group B Streptococcus*, but also consider anaerobes or Staphylococcus.
- *Clinical picture*:

   1. Period of amenorrhea, followed by abdominal pain and vaginal bleeding.
   2. Fever and malodorous vaginal discharge.
   3. Lower abdominal tenderness.

- *Diagnosis*: Cultures from blood, vagina and endocervix.
- *Complications*:

   1. Local: Endo- or myometritis, up to pelvic abscess or peritonitis.
   2. General: DIC, hemolysis, renal failure or even septic shock.

- *Treatment*:

   1. Resuscitation and broad spectrum antibiotics, e.g., Penicillin (Gram positive) plus aminoglycoside (Gram negative) plus metronidazole or clindamycin (Anaerobes).
   2. Evacuate the uterus: Suction or D&C (1st trimester), or using PG or oxytocin (2nd trimester). Complicated cases: Hysterectomy.

Missed Abortion

- *Definition*: Retained products of conception which are no longer viable, a.k.a. *Fleshy mole* or *Bloody mole*.
- *Clinical picture*:

   1. Amenorrhea, followed by minimal dark vaginal bleeding *but no abdominal pain* (*Missed abortion is a painless condition*).
   2. Nipple discharge.

- *On exam*:

   1. Fundal level is *lower* than the period of amenorrhea.
   2. Cervix is *closed,* and there is *a small amount of dark blood*.

- *Complications*: Septic abortion, and DIC (Common after *3–4 weeks*).
- *Diagnosis*:

   1. Elevated B-HCG, *but it does not double every 2 days*.
   2. U/S: Shows *non-moving fetus without cardiac activity*.

- *Treatment*: Uterine evacuation.

Habitual Abortion

- *Definition*: *3 or more successive abortions*.
- *Causes*: Multiple; most important are:

   1. *Patulous internal cervical os*:

      - Congenital, or secondary to obstetric trauma or *use of DiethylStilbesterol (DES) (DES also causes vaginal clear cell adenocarcinoma)*.
      - Abortions occur in *descending* pattern (7 ms in first abortion, 4 ms in second abortion, etc.).
      - Diagnosis: Hysterosalpingography (HSG) shows loss of uterine waist (*Funneling*). Also, a dilator can be passed through the os without resistance.
      - Treatment: *Vaginal cerclage* (Done at 12 weeks gestation).

   2. *Uterine hypoplasia*:

      - Abortions occur in *ascending* pattern (4 ms, 7 ms, etc.).
      - Treatment: Vaginal cerclage.

   3. *Fixed Retroverted Flexed uterus (RVF)*: Abortion here occurs around the 14th to 16th week of gestation. Commonly associated with *urinaryretention*.

Ectopic Pregnancy

- *Definition*: Any pregnancy that implants outside the uterine cavity.
- *Most common site*: *Ampulla* of the Fallopian tube.

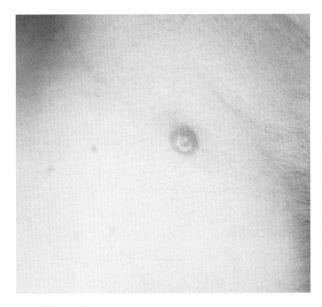

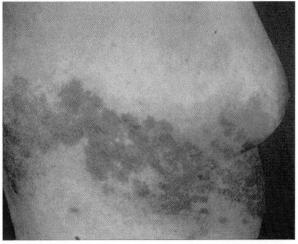

FIG. 2.11 Shingles

FIG. 2.9 Molluscum contagiosum

- **Clinical picture**: Multiple *crops of very painful and tender vesicles* on an erythematous base. During the course of the disease, *which usually lasts around one week*, the vesicles rupture and lesions crust.
- **Treatment**: Systemic *Acyclovir* for 5 days.

Herpes Zoster (refer to Fig. 2.11)

- **Introduction**: Also known as *shingles*. Occurs due to reactivation of a dormant varicella zoster infection, mostly in *dorsal roots*.
- **Risk factors**: Immunocompromised state with a positive history of chicken pox.
- **Clinical picture**:

  1. *Chicken pox*: Caused by varicella zoster. Lesions are arranged in crops of various lesions in different stages of development, *all at the same time,*

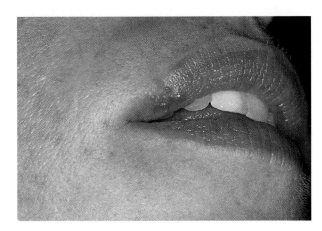

FIG. 2.10 Herpes simplex type I

   i.e.: macules, papules, pustules, vesicles, crusted lesions.
  2. *Shingles (Herpes zoster)*: The key for diagnosis here is the distribution of lesions, which follow *dermatomes*. The disease starts with severe *burning pain and hyperesthesia, taking a dermatomal distribution*, which is then followed by vesicular lesions in a similar distribution and *not crossing the midline*.

- **Complications**: The course of the disease is as long as 3–4 weeks, and is commonly followed by *post-herpetic neuralgia*.
- **Treatment**: Systemic *Acyclovir* for 10 days. Famciclovir and valacyclovir are other options.
- **Notes**:

  1. Vesicular lesions of chicken pox have a *dewdrop on a rose petal* appearance.
  2. Herpetic lesions in the cornea are irregular, *dendritic* and could be seen by slit lamp examination after application of fluorescin dye.
  3. Diagnosis of Herpes viruses: *Tzanck smear*, which shows *multinucleated giant cells, and intranuclear inclusion bodies*.
  4. Treatment of herpes with acyclovir does not cure the rash; it only shortens duration of the rash and decreases the risk of post-herpetic neuralgia.
  5. Acyclovir is not helpful if started after 24–48 hours from the onset of the rash.

Bacterial Infections

Impetigo

- **Introduction**: A *contagious* superficial pyogenic infection.
- **Organisms**: *Staphylococcus aureus* or Streptococci.

- **Risk factors**: STDs (*PID is the most common cause*), tubal surgery and some contraceptives (e.g., *Progesterone pills and intrauterine devices IUD*).
- **Pathology**: During ectopic pregnancy, regardless of the site, the following occurs:

  1. Ovaries: *Corpus luteum* of pregnancy.
  2. Uterus: Increases in size and the endometrium thickens, showing:

     - *Decidual reaction* (*Without* villi)
     - *Arias Stella reaction*: Adenomatous hyperplasia

- **Complications**: Tubal rupture causing intraperitoneal hemorrhage.
- **Clinical picture**:

  1. Amenorrhea: Due to hormones secreted from corpus luteum. *Rarely exceeds 8 weeks in duration.*
  2. Severe lower unilateral abdominal pain: If this radiates to shoulders, think of perforation and diaphragmatic irritation by intraperitoneal blood.
  3. Vaginal bleeding: Mild in amount, and also rarely *decidual casts.*
  4. Pressure symptoms (Dysuria, Dyschezia, Dyspareunia): Suspect pelvic hematocele.

- **On exam**: Cervical motion tenderness (*Jumping sign*), and tender boggy swelling in Cul-de-sac in cases of pelvic hematocele.
- **Diagnosis**: Positive pregnancy test and absence of intrauterine pregnancy by U/S.
- **Treatment**:

  1. *Resuscitation* is the best next step.
  2. If ectopic mass <3.5 cm and *stable*: Abortifacient medications could be used in these cases. e.g., Methotrexate, Prostaglandins or Mifepristone, a.k.a. RU486 (anti-progesterone).
  3. If ectopic mass >3.5 cm or *unstable (e.g., rupture or bleeding)*:

     - Laparotomy or Laparoscopy: Evacuation of fetal sac and membranes.
     - Salpingectomy (Total or partial): If the Fallopian tube is ruptured.

- **Prognosis**:

  1. 50%–60% of patients will have a normal intrauterine pregnancy.
  2. 30%–40% of patients will become infertile.
  3. 10%–15% of patients will suffer another ectopic pregnancy.

- **Note**: *Any female patient of reproductive age who presents with abdominal pain must get a pregnancy test to rule out ectopic pregnancy, even if she insists that she is not pregnant.*

Hydatidiform (Vesicular) Mole

- **Definition**: A *trophoblastic disease* characterized by benign hyperplasia of trophoblast, along with hydropic degeneration of chorionic villi.
- **Risk factors**: Ages >40 or <15, and vitamin A deficiency.
- **Types**: Refer to Table 3.3
- **Pathology**:

  1. Uterus: Studded with *fluid filled vesicles* up to 1 cm in diameter.
  2. Ovaries: *Theca Lutein cysts* (Due to HCG production by trophoblast).

- **Clinical picture**: Amenorrhea, symptoms of pregnancy and uterine bleeding which might contain *vesicles.*
- **On exam**: *Large doughy uterus* with absent fetal heart sounds.
- **Complications**:

  1. *Chorioadenoma Destruens*: Malignant mole that perforates the uterus.
  2. *Choriocarcinoma*: Malignant transformation. Refer to gynecology.
  3. *Thyrotoxicosis*: Due to release of human chorionic TSH.
  4. *Hyperemesis gravidarum*: Due to release of large amounts of HCG.
  5. *Early Pre-eclampsia*: If Pre-eclampsia occurred during *the first half of pregnancy*, think of hydatidiform mole.

- **Diagnosis**:

  1. *B-HCG* will be positive even in the highest dilutions.
  2. U/S of uterus: *Snow storm* appearance.
  3. Doppler: Absent fetal heart sounds.

- **Treatment**: Suction followed by D&C in 2 weeks (*Cluster of grapes inside uterus*).

TABLE 3.3 Hydatidiform mole.

	Complete mole	Partial mole
Incidence	More common	Very rare
Malignant potential	Common (10% chance)	Very unlikely
Karyotype	XX (*All Paternal*)	Triploidy
Contents	Vesicles only	Vesicles + Malformed fetus

- *Follow up*:

  1. Monitoring the HCG levels *weekly for the first 12 weeks* after evacuation (12 weeks is the time HCG needs to fall back to normal values), and *then monthly for 12 months,* to make sure that level of HCG does not rise.
  2. If HCG level does not normalize or starts rising, this suggests Choriocarcinoma.

- *Note*: During the follow up period, *pregnancy is contraindicated*, as that will raise the HCG level and make the follow up difficult.

Antepartum Hemorrhage

- *Definition*: Bleeding from the genital tract after the time of fetal viability (20 weeks), but before full maturation of the fetus (37 weeks).
- *Causes*:

  1. Fetal: Vasa previa.
  2. Placental: Placenta previa or Abruptio placenta.
  3. Local causes: Uterine rupture, due to injury or at the site of a previous scar.

Vasa Previa

- *Mechanism*: Fetal blood vessels present in front of the presenting part of the fetus.
- *Causes*: Velamentous insertion of placenta, and placenta succenturiata.
- *Treatment*: Immediate delivery by C-section.

Placenta Previa

- *Definition*: A placenta that is situated in the lower uterine segment.
- *Degrees*:

  1. 1st degree: Away from the internal cervical os.
  2. 2nd and 3rd degree: Encroaching on the internal os.
  3. 4th degree: Completely covering the internal os.

- *Clinical picture*: *Bright red vaginal bleeding*: Usually related to sexual intercourse or pelvic exam. It is *painless*, recurrent and stops spontaneously.
- *On exam*:

  1. Fundal level and uterine external palpation are normal.
  2. *Pelvic examination is absolutely contraindicated (Fatal bleeding)*.

- *Diagnosis*: Transabdominal (*Not transvaginal*) ultrasound.
- *Treatment*:

  1. Resuscitation is the best next step.
  2. Bed rest and sexual abstinence.
  3. U/S follow-up: The unequal rate of growth of the upper and lower uterine segments can cause the placenta to migrate upwards throughout pregnancy.

- *Indications for immediate termination*: Uncontrolled bleeding or fetal distress.
- *Mode of delivery*:

  1. 1st and 2nd degrees: *Vaginal delivery*.
  2. 3rd and 4th degrees: *C-section*.

Abruptio Placenta

- *Mechanism*: Separation of a normally-situated placenta.
- *Risk factors*: *Hypertension* and *cocaine abuse*. So when you see a pregnant patient in the USMLE who used cocaine and is now presenting with sudden abdominal pain, you know what to think!
- *Types and clinical picture*

  1. *Revealed Abruptio placenta*:

     - Lower margin of placenta separates and blood tracks its way out through vagina.
     - Patient presents with *scanty dark and painful vaginal bleeding* (*It is bright red and painless in placenta previa*).
     - Abdominal examination is normal; however, pelvic exam is contraindicated.

  2. *Concealed Abruptio placenta*:

     - Blood is concealed between placenta and uterus.
     - Patient presents with severe abdominal pain, tenderness and rigidity. (*No vaginal bleeding*).
     - Abdominal examination reveals *board-like abdominal rigidity*, and pelvic exam is still contraindicated.

- *Complications*:

  1. Fetal death: More common in concealed abruptio placenta.
  2. Hemorrhagic shock.
  3. *Couvelaire uterus*: Blood dissects its way through uterus to the peritoneum.
  4. DIC and renal failure.
  5. Postpartum hemorrhage: Might lead to Sheehan's syndrome (Hypopituitarism).

- *Diagnosis*: Transabdominal (*Not transvaginal*) ultrasound.
- *Treatment*: *Immediate termination by C-section.*

Premature Rupture of Membranes (PROM)

- *Mechanism*: Rupture of membranes before the onset of uterine contractions.
- *Causes*: Infections, trauma or iatrogenic (e.g., Cerclage or amniocentesis).
- *Clinical picture*: *Sudden gush of watery fluid from the vagina.*
- *On exam*:

  1. Fundal level is less than period of amenorrhea.
  2. Fetal parts are easily palpated on external uterine palpation.

- *Complications*:

  1. Infection, e.g., Chorioamnionitis: *Group B strept.* is the most common organism.
  2. Abortion and preterm labor.
  3. Prolonged oligohydramnios leading to fetal lung hypoplasia (*Potter syndrome*).

- *Diagnosis*:

  1. U/S: Confirms oligohydramnios.
  2. Sample from the fluid in posterior fornix on a *nitrazine paper gives blue color*. This confirms that the fluid is amniotic fluid (*Amnio dye* or *tampon* test).
  3. Positive *Fern test* (Characteristic pattern of drying on a glass slide).

- *Treatment*:

  1. If >36 weeks: Immediate delivery.
  2. If <36 weeks: Betamethasone for 48 h to accelerate fetal lung maturity, and deliver once lung maturity is proven. Keep a close eye for signs of infection (fever, tachycardia, abdominal pain, vaginal discharge).

- *Note*: PROM is one of the cases associated with accelerated lung maturity; others are pre-eclampsia, intrauterine growth retardation and intrauterine infections.

Pre-Eclampsia

- *Definition*: Pregnancy related *EPH*, i.e., *E*dema, *P*roteinuria and *H*ypertension.
- *Pathology*: Vasospasm and *subintimal* edema.

- *Cause*: Unknown, but most likely due to *prostaglandin imbalance causing endothelial damage.*
- *Risk factors*: *Primigravida*, extremes of age and obese patients.
- *Timing*: A disease of the *second half of pregnancy (20–40 weeks)*. The only conditions in which you suspect this disease in the first half of pregnancy are hydatidiform mole, DM, twin pregnancy and polyhydramnios.
- *Clinical picture and exam findings*: Diffuse body edema and elevated blood pressure more than 140/90 on *more than 2 occasions*.
- *Diagnosis*: Clinical diagnosis, plus elevated urinary protein levels.
- *Complications*:

  1. Eclampsia: *Seizures* associated with a high rate of organ failure and mortality. *Treatment*: Magnesium sulfate IV and immediate stabilization of the mother with subsequent delivery (Mg sulfate is continued for 24 h postpartum). *Signs of magnesium toxicity*: Loss of deep tendon reflexes (*First sign*), and respiratory depression. *Antidote for magnesium*: Calcium gluconate IV.
  2. Placenta: Abruptio placenta.
  3. Cerebral edema or hemorrhage: Headache, blurry vision, nausea and vomiting.
  4. Periportal hepatic necrosis: Jaundice, and elevated bilirubin and transaminases.
  5. Hepatic subcapsular hemorrhage: Epigastric pain.
  6. Renal failure: Oliguria (<500 cc urine output/day), or anuria (<100 cc).
  7. Congestive heart failure and pulmonary edema: Dyspnea, orthopnea and PND.
  8. HELLP syndrome: Microangiopathic hemolysis (H), Elevated liver enzymes (EL), and Low platelets (LP). It carries a very poor prognosis.

- *Treatment of pre-eclampsia*:

  1. *Mild cases*:

     - Control of blood pressure: Best is alphamethyldopa or hydralazine.
     - Betamethasone for 48 h: To accelerate fetal lung maturity.
     - Once fetal lung maturity is achieved, delivery is induced.

  2. *Severe cases, or any signs of organ damage (See complications)*:

     - Immediate termination of pregnancy.
     - Prophylactic magnesium sulfate should be given, and continued until 24 h postpartum.

- *Note*: The one and only definitive cure for pre-eclampsia/eclampsia is *delivery*.

Gestational Diabetes

- **Introduction**: Pregnancy is a diabetogenic state due to placental release of insulinase, and the hyperglycemic effect of hormones, e.g., HPL, Estrogen, Progesterone, Prolactin.
- **Complications**:

  1. Pre-eclampsia and polyhydramnios.
  2. Macrosomia: Neonate weights more than 4 kg, and is fat, with cushingoid features. This occurs *due to the reflex increase in fetal insulin secretion to antagonize the elevated blood glucose levels.* Remember that insulin is an anabolic hormone. Macrosomia has the risks of *post-term labor, C-section, shoulder dystocia* and *brachial plexus injury.*
  3. Congenital anomalies: Due to low levels of arachidonic acid and myoinositol. A rare, but specific, example is *caudal regression syndrome* (Hypoplasia of sacrum and legs), and transposition of great arteries (TGA).
  4. Fetal *hypoglycemia, hypomagnesaemia, hypokalemia* and *hypocalcaemia due to functional hypoparathyroidism.*
  5. Unexplained intrauterine fetal death: Mostly due to *placental insufficiency.*
  6. Hyperviscosity syndrome: Due to *polycythemia,* increasing the risk of renal vein and mesenteric thrombosis.

- **Diagnosis**: *Glucose tolerance test is the test of choice to diagnose gestational diabetes (Done at 26–28 weeks).* Fasting blood sugar is checked ($N < 105$), then the patient is infused with 100 g of glucose, and blood sugar is checked in 1 h ($N < 190$), 2 h ($N < 165$) and 3 h ($N < 145$). If *2 or more* of these numbers are above normal, diagnosis is confirmed.
- **Treatment**: Diet control and insulin therapy. *Oral hypoglycemics are contraindicated during pregnancy due to their teratogenic and hypoglycemic effects.*
- **Note**: Gestational diabetes typically resolves spontaneously after labor. However, patients with gestational diabetes have a higher risk of developing diabetes mellitus (DM) later in life compared to the normal population.

Rh Isoimmunization

- **Mechanism**: Occurs when Rh +ve RBCs are transferred from the fetus to the Rh –ve mother during labor, stimulating the formation of *IgG* antibodies. These antibodies can cross the placenta to hemolyze fetal RBCs, and it usually affects the *next fetus.*

- **Hydrops fetalis**: It is the *most severe* form. Fetus suffers severe hemolysis and diffuse generalized edema a.k.a. *anasarca.* Fetal liver fails to synthesize any proteins. Fetus looks like *Buddha* on ultrasound.
- **Icterus gravis neonatorum**: It is the *most common* form. Significant elevation of bilirubin leads to jaundice and kernicterus (*Remember? Hemolysis increases indirect bilirubin, which cannot pass in the urine or stools, but can easily cross blood brain barrier*).
- **Diagnosis**: In susceptible patients (Rh –ve mother and Rh +ve father, or history of Rh incompatibility), amniocentesis is done at *28 weeks.* The bilirubin level is measured using a spectrophotometer and results are plotted on Liley chart.
- **Screening**: Coombs test and Rh determination should be done at *28 weeks.*
- **Treatment**:

  1. Rh –ve mother should receive *RhoGam at 28 weeks and again during the first 24 h after termination of pregnancy, i.e., Labor, abortion, ectopic, etc...*
  2. For established cases with Rh isoimmunization: depends on Liley chart:

     - Low or midzone (Mild hemolysis): Repeat amniocentesis in 2–3 weeks.
     - High zone: Immediate termination of pregnancy.

Hyperemesis Gravidarum

- **Mechanism**: Severe vomiting during pregnancy, of unknown mechanism. Could be related to *psychological and hormonal* factors.
- **Complications**: Dehydration, hepatic necrosis and renal failure.
- **Treatment**: Conservative using anti-emetics and aggressive hydration. Termination is only indicated for sever cases with organ dysfunction.
- **Note**: Morning sickness is mainly nausea and to a lesser extent vomiting. It occurs mainly *during the 1st trimester* and resolves spontaneously.

Labor

- **Definition**: The end of pregnancy, concluding in expulsion of the fetus and placenta, any time after fetal viability (*20 weeks*).
- **Clinical picture**:

  1. Uterine contractions of *regular pattern* along with hardening of the uterus on palpation.
  2. Dilatation and effacement of the cervix

TABLE 3.4 Stages of labor.

	Duration in nulliparous	Duration in multiparous	Process
1st stage	12–16 h	6–8 h	Cervical dilatation
2nd stage	1–2 h	30 min–1 h	Delivery of fetus: Descent, engagement, flexion, rotation
3rd stage	10 min–30 min	5 min–10 min	Delivery of placenta

- **Stages of labor**: Refer to Table 3.4
- **Bishop score**: Used to assess readiness for labor. Refer to Table 3.5
- **Malpresentations**:

  1. *Face*: Mentum anterior can be delivered vaginally. Mentum posterior presentation must rotate to mentum anterior or C-section will be needed.
  2. *Occiput*: Occipito-anterior can be delivered vaginally. Occipito-posterior presentation must rotate to occipito-anterior or C-section will be needed.
  3. *Brow*: The diameter engaged here is the occipito-frontal diameter (11.5 cm), which is too wide for vaginal delivery, unless rotated to face or occiput presentation.
  4. *Shoulder*: C-section is needed unless rotation to vertex position takes place.
  5. *Breech*: Most common of which is *frank breech* (Flexed hips and extended knees), others include *complete breech* (Hips and knees are all flexed) and *footling*. Most breech presentations are delivered using *C-section*.

- *Notes*:

  1. Prolonged first stage of labor (More than 20 hours in nulliparous and 14 hours in multiparous) is best managed using *meperidine (Demerol)*.
  2. Epidural anesthesia: Prolongs *2nd stage of labor* and increases need for oxytocin.
  3. Paracervical anesthesia: Carries the risk of *fetal bradycardia*.
  4. Intrauterine fetal distress during prolonged labor can be assessed by *Doppler examination*

TABLE 3.5 Bishop score (Normal = 8 or higher).

	0	1	2	3
Effacement	0–30%	40–50%	60–70%	>80%
Dilatation	Closed	1–2 cm	3–4 cm	>5 cm
Consistency	Firm	Medium	Soft	Soft
Station	−3	−2	−1 or zero	+1
Position	Posterior	Middle	Anterior	Anterior

of the fetal renal artery, as well as fetal heart rate monitoring.

Postpartum Hemorrhage

- **Definition**: Hemorrhage (>500 cc) from the genital tract after labor. The most common cause is *uterine atony*, followed by retained placenta.
- **Uterine atony**: Uterus is lax and enlarged.
- **Treatment**:

  1. Resuscitation is the first step.
  2. Bimanual massage of the uterus is effective in most cases.
  3. For resistant cases, oxytocin or prostaglandin F2 could be used.
  4. Last resort (for non-resolving cases): Hysterectomy.

- **Retained placenta**: Treated by manual removal of placental parts from the uterus and curettage.

Amniotic Fluid Embolism

- **Mechanism**: Amniotic fluid enters the maternal circulation during labor.
- **Clinical picture**: Sudden respiratory distress. Just like pulmonary embolism; suspect it when you see a patient in the USMLE who just gave birth few hours ago, now suddenly starting hyperventilating, dropping her oxygen saturation and becoming hemodynamically unstable.
- **Diagnosis**: Clinical diagnosis, confirmed in the postmortem period by presence of *amniotic cells and meconium in the lungs and right side of the heart*.
- **Treatment**: Supportive.

Puerperal Sepsis

- **Definition**: It is infection of the female genital tract after labor.
- **Most common organism**: *Group B hemolytic streptococci*.
- **Clinical picture**:

  1. Fever and leukocytosis.
  2. Lower abdominal pain and tenderness.
  3. Malodorous vaginal discharge. If you see any patient in the USMLE who gave birth very recently, now having fever and lower abdominal pain, you know what to think! *If puerperal sepsis is ruled out, think pelvic thrombophlebitis.*

- *Diagnosis*: Culture of discharge, blood and endocervix.
- *Treatment*:

  1. Broad spectrum antibiotics: Penicillin + Aminoglycosides + Metronidazole.
  2. Evacuation of the uterus.

Miscellaneous Notes

Thromboembolism

- *Introduction*: Pregnancy is a hypercoagulable state, and patients are at high risk for thromboembolic events, e.g., DVT, Pulmonary embolism, etc...
- *Treatment*: Heparin, and continue treatment till *6 weeks postpartum*.
- *Note*: Coumadin is contraindicated during pregnancy due to teratogenicity.

APGAR Score

- *Introduction*: Used to evaluate the cardiopulmonary and nervous system status of the newborn at *1* and *5 min* after delivery.
- *Calculation*: Refer to Table 3.6

Appendicitis During Pregnancy

- *Introduction*: Atypical presentation during pregnancy, as appendix is pushed all the way up to the *right hypochondrium*, so it is often confused with cholecystitis in pregnant patients.
- *Complication*: Higher risk of perforation, peritonitis and abortion.
- *Treatment*: Urgent appendectomy.
- *Note*: Test of choice to diagnose *pancreatitis during pregnancy* is the *amylase/creatinine ratio* (>5–6%)

Pre- and Post-Maturity

- *Pre-maturity*: The most common risk factor for prematurity is *past history of a similar condition*. Fetus is at risk of *sub-ependymal hemorrhage* and *retrolental fibroplasia*.
- *Post-maturity*: The most common cause of postmaturity is *incorrect calculation of dates*. Fetus is at risk of *macrosomia* and *shoulder dystocia*. One of the most important complications of shoulder dystocia is *injury to the brachial plexus, mainly upper trunk*.

Postpartum Changes

- *Menstruation and ovulation*: They re-start around *6–9 months* after labor for breastfeeding patients (*Only after 6 weeks if not breastfeeding*).
- *Lochia*: Discharge from the genital tract after labor; lasts around *3 weeks*. It starts as bloody discharge (*Lochia rubra*), then turns serous (*Lochia serosa*) and finally white (*Lochia alba*).

Caput Succedaneum

- *Definition*: Localized edema of the scalp, mostly due to *venous obstruction*.
- *Causes*: Obstructed labor, or *use of suction cup* during labor.
- *Fate*: *Resolves spontaneously*.
- *Notes*:

  1. *Cephalhematoma* is bleeding that takes place underneath the pericranium, where bleeding characteristically takes the distribution of one or more cranial bones (Unlike caput, Cephalhematoma *does not cross suture lines and is not diffuse*).
  2. Moulding is overriding of fetal skull bones during labor. Complication: Intracranial hemorrhage, mainly from *great cerebral vein of Galen*.

Infections During Pregnancy

- Transmission of hepatitis B from mother to fetus is increased if the mother is positive for the (e) antigen.
- Only 2.5% of neonates born to mothers with positive hepatitis B surface antigen will be infected at birth.
- Gonorrhea during pregnancy is treated using *spectinomycin*.
- HIV transmission from mother to fetus is decreased by using *Zidovudine (AZT)*.

TABLE 3.6 APGAR scoring system (N=7–10 out of 1 0).

	Zero	1	2
Respirations	Absent	Gasping, grunting	Good
Heart rate	Absent	<100 bpm	>100 bpm
Muscle tone	Flaccid	Flexed extremities movement	Active
			Reflexes
Absent		Hyporeflexia	Good
Skin color	Pale	Pink with cyanotic extremities	Pink

Chapter 4
Gynecology

Estrogen

- **Natural**:

  1. Estrone (E1): Estrogen of menopause.
  2. Estradiol (E2): Estrogen of *reproductive age*.
  3. Estriol (E3): Estrogen of *pregnancy*.

- **Synthetic**: Multiple forms and dosages. Note that Diethylstilbestrol (*D.E.S*) is no longer used due to its dangerous effects, e.g., Vaginal adenosis and *clear cell adenocarcinoma*; also incompetent cervix and *abortion*.

- **Sources**:

  1. Graafian follicle: Source of E2 during first half of menstrual cycle.
  2. Corpus luteum: Source of E2 during second half of menstrual cycle.
  3. Placenta: Source of E3 during pregnancy.
  4. Adipose tissue: Peripheral conversion of androgens to estrogen by *aromatase* enzyme.

- **Actions**: Refer to Table 4.1

Progesterone

- **Source**: Corpus luteum and placenta.
- **Actions**: Refer to Table 4.1.

Androgen

- **Sources**:

  1. Ovaries: Secrete Androstenedione and Testosterone.

Table 4.1 Actions of estrogen and progesterone.

	Estrogen	Progesterone
Breasts	• Develop *duct system* • Increase fat deposition	• Develop *acinar* system • Blocks prolactin action on the breast
Kidneys	• Increase salt and water retention	• Induces diuresis
Pituitary	• Feedback inhibition of FSH & LH • When estrogen level exceeds 200 pg/mL, it promotes ovulation by inducing an *LH surge*	• Feedback inhibition of FSH and LH
Genitalia	• Increase epithelial thickness and vascularity. • Induces *copious and alkaline* cervical mucus production. • Inhibits ovulation	• Decrease epithelial thickness and vascularity • Induces *scanty and viscid* cervical mucus production • Regulates formation of mucus plug during pregnancy • Inhibits ovulation • Inhibits uterine contractions • Increase body basal temperature
Miscellaneous	• *Bone*: stimulate osteoblasts, close epiphysis and protects against osteoporosis • *Vascular*: Increase risk of *thromboembolism* and serum HDL	

2. Adrenal glands: Secrete Dehydroepiandroster-one (*DHEA*).
3. Peripheral conversion from one androgen to another.

- *Hyperandrogenism in females*: Anovulation, infertility, hirsutism, clitoromegaly, and increased muscle tone.

Gonadotrophins (Refer to Fig. 4.1)

- *Luteinizing Hormone (LH)*:

   1. Stimulates steroidogenesis by Theca cells.
   2. LH surge stimulates prostaglandins and collagenase enzyme; which induces ovulation by rupture of ovarian follicle.

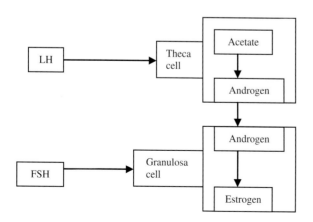

Fig. 4.1 Actions of gonadotrophins

- *Follicle Stimulating Hormone (FSH)*:

   1. Stimulates development of follicles.
   2. Stimulates mitosis of Granulosa cells.

Menstrual Cycle

- *Endometrial and ovarian cycles*: Refer to Fig. 4.2.
- *Cyclic hormonal levels*: Refer to Figs. 4.3, 4.4, 4.5, and 4.6.

Puberty

- *Introduction*: Physical maturity involving sexual and reproductive development. The process *in order of occurrence* includes:

   1. *Thelarche*: Breast development.
   2. *Growth spurt*.
   3. *Pubarche*: Pubic hair development.
   4. *Menarche*: Menstruation.

- *Normal age of puberty*: *9–14 years*.

Precocious Puberty

- *Introduction*: Puberty completion *before 9 years* of age.
- *Types*:

   1. *Isosexual*:

      - *True*: *High FSH, LH and estrogen*. Treatment: Anti-estrogen and GnRH analogues.

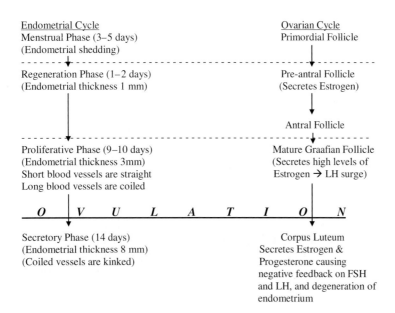

Endometrial Cycle
Menstrual Phase (3–5 days)
(Endometrial shedding)

Regeneration Phase (1–2 days)
(Endometrial thickness 1 mm)

Proliferative Phase (9–10 days)
(Endometrial thickness 3mm)
Short blood vessels are straight
Long blood vessels are coiled

O   V   U   L   A   T   I   O   N

Secretory Phase (14 days)
(Endometrial thickness 8 mm)
(Coiled vessels are kinked)

Ovarian Cycle
Primordial Follicle

Pre-antral Follicle
(Secretes Estrogen)

Antral Follicle

Mature Graafian Follicle
(Secretes high levels of
Estrogen → LH surge)

Corpus Luteum
Secretes Estrogen &
Progesterone causing
negative feedback on FSH
and LH, and degeneration of
endometrium

FIG. 4.2 Endometrial and ovarian cycles

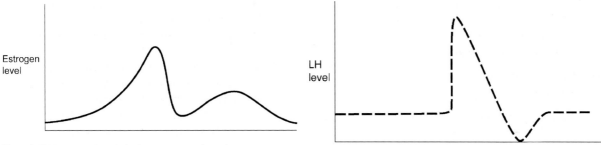

Estrogen
level

FIG. 4.3 Estrogen level during menstrual cycle

LH
level

FIG. 4.5 LH level during menstrual cycle

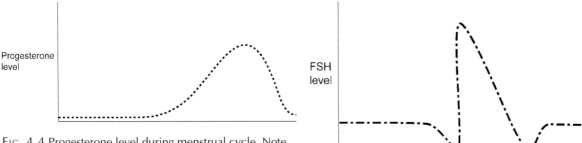

Progesterone
level

FIG. 4.4 Progesterone level during menstrual cycle. Note
that the peak level occurs in the 21st day of the cycle

FSH
level

FIG. 4.6 FSH level during menstrual cycle

- *Pseudo*: *Low FSH, LH and high estrogen.* Estrogen excess either from the ovary or iatrogenic could be the cause, e.g., McCune Albright syndrome (Triad of polyostotic fibrous dysplasia, café au Lait skin patches and autonomous estrogen secretion by the ovaries).

2. **Heterosexual**:

- *Congenital Adrenal Hyperplasia (CAH)*: Due to 21-Alpha Hydroxylase deficiency causing *high androgen* and *low corticosteroid levels*. Suspect it in any female who develops

hirsitism before menarche. Diagnosis: High serum levels of *17-OH progesterone*.
- External androgen source.
- Androgen secreting ovarian tumor.

- *Notes*:

  1. High serum *Testosterone*: *Ovarian* cause.
  2. High serum *DHEA*: *Adrenal* cause.

Menopause

- *Definition*: Permanent cessation of menstruation due to exhaustion of follicles, usually preceded by a period of ovarian functional decline known as *Climacteric*.
- *Normal age of menopause*: Median age of onset in the U.S. is 50 years.
- *Symptoms*:

  1. *Hot flashes* and excessive sweating: Due to *hypothalamic* instability.
  2. Anxiety and depression.
  3. Bone pains and fractures: Due to *osteoporosis*.
  4. Atrophic vulvovaginitis: Vaginal dryness, pruritis and *dyspareunia*.
  5. *UTI* and urinary incontinence.

- *Diagnosis*: Elevated serum *FSH*.
- *Treatment*:

  1. Bone: *Bisphosphonates*, calcium and vitamin D.
  2. Hot Flashes: *Clonidine* or *SSRIs*.
  3. Hormonal Replacement Therapy (HRT): Controversial due to its *thromboembolic* effects, e.g., DVT, CAD, CVA, and increased risk of *breast and endometrial cancer*.

Amenorrhea

- *Introduction*: Few terms you have to be familiar with:

  1. Primary amenorrhea: Absence of menstruation and secondary sexual characters by *age 14*.
  2. Secondary amenorrhea: Cessation of previously normal menstruation for a period of *6 months* or *for 3 successive cycles*.
  3. False amenorrhea (Cryptomenorrhea): Due to cervical atresia, imperforate hymen or transverse vaginal septum. Cryptomenorrhea is characterized by *cyclic pain*.

- *Causes*:

  1. *Physiological*: Pregnancy, lactation or menopause.
  2. *Hypothalamic*: Hyperprolactinemia, or anorexia nervosa.

3. *Pituitary*:

- Hypothyroidism
- Panhypopituitarism, e.g., Postpartum pituitary hemorrhagic infarction a.k.a. *Sheehan syndrome*.
- Levi-Lorain syndrome: Amenorrhea plus *dwarfism*.

4. *Ovarian*: Anovulation, ovarian failure, polycystic ovarian syndrome (PCOS), and Testicular feminization syndrome.
5. *Uterine*:

- Aplasia or hypoplasia.
- Ashermann syndrome: Intrauterine *adhesions*. Diagnosis: Hysteroscopy or hysterosalpingography. Treatment: Dilatation and curettage (D&C).

6. *Others*: Anemia, Debilitating Disease or Endocrinal Disturbance.

- *Diagnosis key*:

  1. Most common cause of primary amenorrhea: *Ovarian,* followed by uterine.
  2. Most common cause of secondary amenorrhea: *Pregnancy*.
  3. Most common cause of postpartum amenorrhea: *Lactation*. Other causes to consider are Sheehan syndrome, prolactinoma and Ashermann syndrome.
  4. *Elevated FSH and LH indicate ovarian failure*.
  5. *Low FSH and LH indicate pituitary or hypothalamic cause*.
  6. *LH: FSH > 3:1 indicates Polycystic Ovarian Syndrome (PCOS)*.
  7. Refer to Fig. 4.7 for an algorithm to approach amenorrhea.

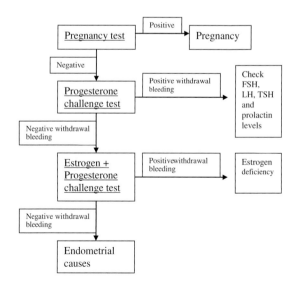

FIG. 4.7 Algorithm for approaching a case of amenorrhea

Polycystic Ovarian Syndrome (PCOS)

- *Introduction*: Also known as *Stein-Leventhal syndrome*.
- *Mechanism*: High LH levels cause increased androgen and estrogen formation, which in turn leads to feedback inhibition of FSH. This leads to arrest of follicular development in various stages, plus the following:

  1. High Androgens: Hirsutism and acne.
  2. High Estrogen: Endometrial and myometrial hyperplasia.

- *Clinical picture*:

  1. Anovulation and infertility: Patient complains of *long periods of amenorrhea interrupted by periods of prolonged bleeding*.
  2. Hirsutism and acne.

- *Diagnosis*:

  1. Serum *LH: FSH ratio >3:1*.
  2. *Elevated serum androgen and estrogen* levels, with *low or no progesterone*.
  3. Laparoscopy: Pearly white ovaries with thick smooth capsules.
  4. Ultrasound: Small ovarian sub-cortical cysts giving *Necklace appearance*.

- *Treatment*:

  1. If the patient desires pregnancy: Induce ovulation by *Clomiphene citrate*.
  2. If the patient does not desire pregnancy: two things you can do:

     - Progesterone supplementation.
     - For hirsutism: Estrogen plus Anti-androgen, e.g., Cyproterone acetate.

  3. Resistant cases: Bilateral wedge resection of ovaries.

Induction of Ovulation

- *Mechanism*: Anti-estrogens, e.g., Clomiphene citrate, Cyclofenil and Tamoxifen, block the negative feedback of estrogen on the pituitary gland. This in turn leads to increase in FSH; stimulating follicular development and ovulation.
- *Side effects*: Tamoxifen can cause *DVT, endometrial cancer* and *hot flashes*.

- *Signs of ovulation*: Pregnancy, *increased body basal temperature*, or an elevation of serum progesterone level.

Dysfunctional Uterine Bleeding (DUB)

- *Introduction*: Any uterine bleeding not related to menstruation.
- *Types*:

  1. *Cyclic*:

     - *Functional*: Short cycles due to short follicular phase. Treatment: Progestins.
     - *Corpus luteum insufficiency*: Premature endometrial shedding causing *premenstrual spotting*. Treatment: Progestins.

  2. *Acyclic*: *Threshold bleeding*: Occurs at extremes of reproductive life due to fluctuations in estrogen levels. Treatment: Estrogen in the first 10 days of the cycle, followed by a combination of estrogen and progesterone in the following 10 days.

- *Diagnosis key for vaginal and uterine bleeding*:

  1. First step: *Pregnancy test. Consider pregnancy and its complications in any female in reproductive age with vaginal bleeding.*
  2. Newborns: Mostly due to *hormonal withdrawal* bleeding. This phenomenon is known as *neonatal crisis*.
  3. Pre-pubertal age: Mostly due to *foreign body*.
  4. Peri-pubertal age: *DUB*.
  5. Childbearing age: Mostly due to *complication of pregnancy*, or a side effect of contraception.
  6. Peri-menopausal:

     - Most common cause: DUB.
     - Most important cause: *Endometrial carcinoma*.

  7. Post-menopausal:

     - Most common cause: Complication of HRT.
     - Most important cause: *Endometrial carcinoma. Any post-menopausal woman with uterine bleeding must get uterine biopsy to rule out endometrial cancer.*

- *Treatment*:

  1. Treat the cause.
  2. If no gross, malignant or pre-malignant lesions: Mostly DUB. Treatment: *Progestins*.

3. Resistant severe cases: Hysterectomy, or hysteroscopic endometrial ablation/resection.

Infertility

- *Introduction*: There are two types of infertility:

  1. Primary: Inability to conceive after 1 year of unprotected sexual intercourse.
  2. Secondary: Inability to conceive for 2 years after a normal fertile life.

- *Causes*:

  1. *Male causes*:

     - Defective spermatogenesis (Normally takes 75 days).
     - Testicular failure: Either primary (*Low testosterone and high FSH*), or secondary (*Low testosterone and low FSH*).

  2. *Female causes*: Ovarian, tubal, uterine or pelvic. Endometriosis causes pelvic adhesions and anovulation *by changing prostaglandin levels.*
  3. *Coital factors*: Dyspareunia, frequent or inadequate sexual intercourse.
  4. *Immunological factors*:

     - Male: Male body forms auto-antibodies against its own sperms. Diagnosis: Agglutination test. Treatment: Steroids.
     - Female: Cervical or serum antibodies against sperms or ova. Diagnosis: Agglutination test and sperm immobilization test. Treatment: Steroids.

- *Diagnosis*:

  1. *Semen analysis*:

     - *Normal semen*:

       1. Character: Viscid and liquefies within 0.5 h.
       2. Volume: 2–4 mL.
       3. Color and Odor: Whitish and odorless.
       4. pH: Alkaline; due to phosphate buffer released by prostate.
       5. Sperm count: 20–200 millions/mL.
       6. Motility: At least 60% of sperms are motile.
       7. Morphology: At least 60% of sperms are normal in shape.

     - *Sources of seminal fluid*:

       1. 60% from seminal vesicles: Releases *fructose* for sperms nutrition.

       2. 20% from prostate: Releases *phosphate buffer* to protect sperms from vaginal acidity.
       3. 10% from Testes.
       4. 10% from other glands.

     - Azoospermia: Absence of sperms. *First thing to do is testicular biopsy*. FSH and LH should also be checked to rule out testicular failure.

  2. *Tests for ovulation and Corpus luteum function*:

     - Ovulation is suggested clinically by regularity of cycles, presence of premenstrual tension syndrome (PMS), ovulation pain, and menstruation.
     - *Tests*:

       1. Rise in body basal temperature.
       2. Vaginal and cervical smears: Scanty secretion, with *negative spinnbarkeit and fern tests.*
       3. Pre-menstrual endometrial biopsy (PEB): Secretory endometrium. *In corpus luteum insufficiency; it shows 3 days lag behind menstrual dates.*
       4. Mid-Luteal serum progesterone level (*Day 21*):

          - 12 ng/mL: Normal ovulation.
          - 3–12 ng/mL: Corpus luteum insufficiency.
          - <3 ng/mL: Anovulation.

  3. *Tests for cervical and vaginal factors*: *Post-Coital test*: Performed 6 h after intercourse, by obtaining a sample of vaginal and cervical mucus:

     - No sperms: Azoospermia.
     - Dead sperms in vaginal drop and no sperms in cervical drop: Vaginal hostility, mostly due to increased acidity or infection.
     - Motile sperms in vaginal drop and dead sperms in cervical drop: Cervical hostility, mostly due to infection.

  4. *Other tests*: Hysterosalpingography (HSG) or hysteroscopy to detect uterine deformities and adhesions. Tubal insufflation to test tube patency (Done 5–7 days post-menstruation).

- *Notes*:

  1. The most common cause of infertility in general: *Male factors.*
  2. The most common cause of infertility in females: *Endometriosis.*

- *Treatment*:

  1. Anovulation: Ovulation induction.
  2. Tubal occlusion: Repeated insufflations, or cutting adhesions.

3. Poor cervical mucus: Estrogen.
4. Immunological: Sexual abstinence for 6 months plus corticosteroids.
5. In Vitro Fertilization (IVF): Ovulation is induced by giving HCG, and intracytoplasmic sperm injection (ICSI) is done.

Contraception

- **Rhythm method**: Intercourse is avoided between *days 10 and 18* of a 28 day cycle.
- **Prolonged lactation**: In a lactating woman, prolactin inhibits release of estrogen and decreases its effects on the uterus preventing conception.
- **Coitus interruptus**: Withdrawal of the penis before ejaculation inside the vagina.
- **Spermicides**: e.g., Non-oxynol 9.

  1. *Advantages*: No medical side effects or contra-indications to this method. Associated with a decreased risk of PID.
  2. *Disadvantages*: Intercourse must occur *within 2 h* of application.

- **Condoms**:

  1. *Advantages*: No medical side effects or contra-indications, decreases risk of STDs, and it *could be used in cases of premature ejaculation*.
  2. *Disadvantages*: High failure rates and may decrease sensation. Latex allergy could be a problem for some patients.

- **Diaphragm/Cervical cap**:

  1. *Advantages*: No medical side effects or contraindications.
  2. *Disadvantages*: Does not decrease risk of STDs. Long term use *may lead to toxic shock syndrome (TSS)*. Mechanism of TSS: Release of the *exotoxin TSST-1*, which stimulates the production of interleukin-1, TNF and *endotoxins*. Prevention: Patients *should not leave the sponge/diaphragm/cervical cap in the vagina for more than 24 h*, or *during menses*. Clinical picture:

     - *Shock*
     - *Rash: Scarlatiniform and diffuse in distribution.*
     - *Diarrhea and electrolyte imbalance.*
     - *Fever and elevated liver enzymes.*

- **Vaginal sponge**: A sponge containing *non-oxynol 9*:

  1. *Advantages*: Easy to use.
  2. *Disadvantages*: *Toxic shock syndrome (TSS).*

- **Intrauterine Device (IUD)**:

  1. *Types*: Inert or coated with copper or progestins.

2. *Mechanism of action*:

   - Aseptic endometritis, leading to phagocytosis of sperms and ova.
   - Histological changes in endometrium; preventing implantation.
   - Copper: Inhibits carbonic anhydrase enzyme (Necessary for implantation).
   - Progesterone: Causes atrophy of endometrium, and *thick cervical mucus.*

3. *Advantages*: Reliable, and may be used for long periods.
4. *Disadvantages*:

   - Spotting: Especially post-insertional.
   - Post-insertion pain and backache: Due to cervical irritation by the threads.
   - Vaginal discharge, infection, expulsion or perforation.
   - Pregnancy: If threads are accessible, remove the IUD. If not, observe for complications. *Septic abortion occurs in 50% of cases.*
   - Ectopic pregnancy: Especially with *progestin coated IUD, because it decreases tubal motility.*

5. *Contraindications*: Uterine malformation or malignancy.

- **Combined oral contraceptive pills (OCPs)**:

  1. *Composition*: Estrogen and progesterone, which suppress FSH and LH. Pills taken in the latter part of the cycle contain more progesterone.
  2. *Mechanism*: They cause endometrial atrophy, and thick cervical mucus.
  3. *Use*: Taken *from 5th day of cycle for 21 days*, then placebo for 7 days.
  4. *Side effects*: Multiple; the most common are:

     - Nausea and vomiting.
     - Salt and water retention: Cyclic weight gain, and hypertension.
     - Acne and hirsutism.
     - Thromboembolic conditions.
     - Cholestasis and rise of liver enzymes.

  5. *Contraindications*: Patients older than 35, smoking, Diabetes mellitus and hypertension.
  6. *Troubleshooting*:

     - Spotting in early part of cycle: Increase estrogen dose.
     - Spotting in late part of cycle: Increase progesterone dose.
     - Breakthrough bleeding (Common in forgetful patients): Stop pills for 5 days then restart, while using backup contraception.

- Missed period: Stop pills and do a pregnancy test in 2 weeks, while using backup contraception.
- Most common cause of OCPs failure: *Incorrect use.*

- **Progesterone only pills**:

  1. *Indication*: Age >45 years, DM, hypertension and lactation.
  2. *Advantages*: Minimal side effects, and no estrogen side effects.
  3. *Disadvantages*: Irregular cycles and spotting.

- **Injectable contraception**:

  1. *Example*: Depot medroxyprogesterone acetate (Depo-provera).
  2. *Indications*: *Forgetful patients*, or the ones with contraindication to estrogen.
  3. *Advantages*: *Improves symptoms of endometriosi.s*
  4. *Disadvantages*: Not immediately reversible, and may cause irregular cycles.

- **Subcutaneous Implants (Norplant)**:

  1. *Six cylinders of levonorgestrel*, implanted in the medial aspect of the arm.
  2. *Advantages*: Slow release of progestin for up to *5 years*, and it can be removed if pregnancy is desired.

- **Postcoital contraception**:

  1. Effective only if done within the *first 72 h after unprotected intercourse.*
  2. *Composition*: *High doses of estrogen,* especially ethinyl estradiol.
  3. *Abortifacients*: e.g., Anti-progesterone known as Mifepristone RU 486.

- **Sterilization**: Tubal ligation and vasectomy are the most common. Indicated for couples wishing *permanent* contraception. Complications include *post-tubal ligation syndrome*; where patients present with *congestive dysmenorrhea* and *menorrhagia*. This syndrome occurs due to interruption of the venous return of fallopian tubes, and is treated with hysterectomy.

TABLE 4.2 Pearl index.

Method of contraception	Pearl index
Combination pills	3
Progestin only pills	3
IUD	3
Norplant	0.2
Sterilization	0.4
Depo-Provera	0.3
Physiological methods	20
Condoms	12
Cervical cap and sponge	18–28

- **Pearl index**: A measure of contraceptive failure rates, presented as the number of pregnancies in *100 women* using a method of contraception *for 1 year*. Refer to Table 4.2 for Pearl index.

Dysmenorrhea

- **Introduction**: Pain related to the menstrual cycle.
- **Types**:

  1. *Spasmodic*:

     - Clinical picture: Colicky pain in the lower abdomen and radiating to the inner thighs and low back. Begins *with the onset of menstruation* and *decreases afterwards,* and is associated with nausea, vomiting and sweating.
     - More common among virgins and nulliparous women.
     - Mechanism: *High levels of prostaglandins ($PGF_{2\alpha}$)* which leads to uterine contraction, or due to failure of the uterus to expel sloughed menstrual tissue secondary to obstruction.
     - Treatment: NSAIDS (PG inhibitor), or OCPs (Inhibit ovulation).

  2. Membranous:

     - Mechanism: *Endometrial hypersensitivity to progesterone.*
     - Clinical picture: Severe lower abdominal and back pain. The pain decreases after passage of *membranous endometrial casts* through the vagina, after which menstruation ensues.
     - Treatment: Progesterone dominant pill to suppress ovulation plus NSAIDs.

  3. Congestive:

     - Clinical picture: Continuous dull achy pain in the lower abdomen and back due to congestion. Begins *3–5 days before menstruation* and subsides with flow.
     - Treatment: Treat the cause of pelvic congestion plus NSAIDs.

  4. *Ovarian*:

     - Clinical picture: Dull aching pain in one or both iliac fossa due to ovarian congestion. Begins a *few days before menstruation* and subsides with flow.
     - Treatment: NSAIDs and glycerine suppositories for congestion.

- **Premenstrual Menstrual Syndrome (PMS)**: Headache, mastalgia, bloating, constipation, joint pains, depression, irritability and nervousness. Etiology is unknown but theories suggest a change in endorphin levels, allergy to ovarian hormones, or vitamin B1 and B6 deficiency. Treatment: NSAIDs (*Ibuprofen*).
- **Mittelschmerz pain**: Mid-cycle pain in *one iliac fossa*, due to *ovulation*.

Endometriosis

- **Introduction**: Presence of *endometrial tissue outside the uterus*.
- **Locations**:

  1. Ovaries: Most common site. Forms *chocolate cysts*.
  2. Myometrium: Either diffuse (*Adenomyosis*), or localized (*Adenomyoma*).
  3. Extra-uterine: Could be anywhere in or outside the pelvis. Nodules could be in a closed organ (*Endometrioma*).

- **Pathology**: Implants are either black active or grey fibrosed lesions.
- **Clinical picture**:

  1. Infertility: *Endometriosis is the most common cause of female infertility*.
  2. *Perimenstrual* lower abdominal and back pain: Due to *spasmodic dysmenorrhea*.
  3. *Dyspareunia* and *menometrorrhagia*.
  4. *Endometriomas* are asymptomatic in most patients.

- **Diagnosis**: U/S of the pelvis is suggestive, but diagnosis is confirmed only by visualizing the *powder burn* implants and *chocolate cysts* during *laparoscopy*.
- **Treatment**:

  1. Create a *pseudo-pregnancy* state using progesterone.
  2. Create a *pseudo-menopause* state using combined anti-estrogen and anti-progesterone, e.g., Gestrinone.
  3. High dose *GnRH* analog: To down-regulate gonadotrophin receptors.
  4. *Androgens,* e.g., Danazol: Acts as an anti-gonadotrophin.
  5. *Surgery*: Reserved for resistant complicated cases.

- **Treatment key**: According to degree of symptoms:

  1. Mild (*Implants without fibrosis*): Hormonal or surgery.
  2. Moderate (*Implants and nodules with fibrosis in the absence of tubal obstruction or ovarian encapsulation*): Hormonal or surgery.

3. Severe (*Implants and nodules with fibrosis plus tubal obstruction or ovarian encapsulation*): Surgery.
4. Extreme (Severe fibrosis leading to *frozen pelvis*): Hormonal. *Surgery is contraindicated.*

Genital Prolapse

- **Introduction**: It is the downward displacement of one or more genital organs.
- **Predisposing factors**:

  1. Weakness of the pelvic floor muscles, e.g., After obstetric trauma.
  2. Increased intra-abdominal pressure, e.g., Chronic cough or constipation.

- **Types**:

  1. *Vaginal*:

     - Anterior wall: Bladder (Cystocele), or urethra (Urethrocele).
     - Posterior wall: Intestine (Enterocele), or rectum (Rectocele).

  2. *Uterine*:

     - 1st degree: Cervix is below level of ischial spines but not past the introitus. *Note that the cervix is normally located at the level of the ischial spines.*
     - 2nd degree: Cervix is protruding outside the introitus, but the uterine body is inside the vagina.
     - 3rd degree (*Procidentia*): The entire uterus lies outside the introitus.

- **Clinical picture**:

  1. *Sense of heaviness with a dragging sensation in the perineum.*
  2. *Backache*: Due to stretching of the uterosacral ligaments.
  3. *Stress incontinence* and incomplete voiding or defecation.
  4. Congestive dysmenorrhea and menorrhagia.
  5. Genital ulcers, infections and vaginal discharge.

- **On exam**: Assess the tone of the levator ani muscle with the patient in the dorsal lithotomy position. If able to approximate fingers behind the prolapsed mass, it is a 3rd degree prolapse.
- **Treatment**:

  1. Treat the underlying cause.
  2. Pelvic floor exercises, and vaginal pessary to support the prolapse.
  3. Surgery: Reserved for complicated cases.

- *Note*: Do not confuse genital prolapse with uterine inversion. In uterine inversion, the fundus is inverted inside the uterine cavity with *the cervix remaining in its normal position*. Treatment of uterine inversion: *Operation of Taxis*; where the cervical ring is cut, uterus is repositioned, then the cervix is repaired.

Retroverted Flexed Uterus (RVF)

- *Introduction*: Normally, the uterus is in *90° of ante-version* and *160° of flexion*.
- *Causes*:

  1. Congenital: *This is the most common cause of RVF uterus.*
  2. Adhesions in Douglas pouch *pulling* the uterus backwards.
  3. Ovarian cyst *pushing* the uterus backwards.

- *Degrees*:

  1. 1st degree: Fundus points to sacral promontory, while the cervix faces downwards and forwards.
  2. 2nd degree: Fundus points toward the body of sacrum, while the cervix faces directly forwards.
  3. 3rd degree: Fundus points toward the tip of coccyx, while the cervix faces upwards and forwards.

- *Clinical picture*: Most cases are *asymptomatic.* Common symptoms include deep dyspareunia, low backache, congestive dysmenorrhea and menorrhagia.
- *Treatment*:

  1. Plication of the *round* or *uterosacral* ligaments.
  2. *Modified Gilliam operation*: Round ligaments are pulled anteriorly from the inguinal ligament and tied to each other in front of the rectus sheath.

Recto-Vaginal Fistula

- *Introduction*: Abnormal communication between rectum and vagina.
- *Cause*: Most common cause is *surgical or obstetric trauma*, e.g., Episiotomy.
- *Clinical picture*: Stool incontinence and vulvovaginitis.
- *On exam*: Wide perineum, bulging rectal mucosa and dimpling on either side of the anus caused by the *torn ends of the anal sphincter*.
- *Treatment*:

  1. Rectal washouts and low residue diet before and after surgery.
  2. Low fistula: *Lawson-Tait operation*.

  3. Middle fistula: *Flap splitting*.
  4. High fistula: *Colostomy, repair the fistula then close colostomy after 2 months*.

Vesico-Vaginal Fistula

- *Introduction*: An abnormal communication between bladder and vagina.
- *Cause*: Most common cause is *surgical or obstetric trauma*, e.g., Hysterectomy.
- *Clinical picture*: Urinary incontinence, and recurrent UTIs.
- *On exam*: Use a *Sims speculum* with the patient lying on her side to visualize the fistula.
- *Diagnosis*:

  1. Urine analysis: *Tthe first step in any patient with urinary incontinence*.
  2. *Methylene blue test*: Insert three pieces of cotton inside the vagina, and fill the bladder with methylene blue:

     - If the cotton pieces remain dry: No fistula.
     - If the cotton pieces are wet and stained blue: Vesico-vaginal fistula.
     - If the cotton pieces are wet and not stained: Uretero-vaginal fistula.

- *Treatment*:

  1. Treat genital and urinary infections.
  2. Small fistulas are treated with *saucerization*. Post-operative urethral catheter and antibiotics are necessary.

Stress Incontinence

- *Introduction*: Escape of a *small amount of urine* that occurs *concomitantly* with any rise in intra-abdominal pressure, e.g., Laughing, coughing.
- *Mechanism*: *Hypermobile bladder neck*.
- *Diagnosis*: *Cystometrogram*: Detects a rise in bladder pressure and activity at the same time as increased intra-abdominal pressure.
- *Treatment*: Bladder training and pelvic floor exercises.
- *Notes*:

  1. In stress incontinence: *Flow rate, residual volume and bladder compliance are all within normal limits*.
  2. In cases of detrusor instability, there is escape of *larger amounts of urine*, occurring *shortly after* a rise in intra-abdominal pressure (Not concomitantly). Treatment: Anti-muscarinics, and tricyclic anti-depressants (TCAs).

3. Anatomical hints:

- Urinary internal sphincter is formed from *3 parts*: Trigonal ring, Posterior loop and Loop of Heiss.
- Urinary external sphincter is formed of *3 muscles*: Sphincter urethrae, Compressor urethrae, and Urethrovaginal muscle.
- The urethra is suspended by the pubourethral ligament; extending from the pubic symphysis to the middle third of the urethra.
- Bladder innervations: Sympathetic (Hypogastric nerve (T10–L2)), parasympathetic (Pelvic nerve (S2, S3, S4)), and somatic (Pudendal nerve).

Genital Infections

- **Introduction**:

1. As a rule, know that the normal vaginal pH is *3.5–4.5*, which is achieved by vaginal flora, namely the *lactobacilli*.
2. All the following infections cause vulvovaginitis, i.e., Painful, red and itchy female genitalia.

Chlamydia

- **Introduction**: *The most common sexually transmitted disease (STD)*.
- **Organism**: *Chlamydia trachomatis*; an *obligate intracellular*.
- **Clinical picture**:

1. *Chlamydia A, B and C*: *Trachoma* and conjunctivitis.
2. *Chlamydia L1, L2 and L3*: *Lymphogranuloma venereum*: Patient presents with *lymphangitis, inguinal lymphadenopathy and proctocolitis*.
3. *Chlamydia D and K*: Urethritis, cervicitis, PID and/or perihepatitis (*Fitz-Hugh-Curtis syndrome*). *Some cases are asymptomatic.*

- **Chlamydia life cycle**:

1. Elementary body – the infective stage – attaches to epithelial cells and is endocytosed. It converts inside the cell to the reticulate body.
2. Reticulate body replicates via binary fission, then reorganizes into elementary bodies.
3. Exocytosis of the elementary bodies which may then re-infect other cells.

- **Diagnosis**:

1. Cytology shows *intracytoplasmic inclusion bodies*, a phenomenon that also occurs in viral infections.
2. *Culture*: For confirmation, and it takes *48–72 h*

- **Treatment**:

1. *Drug of choice: Azithromycin.* Doxycycline is an alternative treatment.
2. Treat all sexual partners.
3. Should also empirically treat *N. gonorrhea*.

Gonorrhea

- **Introduction**: *Second most common STD*.
- **Organism**: Neisseria gonorrhea; *intracellular Gram negative diplococci*.
- **Incubation period**: *7* days in males, and *14* days in females.
- **Clinical picture**: Malodorous *greenish mucopustular* urethral or vaginal discharge. Some cases are asymptomatic.
- **Diagnosis**:

1. *Microscopy*: Intracellular *Gram negative kidney-shaped diplococci*.
2. *Culture*: For confirmation. Media used are Chocolate or Thayer-Martin agars. Culture reveals Gram negative diplococci, with *oxidase positive reaction*.

- **Treatment**:

1. *Drug of choice: 3rd generation cephalosporin. Ciprofloxacin is an alternative treatment.*
2. Treat all sexual partners.
3. Should also empirically treat Chlamydia.

- **Complications**:

1. *Fitz-Hugh-Curtis syndrome*: Peri-hepatitis, caused by gonorrhea or Chlamydia. *Clinical picture*: RUQ abdominal pain, mainly with exertion. *Diagnosis*: Elevated transaminases, and visualization of peri-hepatic adhesions on ultrasound or laparoscopy. *Treatment*: Treat the cause.
2. *Disseminated Gonococcemia*: Occurs when the organisms invade the vascular system. *Clinical picture*: *3(itis)*: Migrating (Fleeting) arthritis, tenosynovitis, and pustular dermatitis. *Note: Blood cultures in these cases are negative*.

Bacterial Vaginosis (BV)

- **Organism**: Symbiotic infection of anaerobic bacteria, e.g., *Gardnerella, Bacteroides, Peptococcus*.

- **Clinical picture**: Thin white/gray vaginal discharge with *fishy odor*.
- **Diagnosis**:

  1. *Whiff test*: Add potassium hydroxide (*KOH*) to discharge, which intensifies the *fishy odor*.
  2. *Clue cells* on wet prep: Clue cells are vaginal epithelial cells coated with coccoid bacteria on their surface.
  3. Vaginal pH >4.5.

- **Treatment**: *Oral metronidazole*.

Pelvic Inflammatory Disease (PID)

- **Introduction**: Ascending genital infection which may include endometritis, salpingitis, hydrosalpinx, and/or tubo-ovarian abscesses.
- **Organism**: Most commonly caused by *Chlamydia trachomatis* D and K and/or *Neisseria gonorrhea*. Any organism mentioned in this chapter may cause PID.
- **Clinical picture**:

  1. Lower abdominal and *bilateral groin pain*.
  2. Purulent vaginal discharge.
  3. Systemic symptoms: Fever, nausea and vomiting.

- **On exam**:

  1. Lower abdominal and *bilateral inguinal tenderness*.
  2. Pelvic exam: *Cervical motion tenderness (Chandelier sign)*.

- **Treatment**: Ceftriaxone or cefoxitin *plus* doxycycline for *2–3 weeks*.
- **Indications for hospitalization**: Pregnancy, pelvic abscess or failure of outpatient therapy.
- **Note**: *Barrier contraception* and *OCPs* decrease the risk of acquiring PID.

Haemophilus Ducreyi

- **Clinical picture**: *Chancroid*; a *painful* genital ulcer with an irregular shape, associated with *painful* lymphadenopathy.
- **Diagnosis**: *Gram negative bacilli* arranged in a *school of fish* pattern.
- **Treatment**: *Ceftriaxone*
- **Note**: *Chancre* and lymphadenopathy in syphilis are *painless*.

Candida Albicans

- **Introduction**: The most common *genital infection*. Note that Chlamydia is the *most common STD*.

- **Clinical picture**: Vulvovaginitis with *white curd-like* vaginal discharge.
- **Diagnosis**: *Pseudo-Hyphae* on microscopic exam.
- **Treatment**: *Local statin cream* and/or *single oral dose of fluconazole*.

Trichomonas Vaginalis

- **Introduction**: *A flagellated organism* causing a post-menstrual infection.
- **Clinical picture**: Vulvovaginitis with *frothy vaginal discharge*.
- **On exam**: Punctate hemorrhages on vagina and cervix (*Strawberry cervix*).
- **Diagnosis**: Microscopy reveals *motile flagellated trichomonads*.
- **Treatment**: Oral *metronidazole*.

Herpes Simplex Virus (HSV)

- **Types**:

  1. Type I: Ophthalmic and oral lesions.
  2. Type II: Genital lesions.

- **Clinical picture**: *Small painful vesicles*, shallow grey ulcers, and tender lymphadenopathy.
- **Diagnosis**: *Tzank smear* shows *multinucleated giant cells, and intranuclear inclusion bodies*.
- **Treatment**: Oral *acyclovir*.
- **Notes**:

  1. Acyclovir is not helpful beyond *24 h* from the start of the rash.
  2. Acyclovir *does not cure the disease*; it only shortens duration of the rash and decreases the risk of complications, e.g., Post-herpetic neuralgia.
  3. If a pregnant patient is having genital Herpes at time of labor, *deliver by C-section* because contact with the lesions in the birth canal may cause neonatal herpes *encephalomyelitis*.

Human Papillomavirus (HPV)

- **Clinical picture**: Lesion starts as a flat wart which later on progress into a verrucous cauliflower-like lesion (*Condyloma accuminatum*).
- **On exam**: *Cobblestoning of the vaginal mucosa*.
- **Diagnosis**: Vacuolated cells with perinuclear halos known as *koilocytes*.
- **Prevention**: Quadrivalent human papillomavirus (Types 6, 11, 16, 18) recombinant vaccine (GARDASIL). Currently approved for females between *9 and 26* years of age.
- **Treatment**: *Cauterization* of the lesions.

Molluscum Contagiosum

- *Organism*: *Pox virus.*
- *Clinical picture*: *Umbilicated pearly white papules.*
- *Diagnosis*: Confirmed by identifying the *inclusion molluscum bodies* upon staining the contents of the lesions with *Wright* or *Geimsa* stains.
- *Treatment*: *Regress spontaneously.* Cauterization is reserved for non-resolving lesions.

Leiomyoma (Fibroids)

- *Introduction*:

  1. A *benign* tumor arising from the uterine *myometrium.*
  2. An *estrogen-dependent* tumor, so more common *in child bearing age* and *rare before puberty or after menopause.*
  3. Fibroids may *grow quickly during pregnancy* and in patients on OCPs, due to *high estrogen levels.*

- *Race*: Fibroids are more common in *African Americans.*
- *Pathology*:

  1. Tumor consists mainly of *smooth muscles* and *fibroblasts.*
  2. Fibroids vary in size, shape and number; however they share the fact that they compress the surrounding myometrium, creating a *false capsule* around them. Luckily, this makes fibroids *easy to be enucleated.*
  3. A fibroid is a firm tumor, however, it gets softer under the following: *Pregnancy*, *degeneration* or if it has undergone a s*arcomatous change.*

- *Types*:

  1. *Corporal fibroids*, i.e., in the uterine corpus: Most common type. Corporal fibroids are mostly interstitial; however they could grow towards the uterine cavity (*Submucous fibroid)*, or towards the abdominal cavity (*Subserous fibroid)*. A subserous fibroid may gain attachment to any abdominal organ and gain blood supply from it, hence the name *parasitic fibroid.*
  2. *Cervical fibroids*: They are *fast-growing* and cause *pressure symptoms.*

- *Clinical picture*:

  1. *The most common presentation is being asymptomatic.*
  2. *Prolonged painful heavy periods are one of the hallmarks of fibroids.* So when you see an African-American female of child-bearing age in the USMLE with very painful heavy periods that last for days, you know what to think!
  3. Pressure symptoms, mainly in cervical fibroids: Urinary frequency, dysuria, dyschezia and dyspareunia.
  4. Subserous fibroids are usually discovered accidentally.

- *Diagnosis*: Ultrasound of the uterus/pelvis.
- *Complications*:

  1. Degeneration:

     - Most dangerous is *red degeneration*; a hemorrhagic necrosis secondary to acute infarction. *Clinical picture*: S*evere abdominal pain*, *fever* and *vomiting. Treatment*: Rest, analgesics and antipyretics.
     - A uterus containing fibroids receives a huge blood supply due to *release of angiogenic factors*; however, the fibroid itself is usually pale and susceptible to degeneration as follows:

       1. *Central part*: *Hyaline* and *cystic* degeneration.
       2. *Peripheral parts*: *Fatty* degeneration and *calcification.*

  2. Sarcomatous change: The incidence is low, approximately *0.5%*; however, the co-incidence of endometrial cancer is around *2%* (*Both are estrogen-dependent tumors*). Sarcomatous change is confirmed microscopically by presence of *more than 10 mitotic figures* per high power field (Normal *<5*).
  3. Torsion and inflammation: Severe abdominal pain, nausea and vomiting.

- *Treatment*:

  1. Supportive: Indicated in mild cases, pregnant or near-menopause patients.
  2. Surgical: Indicated only in severe cases:

     - *Polypectomy and D&C*: For submucous fibroids.
     - *Myomectomy*: A very bloody operation even after ligating the uterine vessels (*At the base of the round ligament*) and ovarian vessels (*In the infundibulpelvic ligament*).
     - *Hysterectomy*: Most common and successful surgery for leiomyoma removal.

Cervical Intraepithelial Neoplasia (CIN)

- *Introduction*: CIN is a *pre-malignant* condition, in which cervical epithelium is replaced by cells having malignant characteristics *without invasion of the basement membrane.*

- **Location**: It starts at the *squamo-columnar junction* of cervix, which is also known as the *transformation zone*.
- **Clinical picture**: Mostly *asymptomatic*.
- **Stages**: Determined by tissue biopsy (*not the Pap smear*):

  1. *CIN I*: Only the deepest *1/3* of the epithelium is involved. Probability of malignant transformation is *15%*.
  2. *CIN II*: The deepest *2/3* of the epithelium is involved. Probability of malignant transformation is *70%*.
  3. *CIN III*: Involves the whole thickness of the epithelium.

- **Diagnosis**: Refer to Fig. 4.8. Microscopic criteria of malignant cells:

  1. Increased nuclear/cytoplasmic ratio.
  2. Pleomorphism.
  3. High number of mitotic figures.
  4. Loss of polarity.
  5. Increased nuclear size and nucleoli.

- **Treatment**:

  1. *CIN I*: Follow up by cytology and colposcopy every *6 months*.
  2. *CIN II and III*: Local destructive surgery, e.g., cautery or laser, however, the lesion must be well-demarcated and the endocervix must be free of disease. If the above conditions are not met, then hysterectomy is indicated.

Cervical Cancer

- **Introduction**: Mostly *ectocervical,* and is *squamous* cell in origin.
- **Predisposing factors**: HPV infection; strains 16, 18, 33, 45 and 56, early sexual intercourse, multiple sexual partners and *multiparity*.

- **Clinical picture**:

  1. The key symptom is *contact bleeding,* e.g., Cervical bleeding after intercourse.
  2. Pain, discharge and metastatic symptoms.

- **Metastases**:

  1. Direct: Surrounding structures.
  2. Blood: Lung, Liver, Bone, Brain, Kidney and Supra-renal glands.
  3. Lymphatic: Paracervical, iliac, and para-aortic L.N.

- **Diagnosis**:

  1. If lesion is grossly visible: Excisional biopsy.
  2. If no visible lesion: Cytology (Pap smear), followed by colposcopy and biopsy.

- **Prevention**:

  1. *Annual pap smears starting the onset of sexual intercourse till 3 successive normal smears, then perform the Pap smear every 3 years.*
  2. GARDASIL: Discussed above. Note that even in immunized patients, Pap smear recommendations should still be followed.

- **Treatment**: Surgery, radiation and chemotherapy: Depending on stage.
- **Notes**:

  1. Most common cause of death in cervical cancer patients is *uremia*.
  2. Types of hysterectomy:

     - *Simple hysterectomy*: Remove uterus.
     - *Extended hysterectomy*: Remove uterus, cervix and vaginal cuff.
     - *Radical hysterectomy*: Remove uterus, cervix, 1/2 vagina, parametrium and lymph nodes.
     - *Exentration*: Radical hysterectomy *plus* organ removal.

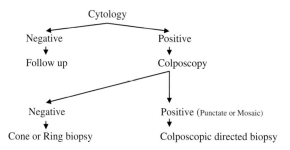

Large loop excision of transformation zone LLETZ

Loop electrosurgical excision procedure LEEP

FIG. 4.8 Pap smear algorithm

3. Most common complication of radical hysterectomy: *Denervation of the urinary bladder, leading to residual urine.*
4. Radiotherapy can flare up pelvic infections and adhesions, causing artificial menopause.

Endometrial Cancer

- *Introduction*: *The most common malignancy of the female genital tract.*
- *Predisposing factors*: Old age, *post-menopausal, low parity, obesity, DM and hypertension.*
- *Pathology*: Mainly an *adenocarcinoma.*
- *Clinical picture*: Key symptom is *post-menopausal bleeding*: So when you see a post-menopausal patient in the USMLE with uterine bleeding, she mostly has endometrial cancer till proven otherwise.
- *Metastases*:

  1. Direct: To surroundings; the *most common metastases of endometrial cancer.*
  2. Blood: Lung, Liver, Bone, Brain, Kidneys and Supra-renal glands.
  3. Lymphatic: *Para-aortic L.N.*

- *Diagnosis*: *Endometrial biopsy* or *fractional curettage*: The best next step in any post-menopausal patient with uterine bleeding. Examine the specimen for the presence of hormonal receptors. If present, post-operative hormonal treatment should be included.
- *Treatment*: Surgery, radiation, chemotherapy and hormonal therapy.
- *Note*: Most common cause of death in endometrial cancer patients is *metastases.*

Ovarian Tumors

Functional Cysts

- *Introduction*: Most common cysts during reproductive age; they are benign.
- *Hallmark*: They never exceed *6 cm* in diameter.
- *Mechanism*:

  1. They occur due to gonadotrophin stimulation.
  2. High *FSH* leads to a *Follicular cyst.*
  3. High *LH* leads to a *Corpus Luteum cyst.* Clinical picture: RLQ or LLQ abdominal pain and *delayed menses.*

- *Treatment*: Observe, as they usually regress spontaneously.

Epithelial Tumors

- *Introduction*: All types have benign and malignant subtypes.
- *Serous tumors*:

  1. *Most common epithelial tumor.*
  2. Formed of low columnar epithelium.
  3. Microscopy: *Psammoma* bodies.
  4. Note: *Psammoma bodies could be seen in (PMS): Papillary carcinoma of thyroid, Meningioma, Serous ovarian cyst.*

- *Mucinous tumors*: Formed of tall columnar epithelium. Could rupture into peritoneum causes *pseudomyxoma peritonei.*
- *Mesonephroid tumors*: Formed of the pathognomonic *Hobnail cells*; cubical cells with clear cytoplasm and hyperchromatic nuclei, over which exists a collapsed cytoplasmic membrane.
- *Brenner tumor*: Transitional epithelium with the nuclei having a characteristic longitudinal groove *(Coffee bean nucleus).*

Sex Cord-Stromal Tumors

- *Granulosa- theca cell tumors*:

  1. Granulosa cell: Polygonal with *coffee bean* nucleus.
  2. Theca cell: *Spindle-shaped and filled with lipid.*
  3. Clinical picture: They are *feminizing* tumors:

     - Pre-pubertal: Precocious puberty.
     - Childbearing age: Amenorrhea and irregular bleeding.
     - Post-menopausal: Bleeding.

- *Sertoli- Leydig cell tumors*:

  1. Sertoli cell: Columnar cell with *cleft nucleus.*
  2. Leydig cell: Polygonal cell with *Crystalloids of Reinke* in cytoplasm.
  3. Clinical picture: These are *virilizing* tumors: Hirsutism, clitoromegaly and deepening of voice.

Germ Cell Tumors

- *Introduction*: Occur mainly in *children and young adults.*
- *Prognosis*: They are *highly malignant* tumors, *except mature teratoma*; however, they are *very sensitive to radiotherapy and chemotherapy.* That leaves germ cell tumors with better prognosis than epithelial tumors.
- *Clinical picture*: *Rapidly growing* tumors, so they present with *abdominal pain.*

- *Dysgerminoma*: Causes *precocious puberty*. Microscopy: Round cells with heavy lymphocytic infiltration.
- *Dermoid cyst (Mature cystic teratoma)*: A thick-walled cyst containing ectodermal, endodermal and mesodermal structures plus a *Rokitansky protuberance*. *Suspect it in the exam in any question describing an ovarian tumor containing hair and teeth.*

Others

- *Krukenberg tumors*: Bilateral in *50%* of cases, they metastasize from stomach cancer and reach the ovary by retrograde lymphatic spread. Microscopy: *Signet ring cells* in fibrous or myxomatous stroma.
- *Ovarian fibroma*: Solitary or as a part of *Meigs syndrome* (Ovarian fibroma (Benign), ascites and right sided pleural effusion).

Clinical Picture

- *Most common presentation is being asymptomatic.*
- Non-specific abdominal symptoms, e.g., Dyspepsia, bloating or pain.

Diagnosis

- *Tumor markers*:

  1. CA-125: Ovarian tumors, *except mucinous cysts*.
  2. Carcinoembryonic antigen (CEA): *Mucinous cyst.*
  3. Lactate dehydrogenase (LDH): *Dysgerminoma.*
  4. Human chorionic gonadotropin (HCG) and Alpha-fetoprotein (AFP): *Germ cell tumors.*
  5. Estrogen and progesterone: *Functioning tumors.*

- *Transvaginal ultrasound*: Excellent in confirming ovarian tumors. Relies on showing tumors and cysts through their *neovascularization*.

Diagnosis Key and Notes

- Most common ovarian tumor in front of uterus: *Dermoid cyst.*
- Most common ovarian tumor behind uterus: *Endometroid cyst.*
- Most common ovarian tumor in children: *Germ cell tumors.*
- Most common ovarian tumor in reproductive age: *Functional cysts.*
- Most common ovarian tumor in menopause: *Epithelial tumors.*
- Benign ovarian swellings: *Unilateral, cystic, mobile and painless.*

- Malignant ovarian swellings: *Bilateral, solid, fixed and painful.*
- Decreased ovulation, e.g., OCPs use, *decreases* risk of ovarian cancer.
- *Peutz-Jeghers syndrome*: A triad of ovarian cancer, familial Adenomatous Polyposis (*FAP*), and circumoral /circumanal pigmentation.

Treatment

- *Surgery*: *Debulking surgeries*, including removal of as much involved tissues as possible. The most important factor determining success in advanced cases is the *residual tumor mass after surgery*.
- *Chemotherapy*:

  1. Epithelial tumors: *Platinum.*
  2. Germ cell tumors: *VBP* (*V*inblastine, *B*leomycin, Platinum) or *BEP* (*B*leomycin, *E*toposide, Platinum) are the most widely combinations.

- *Radiotherapy*: Internal or external: Most beneficial in *germ cell tumors*.
- *Follow up*: Tumor markers, and second look laparotomy.

Notes

- BRCA1 and BRCA2 mutations are associated with high risk of *ovarian and breast cancer.*
- *OCPs decrease the risk of ovarian cancer.*

Choriocarcinoma

- *Introduction*: *Malignant trophoblastic tumor*, usually following a vesicular mole; however, it can follow any form of termination of pregnancy, e.g., Delivery, abortion, ectopic pregnancy.
- *Staging*:

  1. Stage I: Confined to uterus.
  2. Stage II: Extended to pelvic contents.
  3. Stage III: Metastasized to lungs; *Cannon ball metastases.*
  4. Stage IV: Distant extra-pulmonary metastases.

- *Clinical picture*:

  1. Recent history of evacuation of a vesicular mole (or termination of pregnancy), followed by *excessive irregular vaginal bleeding and a pelvic mass.*
  2. CNS metastases could present with headache or dizziness.
  3. Pulmonary metastases present with hemoptysis.

- *Diagnosis*: *Extremely elevated levels of B-HCG.*

- *Treatment*:
  1. *Chemotherapy*: *The mainstay of therapy*. Combinations used are:
     - *Low risk*: Methotrexate + Folinic acid (leukovorin).
     - *High risk*: MAC or EMACO (*E*toposide, *M*ethotrexate, *A*ctinomycin D, *C*yclophosphamide, *O*ncovine (Vincristine).
     - *Criteria for being high risk (3F)*:
       1. Last pregnancy was more than *4* months ago.
       2. Last pregnancy was full term.
       3. B-HCG is higher than *40,000* IU/L.
  2. *Surgery and radiotherapy*: Reserved for resistant cases.
  3. *Follow up*: Serial measurement of B-HCG to detect recurrence.

Non-Neoplastic Epithelial Disorders of the Vulva

- *Squamous cell hyperplasia*: Formerly known as hyperplastic dystrophy. Vulva is thickened, with white patches. Clinical picture: Pruritis of the vulva and dyspareunia. Diagnosis: Biopsy. Treatment: Corticosteroid cream.
- *Lichen sclerosis*: Vulva is atrophic, dry, shrunken and pale white in color.
- *Note*: In a case of vulval *itching* with *white lesions*, consider Lichen simplex chronicus, which is thickening of the vulva due to chronic itching and scratching.

Paget's Disease of the Vulva

- *Introduction*: *Intra-epithelial* neoplasm, which can be associated with an underlying *adenocarcinoma*.
- *Clinical picture*: Intense vulval pruritis and tenderness.
- *On exam*: Vulva is *velvety red*, thickened and covered with white patches.
- *Diagnosis*: Biopsy.
- *Treatment*: *Wide local excision* with close follow up.

Carcinoma of the Vulva

- *Introduction*: A *squamous cell carcinoma*. Usually starts as Vulval Intra-epithelial Neoplasia (*VIN*), which could be detected by the tumor marker *S-100 antigen*.
- *Clinical Picture*: *Painless* vulval swelling, bleeding or discharge.
- *Diagnosis*: Biopsy.
- *Treatment*: *Radical vulvectomy and bilateral lymph node dissection*.

Chapter 5
Surgery

Gastrointestinal System

Pharyngeal (Zenker) Diverticulum

- *Mechanism*: Spasm of cricopharyngeus muscle leads to herniation of pharyngeal mucosa through *Killian's Dehiscence*; a triangle in the posterior pharyngeal wall bound by *oblique fibers of inferior pharyngeal constrictor muscles* and *transverse fibers of cricopharyngeus muscle*.
- *Clinical picture*:

  1. Dysphagia.
  2. Regurgitation of *non-digested* food; especially on lying down.
  3. Neck swelling: Soft, compressible and *gets bigger after meals*.

- *Complications*: Perforation and malignancy.
- *Diagnosis*: Barium swallow is the test of choice (*Esophagogastroduodenoscopy "EDG" might cause perforation*).
- *Treatment*:

  1. Small diverticulum: Repeated dilatation.
  2. Large diverticulum: Diverticulopexy or diverticulectomy.

Congenital Esophageal Atresia

- *Introduction*: Usually associated with *tracheo-esophageal fistula*.
- *Types*: Multiple; the most common is an esophagus with a blind upper pouch, and a *lower pouch connected to the trachea*.

- *Clinical picture*:

  1. Continuous regurgitation of saliva and food *from the first day of life*.
  2. Meconium pneumonia, chemical pneumonitis and bilious sputum: Due to regurgitation of gastric contents into the airways.

- *Diagnosis*: Test of choice is failure to pass a feeding tube from nose to stomach (*Normal = 10 cm*).
- *Treatment*: Urgent surgery involving closing the tracheo-esophageal fistula and connecting the pouches of the esophagus. If the pouches are too far apart, a jejunum or colon segment could be used for anastomosis.

Hiatus Hernia

- *Definition*: Herniation of abdominal contents into the thorax.
- *Anatomy*: Normally, the cardia of the stomach is maintained in place by the *phreno-esophageal ligament*, and it maintains its competence through the acetylcholine release and through the pressure difference between esophagus (*8–25 mmHg*) and stomach (*8 mmHg*).
- *Types*:

  1. Sliding (85%): *Sliding* of the cardia and the stomach into the *posterior* mediastinum.
  2. Para-esophageal (15%): *Herniation* of *greater curvature of stomach* to mediastinum.

- *Causes*: Congenital or acquired, e.g., Obesity, pregnancy, esophagitis.

- *Clinical picture*: Symptoms of Gastro-esophageal Reflux Disease (GERD).
- *Diagnosis*: Barium meal or Esophagogastroduodenoscopy (EGD).
- *Treatment*:

  1. Sliding hiatus hernia: Causes GERD which is treated medically by proton pump inhibitors or H2 blockers (Refer to IM). In young patients with severe disease *resistant to medical treatment, fundoplication* is recommended.
  2. Paraesophageal hiatus hernia: Gastropexy.

- *Notes*:

  1. *Bockdalek hernia*: Hiatal hernia through foramen of Bockdalek; *behind the lateral arcuate ligament*. This is caused by *patent pleuroperitoneal canal*.
  2. *Morgagnian hernia*: Hiatal hernia through foramen of Morgagni; located *between costal and sternal origins of diaphragm*.
  3. *Saint's triad* = Hiatus hernia + Diverticular disease + Chronic cholecystitis.

Post-Corrosive Esophageal Stricture

- *Causes*: Drain liquid, oven cleaner.
- *Clinical picture and complications*:

  1. Severe pain and neurogenic shock.
  2. Edema of airways and esophagus followed by dysphagia and risk of perforation.

- *Treatment*:

  1. *First thing to do*: *Dilution* by ingestion of any liquid, e.g., water.
  2. Antibiotics and steroids: To decrease edema and fibrosis.
  3. Barium swallow in 2 months: Depending on the degree of stricture, the choice is made between dilatation vs Esophagectomy and anastomosis.

Esophageal Cancer

- *Causes*: Smoking, alcohol, Barrett's esophagus, Plummer Vinson syndrome.
- *Types*: Squamous cell carcinoma (90%), while adenocarcinoma is common only in the *lower third* of esophagus; mostly as a complication of *Barrett's esophagus*.
- *Clinical picture*:

  1. Dysphagia:*More to solids* than liquids. *Mirror image of achalasia*.
  2. Regurgitation of meals and loss of weight.

- *Diagnosis*: Test of choice is EGD and biopsy. Barium swallow shows *Rat tail appearance*.
- *Treatment*:

  1. *If small with no metastases*: *Surgery*: Pharyngio-laryngectomy (Upper 1/3), or Esophagectomy (Middle 1/3) or Esophagogastrectomy (Lower 1/3), plus chemotherapy and radiation.
  2. *If large or with metastases*: Chemotherapy (*5-Florouracil and Cisplatinum*) and radiation. No surgery is needed unless it is palliative, e.g., Esophago-gastric bypass.

Congenital Hypertrophic Pyloric Stenosis (CHPS)

- *Mechanism*: Congenital anomaly leading to *hypertrophy of pyloric muscles* and dilatation of the stomach.
- *Clinical picture*:

  1. Vomiting: *Never* at birth (2–6 weeks after birth) and *Never* bilious.
  2. Constipation and failure to thrive.

- *On exam*: *Olive-like mass* in the epigastrium.
- *Labs*: Hypokalemic alkalosis and hyponatremia.
- *Diagnosis*: *Gastrograffin meal*.
- *Treatment*: *Pyloromyotomy*.
- *Note*: Duodenal atresia is the most common congenital cause of congenital intestinal atresia. Vomiting *is since birth* and *is bilious* (Mirror image of CHPS). Diagnosis: *Double bubble sign* on abdominal X-ray. Refer to Fig. 5.1. Treatment: Duodenoje- junostomy.

Stomach Cancer

- *Risk factors*: Atrophic gastritis, *Blood group A*, alcohol and smoked food.
- *Pathology*: Multiple types; the most common is *adenocarcinoma*.
- *Location*: Most common is at the *pylorus*.
- *Metastases*: Multiple; the most striking is the *left supraclavicular lymph node* (*Virchow lymph node*).
- *Clinical picture*:

  1. Dyspepsia: Especially to *meat products*.
  2. Dysphagia, nausea, vomiting and hematemasis.
  3. Fatigue and weight loss.

- *Diagnosis*: Esophagogastroduodenoscopy (EGD) and *biopsy*.
- *Treatment*:

  1. *Upper 2/3 of stomach*: Total radical gastrectomy (Stomach, spleen, pancreas and omenta + Roux en-Y gastrojejunostomy).

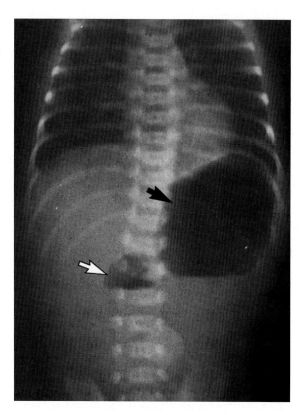

FIG. 5.1 Double bubble sign of intestinal atresia

2. *Lower 1/3*: Lower radical gastrectomy (Lower 2/3 of stomach, spleen, pancreas and omenta + Roux en-Y gastrojejunostomy).

Splenic Rupture

- *Causes*: Closed or open injuries.
- *Clinical picture*:

  1. Pain and rigidity and in the left hypochondrium.
  2. *Cullen sign*: Bluish discoloration around the umbilicus (Remember Pancreatitis?).
  3. *Kehr sign*: Radiating pain in left shoulder due to phrenic nerve irritation.

- *Diagnosis*: Ultrasound of the left hypochondrium, or CT of abdomen.
- *Treatment*: Splenorrhaphy or partial splenectomy. In severe cases, total splenectomy should be done with immunization against *H.influenza B, Meningiococci* and *Strept. Pneumoniae*.
- *Note*: If you see any patient in the USMLE who just had a motor vehicle accident and complaining of abdominal pain, first thing to do is *resuscitation*, followed by CT or US of the abdomen to rule out splenic rupture.

Gall Stones

- *Types*: Mostly *cholesterol* stones, but could also be pigment or mixed stones.
- *Risk factors*: *F*emale, *F*ertile, *F*at, and in her *F*orties
- *Clinical picture*: Asymptomatic vs. Dyspepsia and biliary colic in the right hypochondrium radiating to *right shoulder and right scapula*. Symptoms are commonly associated with ingestion of *fatty food*.
- *On exam*: Pushing on the tip of the right 9th costal cartilage during inspiration elicits severe pain, gasping and guarding rigidity (*Murphy's sign*).
- *Complications*:

  1. Obstruction of biliary ducts.
  2. Cholangitis: Presents with *Charcot's triad* of *fever, pain* and *jaundice*.
  3. Passage of the stone through a fistula into the small intestine causing *obstruction* or *gallstone ileus*. Diagnosis: Abdominal X-ray which shows *air in the biliary tree* and a stone in the right lower quadrant.
  4. Mirrizi syndrome: Stone impaction in the Hartmann's pouch causing fistula formation between the pouch and the *common hepatic duct*.

- *Diagnosis*:

  1. Ultrasound of liver and gall bladder is the test of choice. If that showed dilatation of intrahepatic ducts, next best step is Endoscopic Retrograde Cholangio-pancreaticography (*ERCP*).
  2. *Obstructive (Cholestatic) jaundice*: Stones in CBD cause significant elevation of *alkaline phosphatase* and *direct bilirubin* with only slight elevation of transaminases.

- *Treatment*:

  1. *Gall stones are not treated by cholecystectomy unless they are symptomatic*, or associated with cholecystitis. So, if you see a patient with accidental discovery of gall stones and no symptoms, no treatment is needed.
  2. Cholangitis: Treated with antibiotics, e.g., Cefazolin and Metronidazole.

- *Note*: Most gall stones – unlike kidney stones – are *radiolucent, so X-rays are not very helpful in most cases*.

Cholecystitis

- *Mechanism*: Mostly due to biliary obstruction, e.g., stone, causing stasis of bile and infection ensues.
- *Organisms*: Mostly *Gram negative* organisms, e.g., *E. coli*, Klebsiella. *Clostridium perfringes can cause emphysematous cholecystitis in diabetic patients.*

- *Clinical picture*: Similar to cholangitis, i.e., Fever, pain in right hypochondrium and jaundice.
- *On exam*: Positive Murphy's sign.
- *Diagnosis*: Ultrasound of the gall bladder; typically shows *thickening of gall bladder wall* with *pericystic fluid collection*. If the patient is clinically presenting with cholecystitis but the US did not show any changes, the next step is *HIDA scan* which proves cholecystitis by *failure to visualize the gall bladder* as contrast moves through the biliary system.
- *Treatment*: Cholecystectomy and systemic antibiotics. If the patient is severely symptomatic but is not a candidate for surgery, *cholecystostomy* is done.
- *Note*: Chronic cholecystitis present in the same fashion like acute cases but with more insidious onset and prolonged course. Treated medically except in two situations where it requires cholecystectomy:

  1. Chronic calcular cholecystitis.
  2. Chronic acalcular cholecystitis that failed medical treatment.

- *Note*: One of the rare yet scary complications of chronic cholecystitis is carcinoma of the gall bladder. It is a *squamous cell carcinoma*. Treatment: *Cholecystectomy and wedge liver resection*. Inoperable cases are treated with *radiotherapy*. Remember *Courvoisier's sign*: A palpable gall bladder in any patient with obstructive jaundice is suggestive of malignancy.

Random Biliary Notes

- *Biliary atresia*: Occurs due to failed canalization of biliary tree. Patient presents with hepatomegaly and obstructive jaundice *since birth*, and bilirubin – unlike neonatal hepatitis – *keeps rising*. Extrahepatic types are treated with *hepaticojejunostomy*. Intrahepatic types are treated with *liver transplantation*.
- *Choledochal cyst*: A congenital cystic dilatation of the biliary tree, which may be extrahepatic or intrahepatic, as in Caroli's disease. Treatment: Excision and roux-en-Y anastomosis. Caroli disease is treated with liver transplantation.
- *Cholangiocarcinoma*: Cancer of the biliary tree, with biggest risk factors being infection with *Clonorchis Sinensis (Liver fluke)* and choledochal cyst disease.

Mesenteric Cysts

- *Mechanism*: They are sequestration cysts, e.g., Chylolymphatic or enterogenous.
- *Clinical picture*: Abdominal mass and recurrent attacks of abdominal pain.

- *On exam*: Well-defined abdominal cystic mass; mobile *across root of mesentery*.
- *Diagnosis*: *Ultrasound* or CT scan of abdomen.
- *Treatment*: Resection.

Intestinal Obstruction

- *Mechanism*: Obstruction from *inside the lumen* (e.g., Stools or mass), *in the wall of the lumen* (e.g., Mass), or *due to compression on the lumen from outside* (e.g., Mass or adhesions).
- *Pathophysiology*:

  1. Intestine below obstruction level: *Immobile and collapsed*.
  2. Intestine above obstruction level: *Distended and filled with stools, gas and fluid*.

- *Clinical picture*:

  1. Abdominal pain.
  2. Nausea and vomiting: Early if obstruction is high, late if obstruction is low.
  3. Constipation: Early if obstruction is low, late if the obstruction is high.

- *On exam*:

  1. Abdominal distention and *hyper-resonance or tympanic to percussion*.
  2. Hypoactive or absent bowel movements on auscultation.
  3. Auscultation: *Tinkling* sounds.

- *Complications*:

  1. *Strangulation*: It is interruption of the vascular supply of a segment of intestine leading to interstitial and intraluminal bleeding, gangrene and fatal sepsis.
  2. *Intestinal perforation*: Pathognomonic sign on an abdominal X-ray taken in an upright position is *subdiaphragmatic air*. Refer to Fig. 5.2.

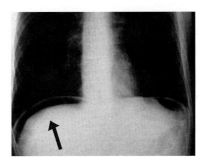

FIG. 5.2 X-ray showing air under diaphragm

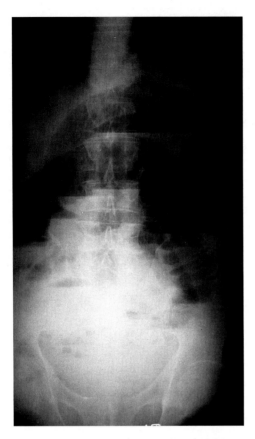

FIG. 5.3 X-ray showing air fluid levels of intestinal obstruction

- **Diagnosis**: Abdominal X-ray in supine and upright positions: *Air fluid levels*. Refer to Fig. 5.3.
- **Treatment**:

  1. Resuscitation: IV fluids and electrolytes correction is the next best step.
  2. Conservative: Nasogastric tube, NPO and await spontaneous resolution.
  3. Surgery: If conservative measures failed. *Exploratory laparotomy* is done, where site and cause of obstruction is identified and repaired.

- **Note**:

  1. Most common cause of intestinal obstruction is *adhesions*.
  2. Ileus: Transient paralysis of the intestine due to *failure of its neurogenic regulation*. Causes: Sepsis, *hypokalemia* or *post-operative* state. Clinical picture and treatment: Similar to obstruction. Abdominal X-ray: *Dilated intestinal loops*.
  3. Acute gastric dilatation is common *2–3 days post-operatively*. Clinical picture: *Persistent hiccough* and huge emesis. Resolves spontaneously.

Volvulus

- **Mechanism**:

  1. Volvulus neonatorum: *Rotation of the midgut loop clockwise instead of counter-clockwise*.
  2. Volvulus in adults: Hiatus hernia or abdominal adhesions.

- **Clinical picture**: *Abdominal pain, constipation* and *bilious vomiting*.
- **Diagnosis**: *Abnormal location of the cecum* on an upper GI series and *Bird beak* appearance on barium enema.
- **Treatment**:

  1. *Best next step*: Rectal tube insertion to deflate the colon.
  2. Surgical untwisting and fixation of the intestine to abdominal wall.

Intussusception

- **Mechanism**: *Invagination of an intestinal loop into another*. Commonly seen in the *ileocecal area*.
- **Clinical picture**: Abdominal pain and *red current jelly* stools.
- **On exam**: An abdominal *sausage-like mass* may be appreciated on palpation.
- **Diagnosis**: Abdominal X-ray shows air fluid levels, while barium enema shows the unique *Claw sign*.
- **Treatment**: Reduction by enema. Surgery and manual reduction if enema fails.

Mesenteric Ischemia

- **Causes**: Arrhythmia, e.g., *A. Fib.*, or atherosclerosis.
- **Clinical picture**:

  1. Abdominal pain only on eating *(Intestinal angina)*.
  2. Ischemic colitis: *Severe abdominal pain* and *bleeding per rectum*.

- **On exam**: The hallmark is abdominal pain *out of proportion* to exam. Meaning the exam is inconclusive, with no major finding to explain patient's pain.
- **Diagnosis**:

  1. Gold standard: *Mesenteric angiography*.
  2. CT abdomen: Shows the pathognomonic *thumb-printing sign*, due to *edema and bleeding in the bowel wall*.
  3. Elevated serum *lactic acid*: Suggestive of ischemic colitis.

- **Treatment**:

  1. *Best next step*: Fluid resuscitation.
  2. Urgent surgery: Exploratory laparotomy, excision of the ischemic segment and end to end anastomosis.

- **Note**: Now when you see a patient in the USMLE who is old and has a history of arrhythmia or severe vascular disease in the heart, brain or legs, and now presenting with abdominal pain, you know what to think!

Acute Appendicitis

- **Location**: The appendix is usually situated *retro-cecally*. However, pre- and post-ileal positions are the most dangerous due to the close proximity to *the ileocolic vein*; hence the potential for *portal sepsis and thrombosis*.
- **Age**: Common in *middle age*, and it is unusual to see appendicitis in extremes of age due to *scanty lymphoid tissue* inside the appendix.
- **Risk factors**: Low fiber and high protein diet, and cecal obstruction, e.g., mass.
- **Causes**: *Lymphoid hyperplasia* is the most common cause followed by *fecolith obstruction*.
- **Organisms**: *E. coli* is the most common organism.
- **Clinical picture**:

  1. Pain: Epigastric or paraumbilical that later migrates towards the *right lower quadrant*.
  2. Fever, nausea, vomiting and constipation.

- **On exam**:

  1. Rigidity, tenderness and rebound tenderness at *McBurney's point*, located *2/3 of the way* along a line between the umbilicus and the right anterior superior iliac spine.
  2. Crossed tenderness and crossed rebound tenderness: Palpation of the LLQ causes tenderness (*Rovsing sign*) and rebound tenderness (*Blumberg sign*) at the RLQ. This occurs due to *displacement of the intestine* towards the RLQ.
  3. *Psoas sign*: Pain in RLQ is increased by right thigh extension.
  4. *Obturator sign*: Pain in RLQ is increased by flexion and internal rotation of the right hip.

- **Diagnosis**:

  1. *CT of the abdomen (Test of choice)*: Thickened wall of appendix with distention of the lumen, and absence of compressibility of the appendix.
  2. CBC: Leukocytosis.

- **Treatment**: *Appendectomy*. The only contraindication for appendectomy is the presence of a mass or abscess as discussed below.
- **Complications**:

  1. *Appendicular mass*: Forms around the *3rd day* after the onset of appendicitis. Formed of edematous cecum and intestinal loops and omentum. Treatment: Keep patient NPO, insert NG tube and start antibiotics and hot compresses, and then plan appendectomy in 3 months. Fate: Resolution or progresses to appendicular abscess.
  2. *Appendicular abscess*: Forms around the *5th day* after the onset of appendicitis. Patient presents with *high fever*, *edema* and *throbbing pain* of RLQ. Treatment: Incision and drainage, then plan appendectomy in 6 months.
  3. Peritonitis: Common in extremes of age, pregnant and diabetic patients.

- **Notes**:

  1. Pelvic and postileal appendix: Presents with diarrhea and urinary frequency and urgency.
  2. Subhepatic appendix: Presents just like cholecystitis, and it is a common presentation of appendicitis during pregnancy, and is associated with *30%–50%* risk of abortion.
  3. Appendicitis in elderly should raise the suspicion of a *mass in the cecum*.

Meckel's Diverticulum

- **Introduction**: It is a remnant of *vitello-intestinal (Omphalo-mesenteric)* duct.
- **Rule of 2s**: Present in 2% of population, 2 feet proximal to ileo-cecal valve, 2 inches long and contains 2 types of epithelium; namely *gastric* and *pancreatic*.
- **Clinical picture**: *Bright red bleeding per rectum, mostly in children*.
- **Diagnosis**: Technetium (*Tm99*) scan; uptake shows a *hot spot*.
- **Complications**: Bleeding, diverticulitis, intussusception or perforation.
- **Treatment**: *Excision*.

Hirschsprung's Disease (Congenital Megacolon)

- **Mechanism**: A congenital disease that occurs *due to presence of aganglionic segment in the colon; lacking Meissner and Auerbach nerve plexuses*. This leads to a *spastic colonic segment*, proximal to which is a transitional zone and a dilated segment.

- **Clinical picture**:

  1. *Constipation since birth*: Newborn passes stools only once or twice a week, but it is huge in amount and extremely malodorous.
  2. Growth retardation.

- **On exam**: Digital rectal exam reveals a spastic segment, and on withdrawal, a *gush of malodorous stool follows*.

- **Diagnosis**:

  1. *Test of choice*: Anorectal biopsy, which shows *absent ganglia and hypertrophied nerve trunks*.
  2. Barium enema *without preparation*: Colon has to be full with stools to visualize the segments described above.

- **Treatment**: Excision of the aganglionic segment and end to end anastomosis of the remaining ends. Complication: *Impotence* in males, due to injury of *pelvic autonomic nerves*.

- **Note**:

  1. Secondary megacolon is a dilated sigmoid colon and rectum all the way down the anal canal *without any spastic segment*. It is mostly due to constipation. Biopsy is normal and treatment entails laxative and regulation of bowel movements.
  2. Secondary megacolon can also be caused by *Trypanosoma cruzi* (*Chagas disease*).

Hemorrhoids

- **Mechanism**: Varicosities of hemorrhoidal venous plexuses. Formed of a small artery surrounded by multiple varicosed dilated veins.

- **Types**:

  1. Internal (*More common*): Located in the lower end of the *rectum* and covered by *mucosa*.
  2. External: Located in the lower end of the *anal canal* and covered by *skin*.

- **Causes**: Chronic straining, or obstruction of superior rectal veins.
- **Location**: Most common at *3, 7 and 11* o'clock positions
- **Degrees**:

  1. *1st degree*: Only *mucosal protrusion* with no hemorrhoidal prolapse.
  2. *2nd degree*: Hemorrhoidal prolapse occurs with defecation and *reduce spontaneously*.

  3. *3rd degree*: Hemorrhoidal prolapse occurs with defecation, but *does not reduce spontaneously. Usually the patient has to push it back in*.
  4. *4th degree*: Hemorrhoidal prolapse that *cannot be reduced*.

- **Clinical picture**:

  1. Painless bright red bleeding per rectum, mostly at the end of defecation. Patient complains "*Small amount of bright red blood in the toilet paper*".
  2. Pruritis and mucus discharge.

- **Diagnosis**: Hemorrhoids can be diagnosed by direct visualization through exam of perineum, proctoscopy or colonoscopy.
- **Complication**: Thrombosis. *Suspect in any patient with hemorrhoids who presents with severe sudden perineal pain*.
- **Treatment**:

  1. 1st and 2nd degrees: Laxatives, decongestant suppositories and minor procedure if necessary, e.g., Cryosurgery, ligation or injection. *Injection causes thrombosis and fibrosis of the hemorrhoids*.
  2. 3rd and 4th degrees: Hemorrhoidectomy.
  3. Hemorrhoidal thrombosis: Urgent hemorrhoidectomy.

Anal Fissure

- **Introduction**: A longitudinal ulcer in the *lower posterior wall* of the anal canal, mostly due to chronic constipation, trauma or ulcerative colitis.
- **Clinical picture**:

  1. Perineal pain during and after defecation.
  2. Bleeding per rectum: Bright red in *streaks* on stools.
  3. Anal mucus discharge.

- **Diagnosis**: On proctoscope or colonoscopy, *hypertrophied anal papilla* is seen proximal to the fissure and a skin tag (a.k.a. *sentinel piles)* distally.
- **Complications**:

  1. Infection: Leads to abscess and fistula formation.
  2. Chronicity: Fissure edges become fibrosed giving it a *Button-hole* appearance.

- **Treatment**:

  1. Acute: Laxatives and anal dilatation.
  2. Chronic: Same as acute plus *fissurectomy and sphincterotomy*.

Anal Fistula

- *Mechanism*: Infection or trauma causing the formation of a fistula that opens externally into the skin and internally into the anal canal.
- *Types*: Multiple; the most common being the *low trans-sphincteric anal fistula*, which crosses through internal and external anal sphincters to open internally at the level of anal valves.
- *Clinical picture*: Anal discharge and pruritis, mainly from the fistula.
- *Diagnosis*: *Fistulogram*.
- *Treatment*: Treat the cause and excise the fistula.
- *Notes*:

  1. Fistulas related to the anterior half of the anal canal have *straight tracks*, while those related to the posterior half have *curved tracks and open into the midline* of the anal canal only.
  2. If you see a patient in USMLE in his 20s or 30s with RLQ abdominal pain, diarrhea, and having a peri-anal fistula, it is Crohn's disease. Refer to IM section.

Ischiorectal Abscess

- *Introduction*: Infection in this fossa is common due *to its poor blood supply*.
- *Clinical picture*: Throbbing pain towards one of the lateral walls of the anal canal.
- *On exam*: Tender *brawny* swelling.
- *Treatment*: I & D via *cruciate incision*.
- *Note*: In the USMLE, a patient with a treated ischiorectal abscess who now has pain on the opposite side of the anal canal likely has another ischiorectal abscess, as these infections crossover easily between both fossae.

Imperforate Anus

- *Mechanism*: Failure of canalization. It could be high, intermediate or low.
- *Clinical picture*: Failure to pass meconium *since birth*.
- *On exam*: A dimple at the anal area which *bulges upon crying*.
- *Diagnosis*: *Invertogram*: *Plain films* in lateral view, upside down and with flexed hips after the anus is labeled with a radiopaque marker. The location of gas bubbles helps to define the level of the atresia.
- *Treatment*:

  1. High: Posterior sagittal anorectoplasty.
  2. Low: Cut-back operation or incision and dilatation.

Pilonidal Sinus

- *Mechanism*: Hair penetration into subcutaneous tissue leads to formation of a sinus, most commonly seen over the *coccyx*.
- *Clinical picture*:

  1. Pain in the buttock area upon sitting.
  2. Discharge from a sinus in the lower back.

- *Diagnosis*: Probing of sinus or fistulogram shows a sinus in the midline of the lower back opening inside into the sacrum.
- *Treatment*: *Elliptical excision of the sinus*.
- *Note*: This disease usually presents in hairy patients sitting for extended periods of time, e.g., Truck drivers, hence it is also known as *Jeep drivers' disease*.

Carcinoid Tumor

- *Introduction*: An *argentaffinoma* that arises from nerve plexuses in *Kulchitsky cells*, most common in the *appendix*.
- *Pathophysiology*: Tumor produces prostaglandin, histamine and serotonin which are then destroyed in the liver. *Liver is the main site of metastases*.
- *Clinical picture*: *Flushing, Diarrhea, Bronchospasm and right-sided heart valve lesions (Tricuspid regurgitation and pulmonary stenosis)*.
- *Diagnosis*: Elevated *5-Hydroxyindolacetic acid (5-HIAA) levels in the urine*.
- *Treatment*: Appendectomy or hemicolectomy depending on extent of the tumor.

Hernia

- *Predisposing factors*: *Chronic* straining increasing intra-abdominal pressure e.g., Heavy lifting, cough.
- *Clinical picture*:

  1. Swelling that gives *expansile impulse on cough*.
  2. Swelling that is *reducible by lying down*.

- *Complications*:

  1. *Strangulation*: A hernia emergency which occurs due to interruption of the blood supply to the herniated intestinal loop. Patient presents with a once reducible hernia that now is *red, warm, tender, tense, irreducible and does not give impulse on cough*.
  2. *Incarceration*: Trapping of the herniated intestine inside the hernial sac, and is a common cause of strangulation. On exam: Failure to reduce the herniated intestine. Treatment: Muscle

relaxants, placement in Trendelenberg position and urgent surgical intervention.
3. Infection or obstruction.

- **Treatment**: Surgical repair. This usually involves reduction of the herniated intestinal segment and covering the defect with a mesh.
- **Inguinal hernia**: Two types:

  1. *Indirect (Oblique)*: Descends into the scrotum, *lateral* to inferior epigastric artery. On exam: Positive internal ring test.
  2. *Direct:* Passes through triangle of Hasselbach, *medial* to the inferior epigastric artery.

- **Femoral hernia**: Common in *females,* where intestine passes down the femoral ring and canal. Swelling is *distal and lateral to pubic tubercle,* and it could be reduced *downwards and medially.* Strangulation is common mainly due to *proximity to lacunar ligament* and to a lesser extent due to the *narrow neck* of hernial sac.
- **Umbilical hernia**:

  1. Congenital (*Omphalocele*): Due to *failure of the midgut to return into the abdomen.* Treatment: Excision of the sac.
  2. Adults: Due to *defect in the linea alba or divarication of recti.*

- **Incisional hernia**: Hernia at the site of an incision, mostly due to *dehiscence of wound layers.* The first sign of abdominal wound dehiscence is *serosanguinous discharge* from the wound.

Random GI Notes

- **Rectal cancer**: Cancer in the upper 2/3 of rectum is treated with *anterior resection,* whereas that of the lower 1/3 is treated with *abdominoperineal resection.*
- **Cancer of anal canal**: Upper 1/2 of anal canal gets *adenocarcinoma,* while lower 1/2 gets *squamous cell carcinoma.* Treatment: *Abdominoperineal resection.*
- **Villous adenoma** (*Carpet tumor*): *Precancerous* adenoma that presents with *watery diarrhea* and hypokalemia. Treatment: Excision and repeat colonoscopy in a few months.
- **Tubular adenoma**: Not precancerous unless it is *bigger than 1 cm* in diameter or it *has a villous component.* Treatment: Excision and repeat colonoscopy in a few months.
- **Duodenal hematoma**: Common after direct injury to epigastrium, e.g., By the steering wheel in a car accident. Diagnosis: *Coiled spring* appearance on X-ray.
- Earliest substrate to be depleted postoperatively is the glycogen.

- The artificial fluid that is closest in composition to small intestinal secretions is lactated ringer, and it has a pH <7. Normal saline combined with D5 as an IV fluid can cause *dilutional acidosis.*

Urinary System

Bladder and Urethra Trauma

- **Anatomical key**:

  1. *Superior surface of bladder*: Urine leaks inside the peritoneum.
  2. *Anterior surface of bladder or urethra above urogenital diaphragm*: Urine leaks into the *retropubic space of Retzius,* which is an extraperitoneal space.
  3. *Urethra below the urogenital diaphragm*: Common in *straddle injury,* and urine accumulates in the *superficial perineal space,* which is bound by *Colle's fascia* and *external spermatic fascia.*
  4. *Penile urethra*: Urine leaks extraperitoneally underneath the *fascia of Buck.*

- **Kidney rupture**: After major abdominal trauma. Clinical picture: Severe flank pain and hematuria. Diagnosis: CT abdomen and pelvis. Treatment: Surgical repair after resuscitation.
- **Urinary bladder rupture**:

  1. Clinical picture: S*trong persistent desire to urinate, but when this is done only a few drops of bloody urine are voided.*
  2. On exam: Prostate is *not* dislocated.
  3. Diagnosis: Ascending cystography: *Tear drop sign.*
  4. Treatment: Surgical closure of bladder. Note: Intraperitoneal rupture will show on abdominal X-ray as *ground glass appearance.*

- **Membranous urethra rupture**: Patient presents with same symptoms as rupture of the bladder above but the prostate here *is dislocated and floating* inside the pelvis. Treatment: Suprapubic cystostomy followed by surgical urethral closure.
- **Penile urethra rupture**: Common in *straddle injury,* e.g., Jumping over a fence or a horse. Clinical picture: *Penile and scrotal swelling, and blood at the external urethral meatus.* Treatment is similar to that of membranous urethra rupture.

Benign Prostatic Hypertrophy (BPH)

- **Mechanism**: Disease of the elderly involving *adenomatous hyperplasia* in the *periurethral zone of the prostate.*

- **Pathology:** *Hyperplastic acini* and *corpora amylacea.*
- **Clinical picture:** *Nocturia, urinary frequency, hesitancy* and *terminal dribbling.*
- **Complications:** Urinary retention and hematuria.
- **On exam:** Rectal exam reveals smooth painless *uniformly enlarged* prostate.
- **Diagnosis:** *Clinical diagnosis,* but can be confirmed using the following:

  1. Transrectal ultrasound and biopsy confirms diagnosis.
  2. IVP: Smooth elevation at the base of urinary bladder.
  3. Prostate specific antigen (PSA): Slightly elevated, but *will not exceed 10 ng/ml.*

- **Treatment:**

  1. Dihydrotestosterone (DHT) antagonists, e.g., Finasteride; *a 5-alpha reductase inhibitor, prevents conversion of testosterone to DHT.*
  2. Surgery, i.e., Transurethral resection of prostate *(TURP)* is reserved for severe resistant cases with complications.

Prostate Cancer

- **Introduction:** *The most common cancer in males.*
- **Location:** *Posterior lobes of prostate,* which are rarely involved in BPH.
- **Most common metastases:** *Spine,* mostly *osteoblastic* lesions.
- **Clinical picture:** Similar to BPH + *Back pain and weight loss.*

- **Diagnosis:**

  1. Transrectal ultrasound and prostate biopsy is diagnostic.
  2. IVP: Irregular elevation at the base of the urinary bladder.
  3. PSA: Elevated – more than 10.

- **Prevention:** Screen by *annual* rectal exam and PSA starting *age 50.*
- **Treatment:**

  1. Hormonal: Through *blocking androgens:*

     - Peripherally: With cyproterone or flutamide.
     - Centrally: With *continuous LHRH stimulation* (Secretion is normally pulsatile rather than continuous).

  2. Surgery: Radical prostatectomy.
  3. Chemotherapy: Using *taxanes.* Only done for cancers resistant to hormonal therapy.

Renal Cell Carcinoma (Hypernephroma)

- **Origin:** *Nephrons;* most commonly *proximal convoluted tubule (PCT).*
- **Pathology:** *Golden yellow* tumor, cells are clear and vacuolated. Refer to Fig. 5.4.
- **Metastases:** Multiple; the most notorious being:

  1. *Cannon ball metastases to lungs.*
  2. Extension to *left renal vein* causing left sided varicocele.

- **Clinical picture:** *Painless hematuria* and *elevated erythropoietin* causing Polycythemia. Refer to IM for clinical picture.

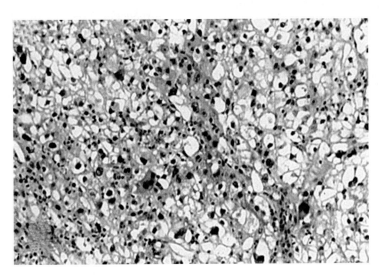

Fɪɢ. 5.4 Renal cell carcinoma

- **Diagnosis**: Test of choice is *Kidney biopsy*. IVP shows *Irregular spider leg deformity*.
- **Treatment:** Nephrectomy and *interleukin* therapy.

Wilm's Tumor (Nephroblastoma)

- **Origin**: *Embryonic nephrogenic cells*.
- **Mechanism**: Deletion of *WT-1 gene* on *chromosome 11*.
- **Clinical picture**: Mostly in children as an *abdominal mass*.
- **Treatment**: A rapidly growing malignant tumor, corrected surgically.
- **Association**: Diseases associated with wilm's tumor can be remembered by GRAWL: *G*enitourinary anomalies, Mental *R*etardation, *A*niridia and *W*ilm's tumor.
- **Note**: Neuroblastoma is a chromaffin tissue tumor that occurs due to a deletion of *chromosome 1* and has *Homer Wright rosettes* on microscopy. Patients with neuroblastomas have high vanillyl mandelic acid (VMA) in their urine. *Suspect this disease in any child with unexplained ecchymosis of eyelids* (Due to *orbital metastases*).

Cancer of the Urinary Bladder

- **Risk factors**: *Dyes* and *smoking*.
- **Location**: Most common in the *base* of the bladder.
- **Type**: Most common is *transitional cell cancer*.
- **Clinical picture**: Non-specific, e.g., Hematuria, *necroturia* (passage of tiny pieces of tumor tissue in the urine) and weight loss.
- **Diagnosis:** Cystoscopy and biopsy.
- **Treatment**:

  1. Radical cystectomy and urinary diversion.
  2. Chemotherapy: Cisplatinum, Methotrexate and Vinblastine.

Horseshoe Kidney

- **Mechanism**: *Fusion of the kidneys at the lower poles during ascent*.
- **Location**: Posterior to *inferior mesenteric artery*.
- **Diagnosis**: IVP shows a *"flower vase"* appearance.
- **Treatment**: Conservative.

Testes

Undescended Testes (Cryptorchidism)

- **Embryology reminder**: Testes develop from the *testicular ridge* (L2 level) and start descent due to *differential body growth*, *high abdominal pressure* and the *pulling effect of gubernaculum*. This descent is completed by the time of birth.
- **Causes**: Hypopituitarism, short spermatic cord or fibrosis.
- **Clinical picture**: Empty and underdeveloped scrotal sac.
- **Complications**: Malignancy (Mainly *seminoma*) and sterility due to high intra-abdominal temperature which destroys testicular cells.
- **Next best step**: CT scan of abdomen and pelvis or laparoscopy to locate the undescended testicle/s.
- **Treatment**: HCG and orchiopexy *if still undescended by 1 year of age*.
- **Notes**:

  1. *Retractile testis*: Sensitive testicle *due to strong cremasteric reflex*. Any stimulus causes retraction of the testicle up to the *superficial subinguinal pouch*. Testes can be felt and easily milked down to the floor of the scrotum.
  2. *Ectopic testis*: Testicle that descends outside its normal line of descent *due to the pulling effect of one of the gubernaculum's tails (Lockwood theory)*. Most common ectopic site is *femoral triangle*. Treatment: Dissection and scrotal replacement.

Epispadius

- **Introduction**: Opening of the urethra into the *dorsum* of the penis.
- **Mechanism**: *Abnormal positioning of the genital tubercle*.
- **Association**: *Exstrophy of urinary bladder*.

Hypospadius

- **Introduction**: Opening of the urethra to the *undersurface* of penis.
- **Mechanism**: *Failed fusion of urethral folds*.
- **Association**: *Bifid scrotum* and *undescended testes*.
- **Clinical picture**: Corpus spongiosum distal to the opening is fibrosed, causing the penis to curve *ventrally*, a condition known as *chordee*.
- **Treatment**: Surgical at the age of *2. Circumcision is contraindicated*.

Varicocele

- **Mechanism**: Dilatation of *pampiniform* and *cremasteric* venous plexuses.
- **Causes**: High venous pressure mostly due to compression, e.g., *Pelvic colon compressing left testicular vein, Superior mesenteric vessels compressing left renal vein*.

- **Clinical picture**: *Dragging pain* in the scrotum, more common on the *left side*.
- **On exam**: *"Bag of worms"* sensation on palpation of scrotal neck, which disappear on scrotal elevation. It also *gives a thrill* on cough.
- **Complications**:

  1. Infertility: Due to thermal effect and *chemical effects of glucocorticoids*.
  2. Thrombosis and hydrocele.

- **Treatment**: Varicosectomy.
- **Notes**:

  1. Retroperitoneal diseases, e.g., Tumor, fibrosis, can compress on testicular veins and present as varicocele.
  2. In the setting of unexplained left sided varicocele, *suspect a renal tumor compressing the left testicular or left renal veins*.

Hydrocele

- **Mechanism**: Fluid collection in the *processus vaginalis*.
- **Causes**: Patent processus vaginalis, varicocele or lymphatic obstruction.
- **Clinical picture**: *Painless cystic translucent* scrotal swelling, more pronounced on standing up and decreased by scrotal elevation.
- **On exam**: *Positive transillumination test*.
- **Complications**: Hematocele, pyocele or testicular atrophy.
- **Treatment**: Eversion or plication of tunica vaginalis.
- **Notes**:

  1. *Congenital hydrocele*: Occurs due to patent processus vaginalis, and the mother will complain of the infant's scrotal swelling *getting bigger towards the end of the day*.
  2. *Encysted hydrocele of the cord*: Due to *non-obliteration of a small segment of processus vaginalis*. Presents as small cystic translucent swelling on

the cord. It is freely mobile, but its mobility is *decreased by pulling down on the testicles*.

Testicular Torsion

- **Mechanism**: Caused by to the high attachment of tunica vaginalis around the distal end of the cord, *a.k.a. Bell Clapper deformity*.
- **Clinical picture**: Sudden severe scrotal pain, especially after trauma or straining, e.g., Heavy weight lifting.
- **On exam**: The testicle is situated *high and horizontally* in the scrotum and extremely tender to touch, plus *blue dot sign*.
- **Diagnosis**: Clinically; however, *venous duplex* should also be done.
- **Complication**: Strangulation and ischemic necrosis of testicle.
- **Treatment**: *Manual detorsion and orchiopexy within 6 hours of presentation*.
- **Note**: Right testicle torsion is usually *clockwise*, while *left is counter-clockwise*.

Epididymorchitis

- **Causes**: UTI, STDs and straining, e.g., Heavy weight lifting.
- **Clinical picture**: Fever and unilateral pain in the scrotum.
- **On exam**: Red, warm, tender and swollen testicle and epididymis.
- **Diagnosis**:

  1. CBC: Leukocytosis.
  2. Urine analysis and intraurethral swab for STDs.

- **Treatment**: Bed rest, scrotal elevation and antibiotics.

Testicular Cancer

- **Types**: Refer to Table 5.1.

TABLE 5.1 Types of testicular cancer.

	Seminoma	Teratoma	Leydig cell tumor	Sertoli cell tumor
Origin	Mediastinum testis; namely the seminiferous tubules	Totipotent cells of the rete testis	Leydig cells	Sertoli cells
Histopathology	Round cells with acidophilic nucleus and clear cytoplasm	Yellow colored cystic tumor engulfed by tunica albuginea	Polyhedral cells with hyaline bodies and cytoplasmic crystalloids of Reinke	Columnar cells with cleft nuclei
Clinical picture	See general clinical picture of tesicular cancer	See general clinical picture	See general clinical picture + Virilization	See general clinical picture + Feminization

- *Clinical picture*:

  1. Painless testicular firm swelling.
  2. *Loss of testicular sensation.*

- *Metastases*: Local, blood and lymphatic, mainly *para-aortic lymph nodes.* Seminoma is famous for sending *cannon ball metastases* to the lungs.

- *Diagnosis*:

  1. Gold standard is *biopsy*, the trick here is that *needle biopsy is contraindicated in the testes,* so an *open biopsy* must be done.
  2. Seminoma: Elevated serum Human Chorionic Gonadotrophins *(HCG).*
  3. Teratoma: Elevated serum *Alpha-fetoprotein (AFP).*

- *Treatment*:

  1. Retrograde orchiectomy.
  2. Chemotherapy: Bleomycin, Etoposide and Platinum *(BEP).*
  3. Radiation therapy: For *seminoma as it is radio-sensitive. Teratomas are radioresistant,* so retroperitoneal lymph node dissection (RPLND) is done.

Breast

Breast Cancer

- *Location*: Most common in the *upper outer quadrant.*
- *Risk factors*: *Age* and *positive family history.*
- *Types*:

  1. *Ductal carcinoma*: The most common type is the *infiltrating adenocarcinoma.*
  2. *Medullary carcinoma*: *Soft and vascular* tumor that occurs at young age, and is characterized by patches of hemorrhage and necrosis under the microscope.
  3. *Colloid carcinoma*: Cystic tumor with *honeycomb appearance* and *signet ring cells.*
  4. *Lobular carcinoma*: Arises from the *terminal lobular ducts,* and is notorious for being *bilateral.*
  5. *Paget's disease*: A slow growing tumor characterized by epidermal hyperplasia, multinucleated vacuolated Paget cells and round cell infiltration of the dermis. Paget's disease might be confused with eczema of the nipple and areola; however, Paget's disease – unlike eczema – is *unilateral, well defined* and *not itchy.*
  6. *Mastitis carcinomatosis*: Aggressive cancer with bad prognosis, common during pregnancy and lactation. It might be confused with lactational mastitis; however, mastitis carcinomatosis – unlike lactational mastitis – affects *more than just one quadrant of the breast, is associated with painless lymphadenopathy and does not respond to antibiotics.*

- *Metastases*:

  1. *Direct*: To breast tissue and skin.
  2. *Blood and transperitoneal,*e.g., *Krukenberg tumor of the ovaries,* now believed to occur via *retrograde lymphatic permeation.*
  3. *Lymphatic*: Subareolar plexus and deep pectoral plexus; both drain to axillary and supraclavicular lymph nodes. Note that medial quadrant's lymphatics cross to the opposite breast. Also the lower quadrants can send metastases to umbilicus (*Sister joseph nodule*).

- *Clinical picture*:

  1. Hard irregular breast mass with ill-defined edge, and lymphadenopathy.
  2. Dimpling and puckering: Due to *contraction of ligaments of Cooper.*
  3. Nipple retraction or inversion.
  4. Peau d'orange: Edema of the breast skin with *pitting* at the sites of hair follicles and sweat glands.

- *Prevention*:

  1. Annual breast exam by a physician starting the age of *20.*
  2. Monthly self breast exam by the patient starting the age of *20 (Controversial).*
  3. Annual mammogram starting the age of *40.*

- *Diagnosis*:

  1. Gold standard is *biopsy.*
  2. Mammogram: *Irregular microcalcifications* are suggestive of malignancy. Refer to Fig. 5.5.

- *Treatment*:

  1. *Surgery*:

     - Stages I and II: Radical mastectomy (Breast, pectoral muscles and axillary lymph nodes are removed) or modified radical mastectomy (Breast, pectoralis minor and axillary lymph nodes are removed).
     - Stage III is treated surgically by simple mastectomy (Breast + axillary biopsy) as a palliative surgery to facilitate radiation and minimize complications.
     - Quadrantectomy and lumpectomy: Indicated for tumors that are *peripheral* in the breast and *smaller than 5 cm* in diameter.

  2. *Radiation therapy*: Used for all patients.

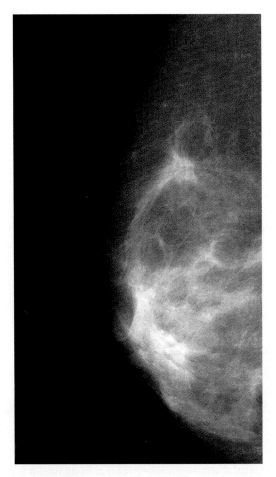

FIG. 5.5 Mammogram showing irregular microcalcifications of breast cancer

3. *Chemotherapy*: Indicated only *if the tumor is bigger than 1 cm* and/or if there is *lymph node involvement*. CMF (Cyclophosphamide, Methotrexate, 5-Florouracil) is a widely used combination.
4. *Hormonal therapy*: Depends on the hormonal receptors found *in the tumor*:

   - Negative hormone receptors: No treatment. However, 10% of patients with negative estrogen receptors still respond to hormonal treatment.
   - Positive hormone receptors in pre-menopausal patient: Tamoxifen for 5 years. Tamoxifen is an estrogen blocker that increases the risk of *DVT, endometrial carcinoma and hot flashes*.
   - Positive hormone receptors in post-menopausal patient: Tamoxifen for 5 years followed by aromatase inhibitor therapy for 5 years.
   - Positive her-2-neu receptors: Treat with *Trastuzumab* (Herceptin).

- *Notes*:

   1. Most important risk factor in breast cancer in females: *Age*.
   2. Most important prognostic factor in breast cancer: *Tumor size* and *lymph node involvement*.
   3. Lobular carcinoma in situ is treated with *tamoxifen*.
   4. Ductal carcinoma in situ is treated with *simple mastectomy* or *local resection*.
   5. Breast cancer in males is treated by *modified radical mastectomy* and *radiation*.

Fibrocystic Disease (Fibroadenosis)

- *Definition*: Changes in the breast that occur due to *evolution and involution*
- *Pathology*: A combination of *fibrotic and cystic* changes.
- *Clinical picture*:

   1. Breast pain and tenderness, *more pronounced around menstruation dates*.
   2. Breast *nodules* and nipple discharge, *more pronounced around menstruation*.

- *On exam*: *Nodular breast diffusely* on palpation.
- *Diagnosis*: *Excisional biopsy is the gold standard*.
- *Complication*: Breast cancer.
- *Treatment*: Supportive, except for large lesions, e.g., Cysts or lumps, which can be excised.

Mastitis

- *Lactational mastitis*: Common in the first few months of lactation. It is mostly caused by *Staphylococcus aureus*, affects *one quadrant* and is treated with *penicillinase resistant penicillin*.
- *Pubertal mastitis*: Common around the age of puberty. So when you get a case in the USMLE about a male teen whose breasts started getting slightly bigger and showing some redness, just reassure the patient that this is *normal*.
- *Neonatal mastitis*: Mostly due to *estrogen withdrawal*, and is associated with nipple discharge a.k.a. *Witch's milk*.

Gynecomastia

- *Definition*: *Painful and tender* enlargement of the *glandular part* of the male breast.
- *Causes*: Liver cell failure or drug induced, e.g., Spironolactone, Cimetidine.

- **Treatment**: Treat the cause. If failed, *subcutaneous mastectomy is done.*
- **Note**: When you get a case in the USMLE about a male teen whose breasts started getting slightly bigger; just reassure the patient that this is normal and will resolve.

Duct Papilloma

- **Clinical picture**: *Multiparous* female with *bloody nipple discharge.*
- **Diagnosis**: Mammogram and cytology of the discharge.
- **Treatment**: *Microdochectomy,* as it is a precancerous lesion.

Fibroadenoma

- **Clinical picture**: *Young nulliparous* female with *firm smooth mobile breast mass.*
- **Complications**: Increase in size, malignancy and myxomatous degeneration.
- **Treatment**: *Inoculation.* If large in size, simple mastectomy can be done.

Traumatic Fat Necrosis

- **Mechanism**: Trauma causing the fat to bind with calcium and form a mass.
- **Treatment**: *Excision.*

Notes

- **Nipple discharge**: Best next step depends on the scenario as follows:

  1. Discharge + breast mass: Next step is *excision of the mass.*
  2. Discharge from a single duct: Next step is *Microdochectomy.*
  3. Discharge from multiple ducts: Next step is *Benzidine test (Detects blood).* If negative, observe the patient. If positive, *ducts excision* is recommended.

- **Duct ectasia:** Breast ductal dilatation along with *plasma cell infiltration.* Clinical picture: *Worm-like structure* extending away from the nipple under the areola. Treatment: *Excision.*
- **Galactocele**: Retention cyst filled with milk. Patient presents with a cyst under the areola which is attached to the nipple *via one point.* Treatment: *Excision.*

Hand Infections

- **Organisms**: Mostly *Staphylococcus aureus*, and to lesser extent streptococcus.
- **Pulp space infection**: Leads to *loss of pulp resilience* and could end up with *necrosis of the distal phalanx in 2 weeks.* Treatment: Incision and Drainage (I&D).
- **Midpalmar space infection**: Leads to *frog hand deformity*, where patient has dorsal hand edema and *loss of palm concavity.* Treatment: I & D.
- **Thenar space infection**: Leads to *ballooning of thenar eminence* with *maintained palm concavity.* Treatment: I & D.
- **Suppurative tenosynovitis**: Patient presents with swollen partially flexed tender fingers. Treatment: I & D and treatment of the cause.

Tongue

Ulcers

- **Herpetic**: Painful and vesicular, affects *only one half of the tongue* and *does not cross the midline.*
- **Syphilitic**: Gummatous ulcer with *punched out edges* and *yellow leather-like sloughed* floor.
- **T.B.**: Multiple *along the edges* of the tongue with *undermined edges.*
- **Dental**: Narrow and long, and rubs against a tooth.
- **Dyspeptic**: Superficial, tender and yellow in color. Heals within *7 days*
- **Post-pertussis**: *Transverse linear* ulcer on the lower surface of the tongue.

Cysts

- **Mucous cyst**: Oval bluish cyst that forms on the floor of the mouth due to retention of secretions of submucous salivary glands. Treatment: Excision.
- **Ranula**: Forms due to *extravasation or retention* of *sublingual* salivary glands. It is also bluish, cystic and in the floor of the mouth. It is different than mucous cyst in being on either side of the frenulum and *never in the midline*, and also being *crossed by the submandibular duct.* Treatment: De-roofing (Marsupialization).

Tongue Cancer

- **Location**: Occurs most commonly in the *anterior 2/3.*
- **Risk factors**: Smoking, alcohol and leukoplakia.
- **Lymphatic metastases**:

  1. *Posterior 1/3: Deep cervical and jugulodigastric lymph nodes.*

2. *Anterior 2/3*:

- Tip: *Submental lymph nodes.*
- Sides: *Submandibular lymph nodes.*
- Center: *Submental and submandibular lymph nodes.*

- **Diagnosis**: *Biopsy.*
- **Treatment**:

1. Anterior 2/3: Radiation needles in the tongue *plus surgery.*
2. Posterior 1/3: Radiation only.

Salivary Glands

Introduction

- **Parotid gland**: Salivary gland around the ear that secretes *serous saliva* inside the mouth through Stensen's duct, which opens at the *upper second molar tooth.*
- **Sublingual glands:** Located just *underneath the tongue,* and secrete *mucous saliva.*
- **Submandibular gland**: Located underneath the ramus of the madible and secretes *mixed saliva (Serous and mucous)*. The duct opens via *Wharton's duct* into the floor of the mouth, just by the *frenulum of the tongue.*

Sialolithiasis

- **Clinical picture**: Pain and swelling of the involved gland. Symptoms *exacerbated by eating*; especially with *sour food or fluids,* e.g., Lemon juice.
- **On exam**: Palpation of the stone in the duct by bimanual palpation.
- **Diagnosis**: X-ray or *sialogram.*
- **Treatment**: Conservative by sialogogues. Sialadenectomy is reserved for severe cases.

Sialoadenitis

- **Mechanism**: Infection of the salivary glands by virus or bacteria, esp. *S. aureus.*
- **Clinical picture**: Gland swelling, warmth and tenderness; *not related to meals.*
- **Treatment**: Best is *penicillinase resistant penicillin.*

Ludwig Angina

- **Mechanism**: *Microaerophilic streptococcal* infection of the *deep* fascia surrounding the *submandibular gland.*

- **Clinical picture**: Fever and *brawny edema* in the submandibular area.
- **Treatment**: *Release incision* of the skin and deep fascia in the submental area, plus systemic antibiotics.

Salivary Tumors

- **Adenolymphoma**:

1. Ectopic salivary tissue in the *superficial layers of the parotid gland.*
2. Adenolymphoma is cystic, benign, painless and *bilateral* tumor, characterized by *big cystic spaces* filled with clear fluid through which *papillae* project.
3. Microscopically shows *palisade* pattern.
4. Diagnosis: *Technetium scan* shows increased uptake with *hot spot.*
5. Treatment: Superficial parotidectomy.

- **Parotid cancer**: *Anaplastic adenocarcinoma* with *facial nerve involvement.* So think of this whenever you see a parotid gland tumor with facial nerve palsy at the same time. Treatment: Total parotidectomy and radiation therapy.
- **Pleomorphic adenoma**: Characterized by *incomplete fibrous capsule.* A benign slow growing tumor that *does not injure the facial nerve* unless it turns malignant. Treatment: Sialadenectomy.
- **Cylindroma**: Characterized by cylinders of cells filled with *mucin.*

Head and Neck

Cleft Lip

- **Mechanism**: Failure of the *maxillary prominences to fuse with medial nasal prominences,* or failure of the *mandibular prominences to fuse with each other.*
- **Cause**: Familial or due to injury during the first trimester, e.g., *Rubella.*
- **Clinical picture**: Cleft lip, usually unilateral and mostly on the *left.*
- **Complications**: Difficulty in feeding.
- **Treatment**: Surgical at age of *10 weeks* by *Millard's operation.*

Cleft Palate

- **Mechanism**: *Failure of fusion of both palatine shelves with either each other, or with the primary palate.*
- **Cause**: Same as cleft lip.
- **Complications**: Difficulty in feeding and speech.

- **Treatment**: Surgical at the age of *10 to 12 months* by *Langenbeck's operation.*
- **Note:** Pierre Robin syndrome is a cleft palate syndrome in which the patient also has *posteriorly displaced mandible (Retrognathia) and tongue.*

Hemangioma

- **Capillary hemangioma**: *Compressible, non-pulsatile hamartoma,* has 3 forms:

  1. *Strawberry*: Present at birth and disappears within first year of life.
  2. *Salmon patch*: Present at birth and disappears within first year of life.
  3. *Portwine stain*: *Does not disappear spontaneously.* Refer to Fig. 5.6. Requires excision and graft. *Sturge-Weber syndrome*: Portwine hemangioma, plus leptomeningeal angiomas causing neurological manifestations, e.g., Seizures, CVAs. Skull X-ray in Sturge-Weber syndrome shows *tram-track like intracranial calcifications.*

- **Cavernous hemangioma**: Ill-defined *bluish* cystic swelling that *does not transilluminate.* Complication: Hemorrhage. Treatment: *No treatment* unless bleeding occurs, then excision is warranted.

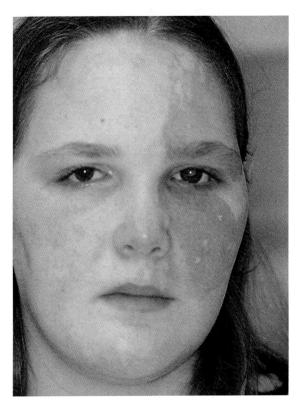

Fɪɢ. 5.6 Portwine hemangioma (Nevus flammeus)

Cystic Hygroma

- **Mechanism**: *Cavernous lymphangioma,* most common in the *lower part of the posterior triangle* of the neck.
- **Clinical picture**: Cystic compressible swelling in the neck; *present since birth.*
- **Treatment**: Excision at *2 years* of age.

Others

- **Frey syndrome**: Excessive *sweating* induced by eating. Mechanism: Injury of *auriculotemporal branch of trigeminal nerve.*
- **Crocodile tears syndrome**: Excessive *lacrimation* induced by eating. Mechanism: *Injury of facial nerve during its course inside the parotid gland.*

Venous System

Varicose Veins

- **Introduction**: The lower limbs drain through 2 systems of veins; superficial and deep. Both systems are connected via *perforators.* This network has valves to guarantee passage of the blood only in one direction; from the superficial system into the deep one.
- **Types and causes**:

  1. *Primary*: Prolonged standing and defective valve system.
  2. *Secondary*: DVT, pelvic tumors and pregnancy. All these factors slow the venous return.

- **Clinical picture**:

  1. Dull aching pain towards the end of the day.
  2. Dilated tortuous veins on the surface of the leg, *more pronounced upon standing and disappear on leg elevation.*

- **Complications**:

  1. Venous ulcer: Due to *liposclerosis.* Occur mainly in the lower leg, just above the ankle and could get deep enough to cause osteomyelitis of the tibia.
  2. Stasis dermatitis: Due to deposition of *hemosiderin.*
  3. Talipus equinus deformity: Due to *contracture of Achilles tendon.* This is induced usually by the patient putting more pressure on his/her frontal part of the foot to avoid pain.

- **Diagnosis**: Duplex ultrasound is the gold standard.
- **Treatment**:

  1. Elastic stockings and treatment of the cause.

2. Injection sclerotherapy: Induces *thrombosis and fibrosis* of varicosities. Used for *localized varicosities only.*
3. Severe cases with complications: Stripping of the varicose veins or multiple ligation of the incompetent areas.
4. Venous ulcer: *Compression*, antibiotics and subfascial ligation of ankle perforators. Another option is excision and grafting of the ulcerated area.

Deep Venous Thrombosis (DVT)

• *Risk factors*:

1. *Previous DVT is the most important risk factor.*
2. Recent prolonged immobilization, e.g., Long car ride, long flight, hospitalization, limb fracture.
3. Medications: *Oral Contraceptive Pills* and Megesterol (Used as appetite stimulant for cancer patients).
4. Hypercoagulable state: Antithrombin III deficiency, Prothrombin gene mutation, Factor V leiden mutation, Protein C or S deficiency, Antiphospholipid antibody syndrome.

• *Pathology*:

1. Virchow's triad = Hypercoagulability + Stasis + Endothelial damage.
2. The blood clot is formed of fibrin and platelets.
3. Most common site is the *lower extremities.*
4. Time frame: Around the *3rd–7th day* after start of immobilization.

• *Clinical picture*:

1. Affected limb is *red, warm, tender and swollen.*
2. *Homan's sign*: Pain in the calf on dorsiflexion of the foot in cases of DVT below the knee.

• *Complications*:

1. Pulmonary embolism (PE): *DVT in the lower extremities is the most common cause of PE.* So keep that in mind when you see any patient with DVT in the USMLE with sudden respiratory distress. Refer to IM section for more on PE.
2. Varicose veins, edema and venous ulcer.

• *Differential diagnosis*: Ruptured baker's cyst or plantaris muscle.
• *Diagnosis*: Gold standard is *venography*. Practically, we use *Doppler ultrasound.*
• *Prevention*: All hospitalized patients get subcutaneous heparin and/or sequential compression devices on their calves during their hospital stay. It is a standard of care.

• *Treatment*: *Heparin IV drip* initially, and then warfarin is started and continued for *3–6 months* maintaining an INR target of *2–3.*
• *Notes*:

1. Inferior Vena Cava filters, e.g., Greenfield filter, are indicated only in 2 conditions:

   • Patients with DVT who have an absolute contraindication to anticoagulation, e.g., GI bleeding.
   • Patients with DVT already on anticoagulation wit therapeutic INR, and yet keep suffering recurrent PE.

2. Thrombophlebitis migrans: *Superficial thrombophlebitis* that lasts for short periods and disappears spontaneously. This is usually a sign of malignancy (*Trousseau's sign*), e.g., Pancreatic cancer. *So, intensive screening for malignancy should be the first next step for any patient with thrombophlebitis migrans.*

Arterial System

Atherosclerosis

• *Pathogenesis*: Thickening of the intima and deposition of subintimal fat forming plaques and calcifications. It occurs mainly in *large arteries.*
• *Clinical picture*: PVD, CAD, CVA.
• *Diagnosis*: Arteriography shows *rat tail* appearance.
• *Treatment*:

1. Treat the cause.
2. Medications: Anti-platelets and vasodilators.
3. Surgery: For complications see below.

Peripheral Vascular Disease (PVD)

• *Causes*: Atherosclerosis, thrombosis, embolism, *smoking.*
• *Clinical picture*:

1. *Acute*: *P*ain, *P*allor, *P*ulselessness, *P*aralysis, *P*arasthesia and *P*oikilothermia.
2. *Chronic*:

   • *Atrophic changes*: Thin skin with loss of hair and possible ulcers.
   • *Intermittent claudications*: *Muscle cramping on exercise that resolves at rest.* This occurs due to accumulation of metabolites due to ischemia, which stimulate the nerve endings.

- *Rest pain*: Due to *ischemic neuritis*. Patient presents with pain in the affected limb even at rest, and tends to keep that limb uncovered and hanging by the side of the bed while sleeping. This is a sign of *impending gangrene*.
- *On exam*: Ankle/Brachial pressure index (ABI) (*Normal >1*). In cases of ischemia, it is expected to be *lower than 1*. In cases of rest pain, *lower than 0.3*.
- *Location*: There are key sites to look for the effects of vascular compromise:

  1. Aorto-iliac: Cramping of *buttocks and thighs and impotence,* a.k.a. *Leriche syndrome.*
  2. Femoro-popliteal: Cramping of the *calf muscles.*
  3. Popliteal: Cramping of the *lower leg and foot muscles.*

- *Diagnosis*: *Arteriography (Digital Subtraction Angiography "DSA") is the gold standard.* Doppler or duplex ultrasound could also be used.
- *Complication*: Gangrene and amputation.
- *Treatment*:

  1. Treat the cause, e.g., *Stop smoking*. Embolic cases should be managed within *6 h* by embolectomy and anti-coagulation, or else gangrene is a risk.
  2. Medications: Anti-platelets and vasodilators, e.g., aspirin, cilostazole.
  3. Surgery: Angioplasty or bypass graft.

Thromboangiitis Obliterans (Buerger's Disease)

- *Pathogenesis*: An atherosclerotic disease that affects entire neurovascular bundles, but mainly targeting *medium and small sized arteries*, leaving them with *intimal proliferation* and a *red thrombus*.
- *Cause*: Strongly linked to *smoking.*
- *Location*: Most commonly *below the elbow and knee.*
- *Clinical picture*: Similar to chronic ischemia. See above.
- *Diagnosis*: *Arteriogram* which shows *patent large vessels* and *occlusion of medium and small sized ones.*
- *Complication*: Gangrene requiring amputation.
- *Treatment*: *Stop smoking*, and start anti-platelets and vasodilators.
- *Note*: *If you see any young or middle aged smoker in the USMLE with severe PVD, it is mostly Buerger's disease, and he should be advised to quit smoking.*

Gangrene

- *Mechanism*: Necrosis and putrefaction of tissues.
- *Causes*: Refer to causes of PVD.

- *Clinical picture*:

  1. Color changes: Brown, green and finally *black*.
  2. Loss of pulse and sensations and function of the affected limb.

- *On exam*:

  1. *Dry*: Bone has a *relatively good* blood supply, so the stump is *conical* in shape, and the demarcation line is formed by an *aseptic* ulcer.
  2. *Moist*: Bone has *poor* blood supply, so the stump is *straight*. The limb is swollen and shows blebs and crepitus. Demarcation line is formed by a *septic* ulcer.

- *Management*: Next best thing to do is *arteriography* to determine the extent of the vascular disease and hence plan for the appropriate level of amputation.
- *Note*:

  1. Gas gangrene: Caused by anaerobic organisms with saccharolytic and proteolytic activity, e.g., *Clostridium*. Wound is characterized by *crepitus* indicating subcutaneous gas. Treatment: *Polyvalent antitoxin* (Anti-gas gangrene serum), *penicillin* and *hyperbaric oxygen* therapy. If failed: Amputation.
  2. Diabetic gangrene: Could be ischemic, infective, neuropathic or mixed.
  3. Bed sore: A form of gangrene characterized by *non-blanching erythema. Prevention*: Frequent positioning of the patient. *Treatment*: Debridement.

Raynaud's Disease

- *Pathogenesis*: Episodic arterial vasospasm of the hands, more common in *females.*
- *Clinical picture*: Sudden *pallor* and pain in the hands, then they turn *blue* and back to normal, all within a *couple of minutes.*
- *On exam*: Radial pulse is within normal limits.
- *Diagnosis*: Clinical, also *immersion of the hands* in cold water triggers an attack.
- *Treatment*:

  1. Avoid cold weather and objects.
  2. *Calcium channel blockers*: Relax vascular smooth muscles.
  3. Sympathectomy is the last resort, which is of 2 types:

     - Cervicodorsal sympathectomy: Removal of *lower half of stellate ganglion*, along with the *2nd and 3rd thoracic* ganglia. This is the type used to treat Raynaud's disease.

- Lumbar sympathectomy: Removal of *2nd, 3rd and 4th lumbar* ganglia. Done for patients with severe lower limb ischemia, where revascularization surgery is not an option.

Crush Syndrome (Traumatic Rhabdomyolysis)

- *Definition*: Ischemic muscle necrosis due to trauma, e.g., Motor vehicle accident, status epilepticus or severe physical exercise.
- *Pathology*: Ischemia causes necrosis of the muscle and release of large amounts potassium and myoglobin from the muscles.
- *Clinical picture*:

  1. Muscle aches.
  2. Acute renal failure (*ATN*): Due to deposition of myoglobin in the tubules (Rhabdomyolysis).

- *Diagnosis*: Elevated serum CPK (*in thousands*), aldolase and urine myoglobin.
- *Treatment*:

  1. *Aggressive fluid resuscitation is the best next step.*
  2. Alkalinization of the urine: Using Bicarbonate drip to help excrete myoglobin without deposition in the tubules.

Thoracic Outlet Syndrome

- *Mechanism*: Cervical rib compressing on 2 main structures; *subclavian artery* and *lower trunk of brachial plexus*.
- *Clinical picture*:

  1. Decreased sensations along the *ulnar nerve* distribution.
  2. *Atrophy of thenar and hypothenar and interossei muscles.*

- *On exam*: *Adson test*: If the patient turns his chin towards the side of the lesion while taking a deep inspiration, the radial pulses in the affected hand will get weaker.
- *Diagnosis*: X-ray of the neck and chest looking for the compressing object.

- *Treatment*: Conservative by physical therapy and exercise. Surgery is reserved for complicated cases with signs of compression, e.g., Muscle wasting.

Lymphatic System

Lymphadenitis

- *Causes*: Infectious or neoplastic.
- *TB lymphadenitis*: Usually affects the *upper cervical lymph node group*, which become *matted* and show *central caseation* surrounded by *epithelioid cells* under microscopy. Complications: *Cold abscess* and *collar stud abscess*, sinus and tract formation.
- *Syphilitic lymphadenitis*: Starts with *chancre*, where patient has *shotty painless* nodes, which usually involves *epitrochlear and posterior cervical* lymph node group.
- *Filariasis*: Patient has high *eosinophilic* count.
- *Malignant*: Aspiration reveals blood and necrotic tissue.

Lymphedema

- *Causes*: Congenital, e.g., Lymphedema congenita, or acquired due to malignancy or infection, e.g., Filariasis, Streptococci.
- *Clinical picture*: Edema mostly of the lower extremities, pitting initially then *non-pitting,* a.k.a. *Elephantiasis.*
- *Diagnosis*: Lymphangiography. *Midnight film is used to diagnose filariasis.*
- *Treatment*: Limb elevation. If resistant, surgery is done to divert lymphatic flow into the deep fascia.

Bones and Fractures

Fracture of the Skull Base

- Refer to Table 5.2 for locations and effects of injury.

TABLE 5.2 Fractured base of the skull.

	Anterior cranial fossa	Middle cranial fossa	Posterior cranial fossa
Effect	• Peri-orbital ecchymosis • Subconjunctival hemorrhage • Epistaxis • CSF rhinorrhea	• Bleeding from the ears • CSF otorrhea	• Bleeding from the mouth • Bruising of the muscles in the back of the neck
Cranial nerves injured	I and II	VII and VIII	IX , X and XI

Rib Fractures

- *Types and clinical picture*:

    1. *Simple*: One or more fractures *at the site of maximum curvature*. Pain is at the fracture site; gets worse by deep inspiration or cough.
    2. *Flail chest*: Multiple fractures *at multiple sites*. Chest wall moves *paradoxically* with breathing, i.e., Moves in with inspiration and out with expiration.

- *Diagnosis*: X-rib in multiple views including *oblique films*.
- *Treatment*:

    1. If no displacement: Pain control, heals spontaneously.
    2. If displaced: Open reduction and internal fixation.

Spondylosis

- *Mechanism*: Degenerative disorder of the spine and intervertebral discs characterized by *osteophytes* formation.
- *Treatment*: Conservative; surgery is only needed if there are signs of cord compression. Refer to internal medicine for more details.

Spondylolysis

- *Mechanism*: *Stress fracture* of the *pars interarticularis*. Occurs mainly in the *lumbar* vertebrae, more common in *athletes*.
- *On exam*: Positive *leg hyperextension test* on exam.
- *Diagnosis:* X-ray; the fracture is *collar-shaped*.
- *Note:* Spondylolithesis is a disorder of the *pedicles* of lumbar vertebrae causing sliding of a vertebral body and lordosis. It is either congenital or secondary to degeneration.

Clavicular Fracture

- *Mechanism*: Occurs at the junction of *medial 2/3* and *lateral 1/3 of clavicle*, mostly due to *fall on outstretched hand*.
- *Clinical picture*: *Step-ladder* deformity and tilt of the head towards fractured side due to contraction of sternomastoid muscle.
- *Treatment*: Closed reduction + Sling (*Figure of eight sling*).

Supracondylar Fracture of Humerus

- *Mechanism*: Fracture of the humerus just above the epicondyles, mostly *due to a fall on the tip of a flexed elbow*.
- *Clinical picture*: Pain and ecchymosis of the antecubital fossa.
- *X-ray*: Positive *fat pad* (*Sail*) sign.
- *Next best step*: *Examine radial pulse*.
- *Complications*:

    1. Injury to brachial artery: Leads to acute ischemia (Remember all the *P*s).
    2. Volkmann contracture: Flexion deformity of the wrist and fingers, mostly *due to ischemia causing muscle fibrosis*.

- *Treatment*: Reduction + immobilization by cast placement.

Nursemaid Elbow

- *Mechanism*: Pulling on the upper limb causing the radial head to be sublaxed off the annular ligament.
- *Clinical picture*: Common in children and the patient presents with *flexed and pronated forearm*.
- *Treatment*: Manual reduction.

Compartment Syndrome

- *Introduction*: Surgical emergency; common after trauma, fracture or severe infection.
- *Clinical picture*: The affected compartment is red, warm, tender and swollen.
- *On exam*: Severe compartmental pain on *passive extension* of the digits.
- *Diagnosis*: Elevated pressure inside the compartment by manometry (*>30 mmHg*).
- *Treatment*: *Immediate fasciotomy*.
- *Notes*:

    1. Structures in anterior compartment of thigh are *femoral artery and nerve*.
    2. Structures in anterior compartment of leg are *anterior tibial artery and deep peroneal nerve*.

Scaphoid Fracture

- *Most common cause*: Fall on an *outstretched hand*.
- *Clinical picture*: Wrist pain and *tender anatomical snuffbox*.
- *Complications*: Avascular necrosis of scaphoid bone in *proximal* fractures.

- *Diagnosis and management*: X-ray does not show the fracture in early stages, so in suspected cases, put a *thumb splint* and repeats the X-ray in *7–10 days*.
- *Remember:* The snuffbox is bounded by 3 *pollicis* tendons: Extensor pollicis longus, extensor pollicis brevis and abductor pollicis longus (The *police* guards the box).

Colle's Fracture

- *Mechanism*: Posterior displacement of distal radius plus *fractured styloid process* of the ulna.
- *Clinical picture*: Pain and palpable fracture in the distal forearm.
- *Diagnosis*: X-ray shows *Dinner fork* deformity.
- *Treatment*: Reduction + immobilization by cast placement.

Dupuytren Contracture

- *Mechanism*: Fibrosis and contraction of palmar aponeurosis.
- *Risk factors*: Alcoholism and liver cirrhosis.
- *Clinical picture: Painless* flexed medial fingers.
- *Treatment:* Physical therapy, surgery is reserved for severe resistant cases.

Miscellaneous Upper Limb Injuries

- *Shoulder dislocation*: Mostly anterior dislocation, injuring the axillary nerve and artery. On exam: *Externally rotated* arm. Treatment: Reduction and sling.
- *Lateral epicondylitis* (*Tennis elbow*): Inflammation of common extensor origin.
- *Medial epicondylitis* (*Golfer's elbow*): Inflammation of common flexor origin.
- *Boxer's fracture*: Fracture of the *head of 5th metacarpal bone*.
- *Gamekeeper's fracture*: Expect it in a patient coming to the ER after *skiing*, complaining of *thumb pain and tenderness*. The pathology is *avulsion of medial collateral ligament* of thumb.
- *Monteggia's fracture*: *Dislocation of radial head* and *diaphyseal ulnar fracture*. Expect it in a patient coming to the ER who was in a fight, and used his forearm to stop an attack by a blunt object.

Femoral Neck Fracture

- *Risk factors*: Elderly women with *osteoporosis*.
- *Clinical picture*: Tender, abducted, externally rotated, and shortened leg.
- *Complication*: Avascular necrosis of femoral head.
- *Treatment*: Open reduction and internal fixation, *unless there is intracapsular fracture, which requires a hemiarthroplasty*.

Knee Injuries

- *Unhappy triad*: The most serious injury after a *lateral* knee injury, which injures 3 structures (*MAM*): Medial collateral ligament, Anterior cruciate ligament and Medial meniscus.
- *Quadriceps tear*: Suspected if you feel a groove above the knee after a knee injury.
- *ACL tear*: Patient hears a popping sound in his knee, usually during *jogging*. On exam: Anterior displacement of tibia on femur with the knee flexed 20° (*Lachmann's test*).
- *Meniscus tear*: Patient develops painful swelling on either side of the knee, usually after *frequent crouching and standing movement, or after a sudden twist injury to the knee*. On exam: Repeated flexion and extension of the knee with internal and external rotation of the ankle reveals *palpable and audible clicking sound* in the knee joint (*McMurray test*).
- *Note*: All knee injuries described above are managed medically with pain control and knee immobilization. *Only if condition is not improving, MRI of the knee is obtained (MRI is the test of choice to visualize cruciate ligaments and menisci)*.

Osgood Schlatter Disease

- *Mechanism*: Common in *soccer players*, due to *avascular necrosis of tibial tuberosity*.
- *Clinical picture*: Pain and swelling below the knee.
- *Note*: Tibial fractures typically do not heal well and there is a possibility of malunion due to the relatively poor blood supply.

Slipped Capital Femoral Epiphysis

- *Introduction*: Common in *obese adolescent African American* children.
- *Clinical picture*: Thigh and knee pain and *limping*.

- **On exam**: Passive hip flexion is associated with an *external rotational* movement.
- **Diagnosis**: *Medio-posterior* displacement of femoral head on *frog leg lateral views* hip X-ray.
- **Complication**: *Avascular necrosis* of femoral head.
- **Treatment**: Surgical fixation.

Miscellaneous Lower Limb Injuries

- **Ankle sprain**: Due to injury of the *anterior talofibular ligament*. No fracture is involved. Treatment: Ice packs and early mobilization.
- **Jone's fracture**: Occurs with foot inversion, where the *5th metatarsal tuberosity is avulsed.*
- **Pott's fracture**: Occurs with foot eversion, where the medial malleolus is avulsed.
- **Lover fracture**: Occurs in patient falling from a height *landing on his heels*. Fracture involves the *calceneous, neck of femur,* and *lumbar vertebrae.*

Osteomyelitis

- **Mechanism**: Infection of the bone, directly from a nearby septic focus or through seeding from the blood stream in cases of bacteremia.
- **Pathology**: Bone death (*Sequesterum*) and new bone formation (*Involucrum*).
- **Most common organism**: *Staphylococcus aureus. Salmonella is common in patients with sickle cell disease, but S. aureus is still the most common organism.*
- **Clinical picture**: Red, warm, tender and swollen limb.
- **Diagnosis**:

  1. Gold standard to diagnose osteomyelitis in general: *Bone biopsy.*
  2. Radiological test of choice for acute cases: *MRI.*
  3. Radiological test of choice for chronic cases: *X-ray*; shows *periosteal elevation.*
  4. Practically: Bone scan – it is very sensitive; however, it is *not specific.*

- **Treatment**: Admit to hospital and start *4–6 weeks* course of intravenous penicillinase resistant penicillin.

Bone Tumors

Refer to Table 5.3 for the most common bone tumors.

Emergencies

Burns

- **Types**: Depends on the surface area involved:

  1. *Minor*: Less than *15%* of body surface area.
  2. *Major*: More than *15%* of body surface area.

- **Degrees**: Multiple classifications exist; the most common are:

  1. *1st degree*: Erythema, e.g., sunburn Heals in one week without scarring.
  2. *2nd degree*: Vesicles, with injury to most of the *dermis.*
  3. *3rd degree*: Injury to the *subcutaneous tissue.*
  4. *4th degree*: Injury to *muscles, ligaments and bones.*

- **Complications**:

  1. Shock: Neurogenic, hypovolemic or even septic shock.
  2. Pulmonology: Edema of the airways.
  3. GI: Stress ulcer of the duodenum (*Curling ulcer*).
  4. Fluid: Dehydration and hemoconcentration.

- **Treatment**: First thing to do is *ABC: A*irway maintenance by intubation, *B*reathing support by mechanical ventilation, *C*irculation maintenance by establishing wide bore IV lines and starting aggressive fluid resuscitation using *6 ratios* of plasma.
- **Notes**:

  1. Plasma ration = Body weight in kg × % of body burned / 2.

TABLE 5.3 Bone tumors.

	Ewing sarcoma	Osteogenic sarcoma	Giant cell tumor
Location	Diaphysis of long bones	Metaphysis of long bones	Epiphyseal end of long bones
Unique feature	Onion skin appearance on X-ray	Sun ray appearance and Codman triangle on X-ray due to elevation of the periosteum	Soap bubble appearance on X-ray
Notes	Translocation t11;22	Most common malignant bone tumor	Benign tumor with spindle shaped and multinucleated giant cells
Treatment	Amputation + Radiation therapy	Amputation + Chemotherapy	Amputation + Radiation therapy

2. Rations are given as 3 in the first 12 h, 2 in the second 12 h, and 1 in the last 12 h.
3. Cleaning of the wounds and grafting if needed.

ABCD of Emergency

- **A (Airway)**: Immobilize the neck, open airway by jaw thrust and clear the airway of any foreign bodies.
- **B (Breathing)**:
  1. If patient is breathing, move to C.
  2. If not breathing, intubate the patient with a cuffed endotracheal tube (*Use uncuffed tube for children below 8 years of age*).
  3. If not breathing and cannot intubate, do *cricothyrotomy*.
- **C (Circulation)**:
  1. Most sensitive indicator for intravascular volume is the *pulse*.
  2. Most sensitive indicator for capillary circulation is the *rate of capillary refill*.
  3. Best place to check for pulse is *carotid artery* (In infants, *brachial artery* is the best).
  4. Wide bore IV line has to be established within *90 seconds*, and CPR (cardiopulmonary resuscitation) should be immediately started if the patient has no pulse.
  5. Best IV fluid is *lactated ringer*; however aggressive hydration is contraindicated for patients with *myocarditis* and *hypoplastic left heart syndrome*.
- **D (Drugs)**: LANE (*L*idocaine, *A*tropine, *N*arcan, *E*pinephrine) could be given through endotracheal tube.

Toxicology

Introduction

- **First aid**: First measure in any patient with any toxicity is securing an *A*irway, maintaining *B*reathing, and establishing *C*irculation (ABC).
- **Activated charcoal**: Helps decrease or even block absorption of toxins in the stomach, and it works for everything except *Lithium, Iron* and *Cyanide* (*LIC*).

Lead

- **Clinical picture**: Patient who just moved to a house with classic old *paints* and *pipe system*, now presenting with *abdominal pain* and *anemia*.

- **Diagnosis**: High blood lead (*>20 mcg/dl*), RBC protoporphyrin and zinc protoporphyrin levels. Also a pathognomonic finding is *basophilic stippling of the RBCs*, which can be detected by *Wright Geimsa* stain.
- **Antidote**: *EDTA* or *Dimercaprol (Succimer)*.
- **Note:** Ethylenedia menetetracetic acid (EDTA) can cause fatal *hypocalcemia* on rapid IV infusion.

Ethylene Glycol (Anti-Freeze)

- **Clinical picture**: *High anion gap metabolic acidosis*, and *oxalate crystals* in urine.
- **Treatment**: *Ethanol and hemodialysis*.
- **Note:** Methanol (Bootleg) (Moonshine) is converted inside the body into formic acid and formaldehyde, which cause *high anion gap metabolic acidosis* and *blindness*, respectively. Treatment: *Ethanol*.

Cyanide

- **Introduction**: Has a *bitter almond* odor, and makes the blood *cherry red* in color.
- **Mechanism**: Inhibits cytochrome oxidase and cellular oxygen uptake.
- **Cause**: Cyanide toxicity is common to happen due to prolonged *Na nitroprusside* infusion.
- **Treatment**: *Nitrites* and *Sodium thiosulfate*.

Organophosphates

- **Introduction**: Present in *insecticides* and *nerve gas*.
- **Mechanism**: Irreversible inhibition of cholinesterase enzyme.
- **Clinical picture**: Cholinergic symptoms, e.g., Salivation, diarrhea, vomiting, miosis.
- **Treatment:** Cholinestrase reactivator, e.g., Pralidoxime.

Arsenic

- **Introduction**: Heavy metal with *garlic* odor that interferes with *oxidative phosphorylation*.
- **Clinical picture**: *Polyneuritis, skin hyperpigmentation*, liver and kidney failure.
- **Treatment**: Gastric lavage, *Dimercaprol* and hemodialysis.

Opioids

- **Clinical picture**: *Pinpoint pupils*, respiratory depression and hypothermia.
- **Antidote**: *Naloxone*.
- **Remember:** BDZ are reversed by Flumazenil, not Naloxone.

Carbon Monoxide

- **Clinical picture**: It is winter time and a family has been spending the entire weekend at home *in front of the fireplace*. Now they *all* presented to the ER with *confusion*, *headache* and *dizziness*. Another classic example is a patient who tried to commit suicide by locking himself in his garage with his car engine running.
- **Treatment:** *Hyperbaric* or *100% oxygen*, and treat the cause.

Mercury

- **Clinical picture**: *Ataxia,* vomiting, diarrhea and renal failure.
- **Treatment**: Dimercaprol or Penicillamine.

Iron

- **Clinical picture**: *Hemorrhagic gastroenteritis.*
- **Treatment**: Iron chelators, e.g., *Desferrioxamine.*

Chapter 6
Pediatrics

Breast Feeding

Introduction

- *Timing:* Most infants start feeding within the *first 6 hours after birth.*
- *Most important factor for efficient breast feeding: Adequate hydration of mother.*
- *Type of milk*: Colostrum is the main breast milk during the *first 7–10 days* after labor, after which it transforms to the established form. Colostrum has a high content of proteins, macrophages, immunoglobulins, epidermal growth factor (*for GI epithelization*), and small amount of calories compared to established milk.

Advantages of Human Milk

- ***Bifidus factor***: A *glycoprotein* that stimulates the growth of *lactobacillus bifidus* and *lactobacillus acidophilus* in the infant's intestine. Lactobacilli convert lactose to lactic acid; which kills pathogens and promotes absorption of *calcium* and *iron.*
- ***Essential fatty acids***: e.g., *Linoleic, linolenic and arachidonic acids.* They are essential for maturation of the CNS.
- ***Iron***: High iron content with high bioavailability, hence, routine iron supplementation is not needed before *6 months* of age in breast fed infants.
- ***Lactoferrin***: Bacteriostatic to *E. coli.* Mechanism: *Iron chelation.*

- ***Immunoglobulins***: Mainly *IgA*, and to a lesser extent IgM and IgG.

Non-Human Milk

- ***Introduction***: Contains more *phosphate* than human milk, *which inhibits iron absorption.*
- ***Cow and buffalo milk***: Most common commercial milk. Cow milk (though rich in *potassium* and *proteins*) causes iron deficiency anemia, allergy, malabsorption, hypocalcemia, and vitamin C deficiency.
- ***Goat milk***: The least allergic; however, it is deficient in *folic acid.*

Forms of Feeding

- ***First 6 months***: Breast feeding.
- ***6–12 months***: Mixed feeding, i.e., Breast milk and solid food.
- ***12 months onwards***: Solid food.

Weight

- ***After birth***: Sudden weight drop, followed by weight gain.
- ***Day 7 to day 14***: Plateau of infant's weight.
- ***Day 14***: A second drop of weight to baseline.
- ***4 months of age***: Normally, weight should be *double the birth weight.*

Troubleshooting

- *Milk engorgement*: Breast is full, tense and tender. *Prevention*: Early and regular breast feeding. *Treatment*: Evacuation, ice packs and NSAIDs.
- *Nipple abnormalities*: e.g., Retracted or inverted nipple. *Treatment*: Manual expression of the milk using suction pump.

Notes

- Best schedule of breast feeding is *on demand,* i.e., Whenever the infant needs to be fed. Another recommended schedule is:

  1. 0–3 months: *6 feeds/day.*
  2. 3–6 months: *5 feeds/day.*
  3. 6–12 months: *4 feeds/day.*

- HIV is a contraindication for breast feeding.
- Hepatitis B is a contraindication for breast feeding, *unless the guidelines are followed,* i.e., The newborn should receive *hepatitis B immunoglobulin and vaccine at birth.*
- Premature milk formulas are rich in *cystine.*
- Iron deficiency is common in infants by *6 months of age* once solid food is introduced; accordingly, *15 mg/day* of FeSO4 starting the *5th month* is necessary. So when you see an infant in the USMLE who is older than 6 months of age and having anemia, you know what to think!

Development

- *Milestones*: Refer to Table 6.1 for developmental milestones.
- *Tanner staging*: Refer to Table 6.2 for Tanner staging.
- *Order of maturation*:

  1. Males: Testes → Penis → Growth spurt → Pubic hair.
  2. Females: Telarche (Breast development) → Growth spurt → Pubarche (Pubic hair development) → Menarche (Menstruation).

Cardiovascular System

Embryology

- *Heart tube*: Two heart tubes form in the *mesoderm.* Lateral folding fuses the two into the *primitive heart tube.* The primitive heart tube gives rise to the *endocardium,* while the mesoderm surrounding the tube gives rise to *myocardium and epicardium.*
- ***The heart tube has 5 dilatations***:

  1. *Truncus arteriosus*: Gives rise to *aorta* and *pulmonary trunk.*
  2. *Bulbous cordis*: Gives rise to the *smooth parts of right and left ventricles* (*Conus arteriosus*) and the *aortic vestibule.*
  3. *Primary ventricle*: Gives rise to *trabeculated parts of both ventricles.*
  4. *Primary atrium*: Gives rise to *trabeculated parts of both atria.*
  5. *Sinus venosus*: Gives rise to *smooth part of right atrium, the oblique vein of left atrium* and the *coronary sinus.*

- *Smooth part of left atrium*: Forms by *fusion of the pulmonary veins and left atrial wall.* Note: The line between the smooth and trabeculated parts of the atria is an important landmark known as the *crista terminalis.*
- *Aorticopulmonary septum*: Formed from the *neural crest* and extends to *separate the aorta and pulmonary trunk.*
- *Atrioventricular (AV) septum*: Formed by *fusion of the ventral and dorsal AV cushions.* Abnormal septum formation results in a *unilateral heart* or *tricuspid atresia.*
- *Interatrial septum*:

  1. Septum primum grows craniocaudally towards the AV septum carrying the foramen primum in its lower edge.
  2. As the septum primum fuses with the AV septum, the foramen primum disappears and foramen secundum forms in the middle part of the septum primum.
  3. The septum secundum grows caudocranially to the right of the septum primum carrying the foramen ovale in its wall.
  4. After birth, septum primum and secundum fuse and the foramen ovale closes.

- *Interventricular septum*:

  1. Muscular part: Grows caudocranially and stops short of the AV septum, leaving a gap.
  2. Membranous part: Fills the gap and joins the muscular portion, completing the IV septum.

- *Timing*: Heart formation is complete and functioning by the *4th week of gestation.*
- *Congenital heart diseases*: Incidence rate is *1%,* which increases to *6% among newborns with family history of congenital heart disease.*

TABLE 6.1 Developmental milestones.

Age	Milestones
1 month	Raising head from prone position, reaction to sounds
2 months	Raising chest from the floor, smiling
3 months	Maintaining "head up" position, cooing
4–5 months	Rolling on the floor, sitting supported
6–7 months	Sitting unsupported, babbling, recognizing strangers
8 months	Saying "papa" and "mama" to anybody
9 months	Creeping, crawling, waves bye-bye
10–11 months	Saying "mama" only to mom, and "papa" only to dad + One new word
12 months	Walking unsupported, Throwing objects, 2 new words
13–14 months	3 new words
15 months	Creeping upstairs, walking backwards, 4–5 new words
18 months	Running, copying others' actions, playing with other children
21 months	Walking upstairs, squatting, asking for food
24 months	Walking upstairs and downstairs, parallel play
30 months	Jumping, holding pen
3 years	Riding tricycle, knowing full name, group play
5 years	Performing complex tasks, e.g., Tying shoes

TABLE 6.2 Tanner staging.

Stage	Breast	Pubic hair	Male genitalia
I	Elevation of nipple	No pubic hair	Small genitalia
II	Breastbud	Sparse fair colored hair, only at base of genitalia	Enlargement of testes and scrotum
III	Increased size of breastbud and areola	Hair gets darker, curlier and starts spreading	Increase in penile length
IV	Further elevation of nipple, a.k.a. secondary mound	Hair is similar to adult type in shape, but there is lack of hair on medial side of thighs	Increase in penile breadth, full development of glans and thickening and darkening of scrotal skin
V	Mature breast	Mature pubic hair Stage VI: Hair grows up linea alba, a.k.a. Male escutcheon	Mature genitalia

- **Shunts**: All congenital heart defects discussed below are *left to right shunts*, except for three (*right to left*): *T*GA, *T*runcus arteriosus and *T*etralogy of Fallot
- **Prostaglandin E1**: Used in cyanotic heart diseases to maintain a Patent Ductus Arteriosus (PDA). If PGE1 is given and the patient develops pulmonary edema, this indicates an *anomalous pulmonary venous return (APVR) with obstruction.*
- **Hyperoxia test**: Administer 100% oxygen and check PO2 on arterial blood gases:

  1. PO2 >200: No congenital heart disease.
  2. PO2 <150: Congenital heart disease.
  3. PO2 <50: TGA, Ebstein anomaly or anomalous pulmonary venous return.

Persistent Truncus Arteriosus

- **Mechanism**: *If the aorticopulmonary septum does not develop completely*, the truncus arteriosus persists with a right-to-left shunt through a *large VSD*.
- **Clinical picture**: *Cyanosis, water hammer pulse* and a *systolic murmur.*

- **Treatment**: *Diuretics* and *digoxin* followed by surgical correction.

Transposition of Great Arteries (TGA)

- **Introduction**: *The most common cyanotic cardiac anomaly.*
- **Mechanism**: *Improper twisting of the aorticopulmonary septum*, leading to the aorta originating from RV, and pulmonary artery from LV.
- **On exam**: Right ventricular heave and harsh pansystolic murmur.
- **Pathology**: These patients have right ventricular hypertrophy giving the heart an "*egg-shaped*" silhouette on CXR.
- **Treatment**: Digoxin, diuretics and *prostaglandin E1 to keep the ductus arteriosus open* until surgical correction is performed.
- **Note**: *Without a PDA, these patients die in a couple of months.*

Tetralogy of Fallot

- **Mechanism**: *Abnormal migration of neural crest cells*, leading to displacement of the infundibular septum.
- **Tetralogy**: Pulmonary stenosis, Right ventricular hypertrophy, Overriding aorta and VSD.
- **Clinical picture**:

  1. Cyanosis: Starts at 3–6 months of age (*Never at birth*).
  2. Cyanotic (Tet) spells: Attacks of infundibular spasm associated with any exercise or infection.

- **On exam**:

  1. Patient is in *squatting position*: Increases venous return, hence decreases hypoxia.
  2. Systolic murmur at the left sternal border.

- **CXR**: *Boot shaped heart*.
- **Treatment**: Surgical correction, e.g., Blalock Taussig.
- **Treatment of tet spells**: Put the patient in squatting (or knee-chest) position and administer IV fluids, beta blockers, morphine to decrease ventilations and phenylephrine to increase SVR. Oxygen is only minimally effective since the problem is decreased pulmonary blood flow.

Ebstein Anomaly

- **Mechanism**: *Prolapse of the tricuspid valve into a hypoplastic right ventricle.*
- **Pathology**: Patients have *patent foramen ovale*, resulting in *dilated left atrium*.
- **Complications**: *Supraventricular tachycardia* and *Wolf Parkinson White syndrome*.
- **Treatment**: *Digoxin, diuretics* and *prostaglandin E1.*

Ventricular Septal Defect (VSD)

- **Mechanism**: *Failed fusion of the right and left bulbar ridges with the AV cushions.*
- **Location**: Most commonly in the *membranous part* of the IV septum.
- **Pathology**: Begins as a left-to-right shunt at birth but the shunt reverses due to pulmonary hypertension. This shunt reversal is known as *Eisenmenger syndrome*.
- **Clinical picture**: Cyanosis and *recurrent chest infections*.
- **On exam**: *Harsh pansystolic murmur* all over the precordium.
- **CXR**: Biventricular enlargement and left atrial dilatation.

- **Treatment**: The defect usually closes spontaneously by *age 7*; otherwise, surgical correction is required.

Atrial Septal Defect (ASD)

- **Mechanism**: *Persistent ostium secundum* or less likely an ostium primum defect.
- **Clinical picture**: Most cases are asymptomatic and have a *wide fixed and split S2*.
- **CXR**: Right atrium and right ventricle dilatation.
- **Treatment**: Most cases do not require treatment. Complicated cases are treated surgically by closing the defect with a pericardial patch.
- **Note**: *Holt-Oram syndrome: ASD + Multiple congenital skeletal anomalies.*

Patent Ductus Arteriosus (PDA)

- **Pathology**: Ductus arteriosus normally closes *2 weeks after birth*. PDA is more common in *premature infants* and in *congenital rubella syndrome*, due to *high prostaglandin E levels*.
- **Clinical picture**:

  1. Hyperdynamic circulation.
  2. *Wide pulse pressure*, i.e., High systolic and low diastolic pressure.
  3. *Machine-like murmur* heard best on the pulmonary area (*Left 2nd space*).

- **Treatment**: Anti-prostaglandin, e.g., *Indomethacin*.

Hypoplastic Right Heart Syndrome

- **Causes**: Tricuspid atresia, or pulmonary atresia with an intact septum.
- **Pathology**: Most cases also have VSD, ASD or PDA, resulting in *left* ventricular hypertrophy.
- **Treatment**: *Prostaglandin E1* until surgical correction can be performed.

Hypoplastic Left Heart Syndrome

- **Introduction**: *Most common congenital heart disease to cause death in the first month of life.*
- **Pathology**: Hypoplastic left ventricle, along with mitral and aortic atresia.
- **Association**: PDA and ASD to maintain circulation through a left to right shunt.
- **Treatment**: PGE1 and heart transplant.

Respiratory System

Hyaline Membrane Disease (Respiratory Distress Syndrome)

- *Mechanism*: Deficiency of surfactant secreted by *type II pneumocytes*.
- *Incidence*: More common among *premature* and *low birth weight* infants.
- *Pathology*: Surfactant production is suppressed by *asphyxia* and increased by *thyroxin and cortisol*.
- *Clinical picture*: *A newborn in respiratory distress and cyanosis due to collapsed alveoli.*
- *CXR*: Diffuse *ground glass appearance*. Refer to Fig. 6.1.
- *Detection*: Amniotic fluid's *Lecithin/Sphingomyelin ratio <1.5.*
- *Complication*: Bronchopulmonary hypertrophy and squamous dysplasia.
- *Treatment*:

    1. Steroids (Betamethasone) to mother before premature delivery to accelerate fetal lung maturity.
    2. Mechanical ventilation and artificial surfactant.

Cystic Fibrosis

- *Mechanism*: Mutation of *CFTR gene* on the long arm of *chromosome 7, which controls chloride channels*. It is an *autosomal recessive* disease, due to *3 base deletion of phenylalanine*.
- *Clinical picture*:

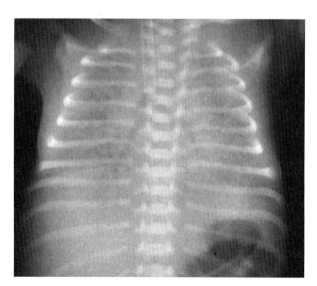

FIG. 6.1 CXR showing hyaline membrane disease (Neonatal RDS)

1. Recurrent respiratory infections: Mainly *Pseudomonas cepacia* and *Staphylococcus aureus*.
2. Malabsorption and steatorrhea: Deficiency of vitamins *A, D, E and K*.
3. Infertility and meconium ileus: Due to viscid secretions.
4. Dehydration: Hyponatremia and metabolic alkalosis.

- *On exam*: Clubbing is present in all cases.
- *CXR*: *Bleb sign*.
- *PFTs*: Mixed obstructive and restrictive pattern.
- *Diagnosis*: *Sweat chloride test*; level of more than *60 meq* is diagnostic.
- *Treatment*: Chest physiotherapy, antibiotics and pancreatic enzymes.

Alpha-1 Anti-Trypsin Deficiency

- *Mechanism*: Inherited deficiency leading to *congenital panacinar emphysema*.
- *Pathology*: Emphysema is dilatation of the airspaces *distal to terminal bronchioles*, and is normally centroacinar, except in this disease where it is *panacinar*.
- *Clinical picture*:

    1. Congenital dyspnea and wheezing.
    2. Recurrent hepatitis. So keep your eyes open in the USMLE for this patient who was born with emphysema and is presenting with elevated transaminases.

- *Diagnosis*:

    1. Low or undetectable alpha-1 anti-trypsin level.
    2. PFTs: Show obstructive picture ($FEV1/FVC <80$).
    3. Chest X-ray: Hyperinflated lungs and flattened diaphragm.

- *Treatment*: Alpha-1 anti-trypsin replacement.
- *Note*: Patients with emphysema have a tendency to form bullae. The bullae here are mainly *basal*, while in acquired emphysema or COPD, they are apical.

Kartagener's Syndrome (Immotile Cilia Syndrome)

- *Pathology*: Ciliary dysmotility due to a *defective dynein arm*.
- *Clinical picture*: SSSS: Recurrent *S*inusitis, *S*terility, *S*itus inversus, e.g., Dextrocardia and Bronchiectasi*S*.

Infectious Diseases

Croup

- *Cause*: Multiple, but most common is *parainfluenza-1*.
- *Clinical picture*: Croup is *laryngo-tracheo-bronchitis*, as follows:

  1. Laryngitis: Hoarseness of voice.
  2. Trachiitis: Retrosternal pain and *brassy, metallic barking cough*.
  3. Bronchitis: *Barking cough* and expectoration.
  4. Stridor: It is *noisy inspiration* due to *upper airways* narrowing (*Note: Asthma and emphysema cause noisy expiration "wheezing" due to lower airways narrowing*).

- *Diagnosis*: Neck X-ray: *Subglottic narrowing (Steeple sign)*. Refer to Fig. 6.2.
- *Treatment*:

  1. Supportive treatment till viral infection resolves.
  2. Stridor: *Racemic epinephrine nebulizer inhalation*.
  3. Oxygen and systemic steroids are reserved for severe cases.

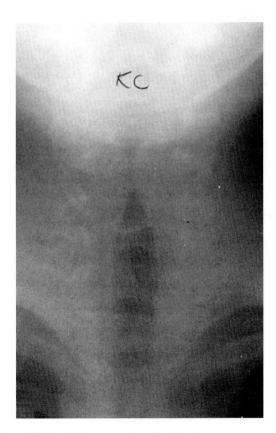

FIG. 6.2 Neck X-ray showing steeple sign

- *Note*: Vascular rings also cause barking cough, but examination of the patient and radiological work up is completely normal.

Epiglottitis

- *Cause*: Multiple, but most common is *Haemophilus influenza B. This organism grows only in the presence of NAD and hematin (Factors V and X)*.
- *Clinical picture*:

  1. Fever.
  2. *Hyperextended neck with the patient leaning forwards (Dog sniffing position)*.
  3. *Persistent copious drooling*.
  4. Sore throat and hoarseness of voice (*Hot potato voice*).
  5. Stridor and respiratory distress in severe cases.

- *Diagnosis*:

  1. Lateral view neck X-ray: Edematous epiglottis (*Thumbs-up sign*). Refer to Fig. 6.3.
  2. Definitive diagnosis is through direct visualization of a *swollen cherry red epiglottis*; however, *examination of the oropharynx in any case suspicious for epiglottitis is contraindicated,* unless it is done in the operating room, with easy access to cardio-pulmonary support measures. The concern here is how easy these patients can have *laryngospasm* and complete airway obstruction by any minimal manipulation of the oropharynx.

- *Treatment*:

  1. First thing to do is *secure an airway* by intubating the patient. If in emergency situation, and the airway has collapsed, do *cricothyrotomy*.
  2. Antibiotics: Drug of choice is *3rd generation cephalosporins, e.g., Cefuroxime*.

- *Note*: Hot potato voice is also a sign of *peri-tonsillar abscess*. Clinical picture: Sore throat, odynophagia and hot potato voice, *but no hyperextended neck, drooling or stridor*.

Bronchiolitis

- *Age*: 4 months–18 months (*Rare in patients older than 18 months*).
- *Cause*: Multiple, but most common is *Respiratory Syncytial Virus (RSV),* followed by *mycoplasma*.
- *Pathology*: Inflammation of the *respiratory bronchioles*, along with excessive secretions and wall edema, leading to airway narrowing.

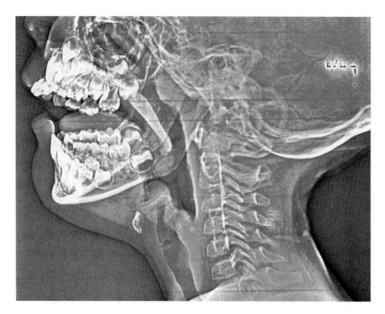

FIG. 6.3 Thumb up sign of epiglottitis

- **Clinical picture**: Cough and expectoration.
- **On exam**: Crackles and wheezing on chest auscultation.
- **CXR**: *Hyperinflated chest.*
- **Complications**: Respiratory failure and apnea.
- **Treatment**:

  1. Hospitalization, IV fluids and oxygen.
  2. Anti-viral: Best for RSV is *Ribavirin*, and for mycoplasma is *erythromycin*.

Whooping Cough (Pertussis)

- **Cause**: Bordetella pertussis.
- **Mechanism**: Toxin activates *cAMP (Through ADP ribosylation, by inhibiting Gi protein)*. This stimulates the release of *histamine* and *insulin*, and *inhibits phagocytosis*.
- **Clinical picture**:

  1. Catarrhal phase (1–2 weeks): Fever, cough and expectoration.
  2. Paroxysmal phase (4–8 weeks): Paroxysms of cough followed by a stridor, a.k.a. *inspiratory whoop*. The pathognomonic feature is *vomiting immediately following these paroxysms*.
  3. Convalescent phase (Months): Mild cough that resolves gradually.

- **Complication**:

  1. Bronchopneumonia: *It is the most common complication.*
  2. Bronchiectasis: It is the second most common, however, *very specific*.

- **Diagnosis**: Unique presentation, plus:

  1. Leukocytosis: Namely *atypical lymphocytosis*.
  2. Sputum culture: Bordetella pertussis grows on *Bordet Gengou agar*.
  3. Normal ESR.

- **Treatment**: *Erythromycin for 14 days.*
- **Notes**:

  1. There is *no transplacental immunity* against pertussis. Immunity against pertussis is only cell mediated, while the transplacental immunity is humoral.
  2. There is *no post-infectious immunity* against pertussis.
  3. *B. Pertussis* and *C. Diphtheria* are both ex*tracellular* organisms releasing ex*o*toxins.

Scarlet Fever (Scarlatina)

- **Cause**: *Group A beta-hemolytic streptococcus.*
- **Clinical picture**:

  1. Scarlet rash: *Sandpaper-like punctate erythematous rash.* It starts in the neck, axilla and groin. Fate of rash: Desquamation; starts in fingers and toes.
  2. Fever: High grade.
  3. Swollen erythematous tonsils, covered by pus and exudates.
  4. *Strawberry tongue*: Starts *white with red dots*, then becomes *red with white dots*.
  5. Flushed cheeks with *circum-oral pallor*.
  6. *Pastia lines*: Erythematous lines in skin creases.

- **Complications**: Post-strept. glomerulonephritis and rheumatic fever.
- **Diagnosis**: Oropharngeal swab to check for strepto-coccal antigens.
- **Treatment**: *Penicillin 40 mg/kg/day for 10–14 days.*
- **Note**: If patient is allergic to penicillin, the alternative is *erythromycin.*

Botulism

- **Cause**: Clostridium botulinum; a Gram-positive, spore forming anaerobe.
- **Mechanism**: Toxins prevent acetylcholine release at neuromuscular junction.
- **Source**: Canned foods and honey. A typical case in the USMLE is for an infant whose parents put honey in his milk bottle.
- **Clinical picture**:

  1. Flaccid paralysis: *Descending marsh from head to toe*, a.k.a. *Floppy baby.*
  2. Ds: Dilated pupils, Diplopia, Dysphagia, Dysar-thria, Diminished gag reflex.

- **Diagnosis**: Detection of toxins in *stools (Best)* or serum.
- **Treatment**:

  1. First next step is to *secure an airway by intubating the patient.*
  2. Botulinum antitoxin: Even before confirming the diagnosis.

Diphtheria

- **Cause**: Corynobacterium diphtheria; a *non-spore forming bacillus.*
- **Mechanism**: Colonizes in the *pharynx* releasing *exo-toxins* targeting CVS & CNS.
- **Clinical picture**: Fever, chills, sore throat and bark-ing cough; often confused with croup.
- **On exam**: *Grey pseudomembrane* on pharynx. His-tologically, it is formed of C. Diphtheria, necrotic tissue, WBCs and fibrin.
- **Diagnosis**: Culture on *Loeffler* or *Tellurite* media.
- **Complications**: Respiratory failure, myocarditis, bulbar palsy or even LMNL (Combined motor and sensory loss).
- **Treatment**: Treat Diphtheria with (*DAD*):

  1. *Diphtheria antitoxin.*
  2. Antibiotics: *Penicillin is the drug of choice.* If PCN allergy exists, erythromycin.
  3. DPT vaccination: As there is *no post-infectious immunity.*

- **Notes**:

  1. Diphtheria toxins can only be produced in patients *with iron deficiency.*
  2. Exotoxin of Diphtheria works through its (A) portion by inhibiting *Elongation Factor 2 (EF2)* and protein synthesis. This is achieved by *ADP ribosylation.*
     Factor 2 (EF2) and protein synthesis. This is achieved by *ADP ribosylation.*

Lyme Disease

- **Cause**: *Borrelia Burgdorferi; a spirochete.*
- **Transmission**: *Ixodes tick (Deer tick).*
- **Clinical picture**:

  1. Stage 1: *Erythema Chronicum Migrans* (ECM). Ring-shaped lesion with central clearing. Refer to Fig. 6.4.
  2. Stage 2:

     - Arthralgias and arthritis.
     - CVS injury, e.g., Myocarditis, A-V block.
     - CNS injury, e.g., Meningitis, bilateral Bell's palsy.

  3. Stage 3: Chronic arthritis and encephalopathy.

- **Prevention**: Vaccination, e.g., Lymerix, Immulyme, before going to infested areas, i.e., *Northeast, Mid-west and west coast.*
- **Diagnosis**: *Clinical*, as antibodies against Borrelia Burgdorferi cross react with other organisms.
- **Treatment**:

  1. Less than 8 years of age: *Oral amoxicillin for 21 days.*
  2. Older than 8 years of age: *Oral doxycycline for 21 days.*
  3. If CNS or CVS injury: *Parenteral ceftriaxone or penicillin G for 21 days.*

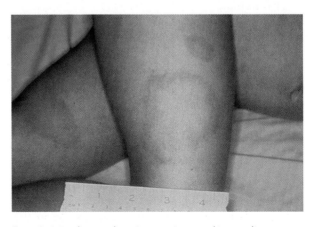

Fɪɢ. 6.4 Erythema chronicum migrans of Lyme disease

Rocky Mountain Spotted Fever

- *Cause*: *Rickettsia rickettsii.*
- *Geographical distribution*: *Southeast, and ohio river valley.*
- *Clinical picture*: Fever and *petechial* (Spotted) *rash, starting at wrists and ankles,* and spreading proximally.
- *Complications*: Thrombocytopenia, CVS or CNS injury.
- *Treatment*: *Tetracycline.* Must be started within *5 days* from onset of symptoms.

Infectious Mononucleosis

- *Cause*: *Epstein Barr virus (EBV),* and less likely Cytomegalovirus (CMV).
- *Transmission*: Mostly through saliva, hence the name *kissing disease.*
- *Clinical picture*: Fever, chills, fatigue, sore throat due to pharyngitis and abdominal pain due to splenomegaly.
- *On exam*:

  1. *Petechiae* on hard and soft palate.
  2. Multiple enlarged and tender cervical lymphadenopathy.
  3. *Splenomegaly*: Lower edge is palpated just below the costal margin.

- *CBC*: *Atypical lymphocytosis,* and *anemia due to antibodies against Li antigen of RBCs.*
- *Diagnosis*: *Monospot test*: Positive heterophil antibodies against sheep RBCs.
- *Contraindication*: Penicillin causes rash in these patients.
- *Complication*: Splenic rupture. So when you see a patient in the USMLE with features of mononucleosis who goes to wrestle, and then comes to the ER with excruciating abdominal pain, you know what to think!
- *Treatment*: Self resolving.

Measles

- *Early clinical picture*:

  1. *CCC*: Cough, coryza and conjunctivitis.
  2. *Koplik spots*: Red lesions with white center on buccal mucosa.

- *Late clinical picture*: Rash: Maculopapular and confluent, starts behind the ears and descend downwards. It heals with branny desquamation in the same fashion, i.e., From the top downwards.

- *Complications*:

  1. *Most common*: Pneumonia. Early due to measles, or late due to secondary bacterial infection.
  2. *Most specific*: Subacute sclerosing pan-encephalitis (*SSPE*).

- *Note*: Measles is a predisposing factor for *vitamin A deficiency.*
- *Rubella*: Known as *German measles* or *3 days measles.* Also starts with cough, coryza and conjunctivitis and the rash has a descending marsh. The differentiating points are:

  1. Koplik spots are pathognomonic for measles, while *post-auricular* and *posterior cervical lymphadenopathy* is pathognomonic for rubella.
  2. Rash of measles is confluent, while that of rubella is not.

Mumps

- *Clinical picture*: Swollen salivary glands, mainly the *parotids*
- *Complications*:

  1. *Most common*: Pancreatitis.
  2. *Most dangerous*: Endocardial fibroelastosis.
  3. *Orchitis*: Might cause testicular atrophy and sterility.
  4. *Sensorineural* hearing loss.

Roseola Infantum (Exanthem Subitum)

- *Cause*: *Human Herpes virus 6.*
- *Clinical picture*: *High grade fever,* followed by rash on the trunk which *spreads distally* towards the extremities as it fades away.

Erythema Infectiosum (Fifth Disease)

- *Cause*: *Parvovirus.*
- *Clinical picture*: *Slapped cheeks* appearance and maculopapular rash that *starts in the arms,* and spreads *proximally* to the trunk then to lower extremities.

Chicken Pox

- *Cause*: *Varicella zoster virus.*
- *Clinical picture*: *Crops of lesions* in various stages of development at the same time, i.e., Macules, papules, crusted, healing. Rash is *vesicular* and is characterized by the pathognomonic *teardrop-shaped vesicles (a.k.a. Dew drops on a rose petal).* Refer to Fig. 6.5.

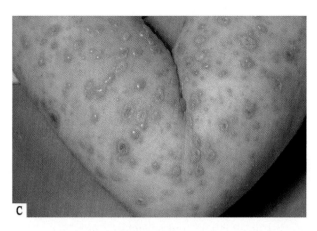

FIG. 6.5 Rash of Chickenpox

- **Complication**: Extension to *cerebellum*. So, when you see a patient with chicken pox in the USMLE who suddenly started developing ataxia and incoordination, you know what to think!
- **Note**: If a patient who just gave birth has a chicken pox for less than 2 days, isolate the neonate and give him varicella zoster immunoglobulin. If more than 2 days, it is too late to intervene.

Syphilis

- **Cause**: *Treponema pallidum*.
- **Incubation period**: *6 weeks*.
- **Congenital syphilis:** Transmits to fetus *after the 4th month of gestation*:

  1. *At birth*:
     - Atrophied dried nasal mucosa (*Snuffles*).
     - Hepatosplenomegaly.
     - Maculopapular rash and *severe periostitis*.

  2. *Childhood form*: Characterized by multiple pathognomonic findings:
     - E.N.T.: *Saddle nose* (Destroyed nasal bridge), *Hutchinson teeth* (Separated and notched upper central incisors), *Mulberry molars* (Molars with too many cusps) and *raghades* (Linear scars around the mouth).
     - Bone: *Sabre shins* (Inflamed bowed tibiae), *Clutton joints* (Painless effusion) and destruction of medial proximal tibial metaphysis (*Wimberger sign*).

- **Adulthood syphilis**:

  1. *Primary (6 weeks)*: Characterized by *painless chancre* and *painless lymphadenopathy*. Chancre is a *well demarcated* ulcer with *indurated base*, and it resolves spontaneously *without scar* formation.

  2. *Secondary*:
     - Rash: All forms *except vesicular*, i.e., Macular, papular, pustular, mixed, but *never vesicular*. Rash is more prominent *in palms and soles*.
     - Condyloma lata: Wart-like lesions on moist surfaces, e.g., Lips. *Highly contagious lesions*.

  3. *Latent*: 25% of patients have relapse during that period.
  4. *Tertiary*:
     - *Gummas*: Occur in skin (*Painless*) or bones (*Painful*).
     - CVS: Injury to vasa vasora of aorta, leading to *aortic aneurysm* and *aortic dissection*. Also causes coronary obstruction and aortic regurgitation.
     - Neurosyphilis: Multiple forms ranging from asymptomatic, to meningitis or even infarction. Pathognomonic presentations are:
       a. *Tabes dorsalis*: As explained in neurology, it targets the *dorsal column* (Causing ataxia), and *dorsal roots* (Causing loss of reflexes, pain and temperature sensation).
       b. General paresis of insane: Aphasia, confusion and seizures.
       c. *Argyl-Robertson pupil*: As explained in neurology, it *accommodates to near vision, but never reacts to light*.

- **Diagnosis**:

  1. Dark field microscopy: *Corkscrew movement*.
  2. Serology: Venereal Disease Research Laboratory (VDRL), Rapid Plasma Reagin (RPR), Treponema pallidum immobilization test (TPI) or *the most specific test Florescent Treponemal Antibodies (FTA)*.

- **Treatment**: *Penicillin* is the drug of choice for all patients, as follows:

  1. Congenital syphilis: Benzathine penicillin G for 10 days.
  2. Primary, secondary and early latent syphilis: Benzathine penicillin G 2.4 million units IM, *only once*.
  3. Late latent syphilis: Benzathine penicillin G 2.4 million units IM *weekly for 3 weeks*.
  4. Neurosyphilis: Procaine penicillin G 2.4 million units IM daily + Probenecid for *14 days*.

- **Notes**:

  1. Patients with penicillin allergy must get *desensitization*.
  2. *Jarish Herxheimer?s reaction*: Few days after starting treatment, patients develop sudden spike in temperature and worsening symptoms. This occurs

due to release of pyrogenes from killed bacteria. Treatment: Supportive, and continue treatment.

3. Indication of cure from syphilis: *fourfold decrease in titers.*

Herpangina

- *Cause*: Coxsackie A16 virus.
- *Clinical picture*: Sore throat and painful erythematous ulcers on corners of mouth.
- *Complication*: Spread of lesions to hand and feet (*Hand-foot-mouth syndrome*).

Immunization

- *Schedule*: Refer to Table 6.3 for the latest immunization guidelines.
- *Side effects of vaccines*:

  1. Pain, redness and swelling around injection site.
  2. Low grade fever.
  3. MMR: Rash, arthralgia, arthritis and mild parotid enlargement.

- *Note*:

  1. Polio vaccine is stored in very low temperature to remain active. Breast feeding is contraindicated 2 hours before and after polio immunization.

2. Diphtheria and tetanus vaccines are *toxoids*.
3. MMR is a *live attenuated vaccine*.
4. H. Influenza B is a *polysaccharide protein vaccine*.

Neurology

Cerebral Palsy

- *Definition*: Central *motor* deficit that occurs during brain formation.
- *Causes*: Multiple, the most common of which are *fetal hypoxia* (e.g., Placental insufficiency or obstructed labor), and *intrauterine infections*.
- *Clinical picture*:

  1. Paralysis: One or more or all limbs. *Again, pure motor paralysis, with no sensory deficits.*
  2. Hypertonia with spasticity: Affects *flexor muscles of upper limbs*, and *extensor muscles of lower limbs*.
  3. Hyperreflexia and *clonus*.
  4. Scissoring of lower limbs, arched back and contracture of Achilles tendon.
  5. Extra-pyramidal injury: Chorea and athetosis.

- *Treatment*: Physical, occupational and speech therapy.

TABLE 6.3 Immunization schedule.

Vaccine	Schedule
Hepatitis B	• Monovalent hepatitis B vaccine is given in a series of 3 shots: 0, 1 and 6 months of age If mother is hepatitis B positive, the newborn should receive the monovalent vaccine and hepatitis B immunoglobulin within the first 12 hours after birth
Hepatitis A	• A series of 2 shots: 12 and 18 months of age
Rotavirus	• A series of 3 shots: 2, 4 and 6 months of age

Diphtheria, Tetanus and Pertussis (DTaP)	• A series of 5 shots:
	  1. First three: 2, 4 and 6 months of age
	  2. Fourth shot: 18 months of age (12 months after the third dose)
	  3. Fifth shot: 5 years of age
	
	Booster: 11–12 years of age, and every 10 years from then onwards

Hemophilus influenza B (HiB)	• A series of 4 shots:
	  1. First three: 2, 4 and 6 months of age
	  2. Fourth shot: 12 months of age

Pneumococcal	• Similar to HiB

Inactivated polio	• A series of 4 shots:
	  1. First three: 2, 4 and 6 months of age
	  2. Fourth shot: 4 years of age

Measles, Mumps and Rubella (MMR)	• A series of 2 shots:
	  1. First shot: 12–15 months of age
	  2. Second shot: 4–6 years of age

Varicella	• Similar to MMR

Human Papilloma Virus (HPV)	• A series of 3 shots, approved for females only at this time:
	  1. First shot: 11 years of age
	  2. Second shot: 2 months after first shot
	  3. Third shot: 6 months after second shot

Meningococcal vaccine	• One shot at age 11–12 years

Craniostenosis

- **Definition**: Premature closure of one or more of the cranial suture lines.
- **Clinical picture**:

  1. Abnormally shaped skull.
  2. Increased intracranial pressure: Headache, blurry vision, nausea and vomiting.
  3. Ophthalmology: Optic atrophy and blindness.

- **Diagnosis**: Palpable ridge over the prematurely closed suture line. Skull X-ray shows *Silver beaten appearance*.
- **Types**:

  1. Acrocephaly: Due to premature closure of *coronal* and *lambdoid* sutures.
  2. *Scaphocepahly*: Due to premature closure of *sagittal* suture.
  3. Plagiocephaly: Due to unilateral closure of *coronal* suture.

- **Treatment**: Craniotomy and opening of the suture.

Febrile Convulsions

- **Definition**: *Tonic clonic seizures* due to *sudden rise* of body temperature above *38.5 °C*.
- **Mechanism**: Irritation of brain cells due to hyperthermia.
- **Diagnostic criteria**:

  1. Patient: *6 months–6 years old* with *normal CNS*.
  2. Fever: *Rapid* rise above *38.5 °C*.
  3. Convulsions: Tonic clonic, *less than 15 min in duration*, and is *recurrent*. After the seizure, the patient regains full consciousness and has no residual neurological deficits. *Accordingly, it is very easy to differentiate from epileptic seizures, as the latter are followed by a postictal state (Confusion, neurological deficits, Todd's paralysis)*.

- **Treatment**:

  1. Urgent decrease of body temperature.
  2. *Phenobarbitone*: Drug of choice if patient is still having seizures after controlling body temperature.

- **Notes**:

  1. Febrile convulsions is a *familial disease*.
  2. EEG is completely normal *2 weeks* after the attack.
  3. Of these patients, *2%* end up suffering from epileptic seizures later in life.

Retinoblastoma (Cat Eye)

- **Incidence**: Most common ocular malignancy in children.
- **Mechanism**: *Mutation of the RB gene, due to deletion of long arm of chromosome 13)*. This activates binding of a dephosphorylated protein to transcription factor E2F, causing *G1 arrest*.
- **Clinical picture**: White pupil (Leukocoria).
- **Treatment**: Surgical plus chemotherapy and radiation.
- **Notes**:

  1. Cataract is the most common cause of white pupil.
  2. Causes of congenital cataracts are toxoplasmosis, galactosemia and Down syndrome.

Retinitis Pigmentosa

- **Mechanism**: *Genetic, but could also occur due to abetalipoproteinemia*
- **Clinical picture**: *Tubular vision* and *night blindness*.
- **Treatment**: Supportive and vitamin A in abetalipoprotenemia.

Miscellaneous

- *Buphthalmos* (Congenital glaucoma): Either genetic or secondary to *congenital rubella syndrome*. The eyes and pupils are usually enlarged with deep anterior chambers and impending damage to the optic nerve.
- *Retrolental fibroplasias*: Oxygen induced retinopathy in premature infants.
- *Coloboma iridis*: Defect in the iris due to *failure of closure of choroid fissure*.
- *Retinal detachment*: Usually occurs between *pigment* and *neural* layers.

Musculoskeletal System

Duchenne Muscular Dystrophy (DMD)

- **Mechanism**: X-linked disease, as the *DMD gene* is located on the short arm of X chromosome on location *(Xp21)*.
- **Defect**: Lies in the *lack of*:

  1. *Dystrophin* protein: Regulates *calcium channels of muscles*.
  2. *Actin*: Anchors the extracellular matrix.

- **Clinical picture**:

  1. *Pseudohypertrophy* of muscles: Most pronounced in *calf muscles*, and occurs due to deposition of *connective and fibrous tissue*.

2. Muscle weakness and hyporeflexia: *Proximal more than distal.*
3. *Gower sign*: Patients use their arms to rise from the floor.
4. Cardiomyopathy and sudden death.

- *Diagnosis*: High serum levels of CK-MM, aldolase and LDH. *EMG and muscle biopsy are diagnostic.*
- *Notes*:

1. Duchenne is the most common cause of thoracolumbar scoliosis in children.
2. Becker muscular dystrophy is similar to DMD, except for the fact that *dystrophin is present but small in quantity.* The disease in Becker is milder and slower in progression.

Marfan Syndrome

- *Mechanism*: *Autosomal dominant* disease resulting in defective *Fibrillin-1.*
- *Clinical picture*:

1. Very tall patient *with arm span exceeding height,* and elastic joints.
2. *Dilated ascending aorta, aortic regurgitation* and *mitral valve prolapse.*
3. *Thoracic aortic aneurysm* due to *cystic medial necrosis.*

- *Complication*: *Aortic dissection.* So when you see a patient in the USMLE with features of marfan presenting with tearing chest pain radiating to his back, and big difference of blood pressure between right and left arms, you know what to think!

Ehler-Danlos Syndrome

- *Mechanism*: *Autosomal dominant* disease resulting in *defective collagen*, mainly types I and III. Underlying disorder is *failed hydroxylation of collagen's lysine.*
- *Clinical picture*: Hyperelastic skin and joints.

Osteogenesis Imperfecta

- *Mechanism*: Deficiency of *type 1 collagen*, due to mutation of *COL1A1 gene.*
- *Clinical picture*: Fragile bones with multiple fractures and *blue sclera* due to thin connective tissue.

Developmental Dysplasia of the Hip (DDH)

- *Definition*: Congenital dislocation of the hip.

- *On exam*:

1. *Ortolani test*: Abduction of the hip results in a click of relocation.
2. *Barlow test*: Abduction of the hip along with pressure leads to poster-superior dislocation.

- *Diagnosis*: Hip X-ray shows *false acetabulum.*
- *Complication*: *Avascular necrosis of femoral head.*
- *Treatment*: Heals spontaneously in *4 weeks.* If it did not heal, keep the thigh in an *abducted flexed position using a harness.*

Achondroplasia

- *Mechanism*: *Mutation of fibroblast growth factor (FGF-3).*
- *Clinical picture*: Newborn born as a dwarf with *short limbs* and *normal IQ.* Refer to Fig. 6.6.

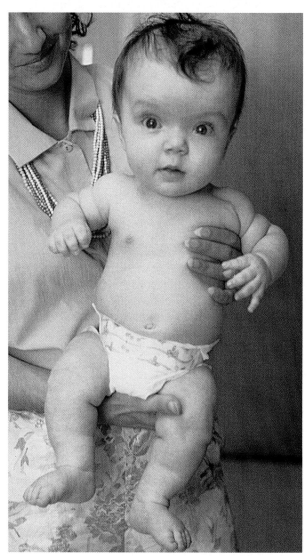

Fɪɢ. 6.6 Achondroplasia

- *Complication*: Neck X-ray is important to rule out *odontoid process hypoplasia;* a risk factor for subluxation and spinal cord compression.

Congenital Absence of Muscles

- *Poland syndrome*: Defect in formation of the *pectoralis major* muscle.
- *Prune belly syndrome*: One or more *abdominal muscles* are absent; usually associated with *hydronephrosis and undescended testes.*

Genetic Disorders

Down's Syndrome (refer to Fig. 6.7)

- *Mechanism*: *Trisomy of chromosome 21.* Most common underlying mechanism is *nondisjunction*, and less commonly translocation *(t14:21)* and mosaicism.
- *Clinical picture*:

  1. Head: Microcephaly with flat occiput and flat nasal bridge.
  2. Eyes: *Medial epicanthal folds* and *speckled iris* (Brushfield spots).
  3. Mouth: Small mandible (Micrognathia) and small mouth (Microstomia).

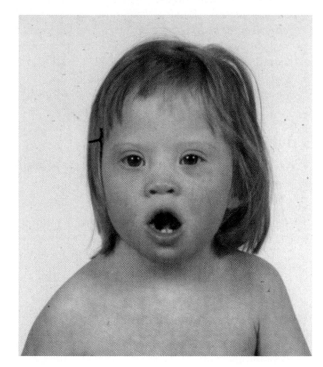

Fig. 6.7 Down syndrome

4. Upper limbs: Short broad hands (*Brachydactyly*) with a *simian crease.*
5. Genital: Cryptorchidism and infertility.
6. Lower limbs: Gapping between toes (*Sandal gap toe*).
7. Impaired phagocytic system: Frequent and recurrent infections.
8. Congenital anomalies: *The most common in descending order are*:

   - *Endocardial cushion defects* = VSD + ASD + Common A-V canal.
   - *Annular pancreas* and *duodenal atresia.*

- *Ultrasound*: Suspected in the first trimester by presence of *nuchal translucency.*
- *Antenatal diagnostic criteria for Down syndrome*:

  1. *Low alpha-fetoprotein level: MSAFP <0.4 mom.*
  2. *Low estrogen (E3) level.*
  3. *Elevated B-HCG level.*

- *Notes*:

  1. *Down syndrome is the most common cause of congenital mental retardation.*
  2. Down syndrome patients also have high risk of developing *acute lymphoblastic leukemia (ALL)* and *Alzheimer's dementia at an early age.*

Edward's Syndrome

- *Mechanism*: *Trisomy of chromosome 18.* Most common underlying mechanism is *nondisjunction.*
- *Clinical picture*: Mental and growth retardation, and multiple congenital anomalies with some unique features:

  1. *Hypertonia, prominent occiput, clenched hands* and *rocker-bottom feet.*
  2. *Choroid plexus cysts.*
  3. Intrauterine: *Single umbilical artery.*

- *Antenatal diagnostic criteria for Edward's syndrome*:

  1. *Low alpha-fetoprotein level: MSAFP < 0.4 mom.*
  2. *Low estrogen (E3) level.*
  3. *Low B-HCG level.*

Patau's Syndrome

- *Mechanism: Trisomy of chromosome 13.* Most common underlying mechanism is *nondisjunction.*
- *Clinical picture*: Mental and growth retardation, and multiple congenital anomalies with some unique features:

1. *Colobomas:* Erosions in the iris.
2. *Cleft lip* and/or *cleft palate*.
3. *Polydactly.*

Turner Syndrome

- *Mechanism*: *Monosomy (45X) or isochromosome of long arm of X chromosome.*
- *Barr bodies*: Buccal smear in these patients shows *no Barr body*.
- *Clinical picture*:

    1. Spontaneous abortion: Usually occurs when the fetus has Turner syndrome, as she develops *hydrops fetalis* or *cystic hygroma*.
    2. Short stature.
    3. Head: Low posterior hair line and low set ears.
    4. Mouth: Straight lower lip and curved upper one (*Shark mouth*).
    5. Neck: *Webbing*.
    6. Chest: Underdeveloped breasts with *widely spaced nipples (Shield chest)*.
    7. Extremities: Cubitus valgus and short metacarpal bones.
    8. Congenital anomalies:

        - CVS: *Coarctation of the aorta.*
        - GU: *Fibrosed ovaries* and *horseshoe kidneys*.
        - GI: *Colonic telangiectasia.*

- *Management*: Patients with Turner syndrome should receive screening for all the congenital anomalies and receive hormone replacement therapy.

Klinefelter Syndrome

- *Mechanism*: *Extra X chromosome causing trisomy (47XXY)*.
- *Barr body*: Buccal smear in these patients shows *at least one Barr body*.
- *Clinical picture*:

    1. Tall stature with *eunuchoid* features.
    2. GU: Small penis, scrotum and testicles.
    3. Infertility: Due to an *occluded genital ductal system*.

- *Management*: Patients with Klinefelter syndrome should receive testosterone replacement therapy.

Fragile X Syndrome

- *Mechanism*: *X-linked recessive* disease.
- *Disorder*:

    1. *Fragile site on the long arm of the X chromosome.*

2. Fragile site is due to an abnormal number of *CGG repeats*.
3. This leads to decreased expression of the *FMR1 gene*, which normally produces a protein needed for brain functioning.

- *Clinical picture*:

    1. Head: *Long face, big ears and big jaw.*
    2. GU: *Big testicles.*
    3. Development: Autism and mental retardation.

Ornithine Transcarbamoylase Deficiency

- *Mechanism*: *X-linked recessive.*
- *Pathology*: This enzyme normally binds *ornithine* to *carbamoyl phosphate* to form *citrulline* inside the mitochondria during the *urea cycle*.
- *Clinical picture*: Vomiting, headache, lethargy and seizures *after ingestion of high protein diet*, mainly due to *hyperammonemia and hypernitrogenemia*.
- *Diagnosis:* High *orotic acid* levels in the urine.
- *Treatment*: Nitrogen excretion using benzoic acid and phenylacetate.

Alport Syndrome

- *Mechanism*: *X-linked dominant*, however in a minority of cases AR or AD.
- *Disorder*: Defects in *type IV collagen*; a component of basement membranes.
- *Clinical picture*: *Painless hematuria, cataract and sensorineural hearing loss*. So when you see a child in the USMLE who is deaf and having painless hematuria, you know what to think!
- *Complication*: Chronic kidney disease, and End Stage Renal Disease (ESRD).

Cri-du-Chat Syndrome

- *Mechanism*: *Deletion of the short arm of chromosome 5* (5p-).
- *Clinical picture*:

    1. Mental and growth retardation, and multiple congenital anomalies.
    2. *Moon face* and *cat-like cry*: Due to *laryngeal hypoplasia*.

Wolf-Hirshhorn Syndrome

- *Mechanism*: Partial *deletion of the short arm of chromosome 4* (4p-).
- *Clinical picture*:

1. Prominent forehead and nose, *frequently compared to a warriors helmet.*
2. Short philtrum of the upper lip.

Prader-Willi Syndrome

- **Mechanism:** *Deletion of the long arm of chromosome 15* (15q-).
- **Source:** Deletion here occurs by *paternal* imprinting *due to methylation of cytosine during gametogenesis.*
- **Clinical picture:**

1. Short, obese patient with small hands and feet and *almond-shaped eyes.*
2. *Hyper*phagia and *hypo*gonadism.

Angelmann Syndrome (Happy Puppet Syndrome)

- **Mechanism:** *Deletion of the long arm of chromosome 15* (15q-).
- **Source:** The differentiating point from Prader-Willi is that the imprinting here is *maternal.*
- **Clinical picture:** Mental retardation, and continuous laughing and smiling (*Like a happy puppet*).

DiGeorge's Syndrome

- **Mechanism:** *Deletion of long arm of chromosome 21* (21q-).
- **Pathology:** This leads to defective development of the *3rd and 4th pharyngeal pouches;* accordingly, *parathyroid glands and thymus are absent.*
- **Clinical picture** (*George always shows TLC*):

1. Tetany: Due to *hypocalcemia,* caused by *lack of parathyroid hormone.*
2. Lack of *thymus:* Leads to recurrent infections.
3. Cardiovascular anomalies.

- **Treatment:** Thymus and bone marrow transplantation.

Von Hippel Lindau Syndrome (VHL)

- **Mechanism:** *Deletion* of VHL gene on chromosome 3.
- **Clinical picture:**

1. Hemangioblastomas everywhere, e.g., Cerebellum, retina.
2. Malignancy: VHL is normally a tumor suppressor, so these patients are at risk of developing *renal cell cancer.*

Phenylketonuria (PKU)

- **Mechanism:** *Autosomal recessive* disease.
- **Disorder:** *Absence of phenylalanine hydroxylase* enzyme which normally converts phenylalanine to tyrosine.
- **Clinical picture:**

1. Fair skin, hair and eyes: Due to decreased *melanin* synthesis.
2. Microcephaly and mental retardation: Due to accumulation of phenyl-pyruvate, -lactate and -acetate.
3. Hypertonia and seizures: Due to accumulation of *serotonin.*
4. Musty odor: Due to accumulation of *phenylacetate.*

- **Diagnosis:**

1. Measuring the activity of phenylalanine hydroxylase enzyme.
2. Elevated serum levels of phenylalanine >20%.
3. Elevated urine levels of phenyl-pyruvate, -lactate and -acetate.

- **Treatment:** *Dietary restriction of phenylalanine and aspartame* (Aspartame releases phenylalanine when digested).
- **Note:** Do not confuse PKU with homocystinuria, as the latter also causes congenital fair skin, hair and eyes, and some features of Marfan syndrome *plus multiple recurrent thromboembolic phenomena.* Homocystinuria is treated by restriction of diet rich in sulfhydryl groups.

Galactosemia

- **Mechanism:** *Autosomal recessive* disease.
- **Types and clinical picture:**

1. *Type I:*

   - Disorder: Absence of *galactokinase* enzyme, which normally converts galactose to galactose-1-phosphate.
   - Clinical picture: Cataracts and galactosuria.

2. *Type II:*

   - Disorder: Absence of *galactose-1-phosphate uridyltransferase* enzyme, which normally converts galactose-1-phosphate to glucose-1-phosphate.
   - Clinical picture: *Cataracts, galactosuria* and:

     1. CNS: Microcephaly and mental retardation.
     2. GI: Hepatosplenomegaly and liver cirrhosis.

3. GU: Fanconi's syndrome = Glucosuria, phosphaturia and aminoaciduria.
4. Metabolic: Hypoglycemia due to inhibited *glycogenolysis* enzymes.

- **Treatment**: *Restricting galactose in the diet.*

Albinism

- **Mechanism**: *Autosomal recessive,* but can also be inherited as AD or XLR.
- **Disorder**: Absence of *tyrosinase* enzyme, which normally converts tyrosine to melanin.
- **Clinical picture**:

1. Depigmented skin, hair, iris and retina.
2. High risk of *blindness* and *skin cancer.*

Apert Syndrome

- **Mechanism**: *Autosomal dominant* syndrome.
- **Disorder**: Mutation occurs in the gene of *fibroblast growth factor (FGF-2).*
- **Clinical picture**: *Craniostenosis* and *fused digits.*

Neurofibromatosis

- **Mechanism**: *Autosomal dominant* syndrome.
- **Types and clinical picture**:

1. *Type I* (Von Recklinghausen's): Inherited on *chromosome 17.*
   - Skin: *café-au-lait patches. Refer to Fig. 6.8.*
   - *Lisch nodules:* Pigmented iris nodules.

2. *Type II* (Central neurofibromatosis): Inherited on *chromosome 22.*
   - Bilateral *acoustic neuroma*: Acoustic neuroma is a *schwannoma* with *Antoni A* and *Antoni B* bodies.
   - Astrocytoma.

Tuberous Sclerosis

- **Mechanism**: *Autosomal dominant* syndrome.
- **Clinical picture**: Multiple *hamartomas* plus 4 pathognomonic signs:

1. *Ash leaf spots*: Flat, hypopigmented skin lesions.
2. *Shagreen patches*: Areas of increased skin thickness.
3. Subungual fibroma.
4. *Periventricular tubers*: Causing *mental retardation* and *seizures.*

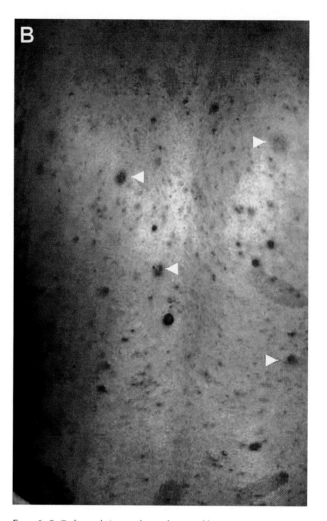

FIG. 6.8 Cafe au lait patches of neurofibromatosis

Xeroderma Pigmentosum

- **Mechanism**: *Breakage* disorder.
- **Pathology**: Ultraviolet light causes *failure of the DNA repair* mechanism, namely the *ultraviolet endonuclease*, which in turn leads to accumulation of *pyrimidine dimers.*
- **Clinical picture**: Multiple skin lesions, and skin cancer.

Hereditary Non-Polyposis Colon Cancer (HNPCC)

- **Mechanism**: *Mismatch repair secondary to microsatellites. MSH2 gene is blamed in most HNPCC cases.*
- **Clinical picture**: HNPCC (Lynch syndrome) is a familial form of colon cancer. Involves the following diagnostic criteria *(3,2,1)*:

1. Occurrence of colon cancer in at least 3 *first degree relatives*.
2. These cancers occur over a period of at least 2 *generations*.
3. At least *one* of these 3 relatives is less than *50 years of age*.

- *Note*: Women in families with HNPCC are at high risk of *endometrial* and *ovarian* cancer as well.

Leber's Optic Neuropathy

- *Mechanism*: *Mitochondrial* inheritance.
- *Disorder*: Mutation of *ND4 gene* which is normally responsible for:

1. Regulation of the conversion of *arginine* to *histidine*.
2. Encoding *NADH dehydrogenase*, which regulates ATP and electron transport.

- *Clinical picture*: *Loss of central vision*, and maintaining a *peripheral tubular visual field*.
- *Complication*: *Optic nerve degeneration and blindness*.

Spotlight on Famous Oncogenes

- *BRCA*: Mutation leads to *br*east and ovarian *ca*ncer.
- *p53*: Mutation of this gene on chromosome *17* leads to cancer.
- *Rb1*: Mutation of this gene leads to *retinoblastoma*.
- *APC:* Mutation of this gene leads to *familial adenomatous polyposis*.
- ras: This gene is associated with *colon cancer*.
- *c-myc, t8:14*: This gene is associated with *Burkitt's lymphoma*.
- *Bcl-2, t14:18*: This gene is associated with *follicular lymphoma*
- *Bcr/abl*: This gene is associated with *chronic myeloid leukemia* (CML).
- *Philadelphia chromosome (t 9:22)*: This translocation is pathognomonic for *CML* and its presence is associated with a *good prognosis*.
- *t15:17*: This translocation is pathognomonic for *AML*, and its presence is associated with a *good prognosis*.
- *Human Herpes Virus (HHV-8)*: Kaposi sarcoma.
- *Human Papilloma Virus (HPV)*: Cervical cancer.
- *Epstein Barr virus (EBV)*: Burkitt's lymphoma and nasopharyngeal cancer.
- *Hepatitis viruses B and C*: Hepatocellular cancer.
- *Note*: DNA mutations can be diagnosed using Single Stranded Conformational Polymorphism (*SSCP*), which shows *2 bands for homozygous* mutations, and *4 for heterozygous* ones.

Immunological Diseases

Introduction

- *Fact*: Know the following as a rule:

1. Failure of cell mediated immunity (CMI): Leads to infection by *viruses and intracellular bacteria*.
2. Failure of humoral immunity: Leads to infection by *extracellular bacteria*.

Bruton's Agammaglobulinemia

- *Mechanism*: *X-linked recessive* disease, where there are no or low gammaglobulins due to deficiency of the tyrosine kinase needed for maturation of B lymphocytes.
- *Pathology*: Patient *does not have tonsils or germinal centers in the lymph nodes*.
- *Clinical picture*: Patient is usually 6 months of age or older presenting with recurrent *extracellular* bacterial infections and *absent tonsils*.
- *Diagnosis*: Very low *IgG* level and absence of all other immunoglobulins.

Selective Ig Deficiency

- *Mechanism*: Deficiency of one or more Ig, most common is selective *IgA* deficiency.
- *Clinical picture*: Frequent upper and lower *respiratory tract infections*, allergies, diarrhea, or could even be asymptomatic.

Wiskott-Aldrich Syndrome

- *Mechanism*: *X-linked recessive* disease.
- *Defect*: Defect in *T cells* and *IgM* only.
- *Clinical picture*: Triad:

1. Thrombocytopenia and bleeding.
2. Eczema.
3. Combined T and B cell deficiency causing recurrent infections.

- *Historically*: Thought to be caused by a *defective IgM response to capsule polysaccharides*, such as pneumococcus.
- *Note*: The gene for the *Wiskott-Aldrich syndrome protein* (WASP) has now been isolated and it plays a role in many immune functions.

Severe Combined Immunodeficiency (SCID)

- *Mechanism*: Absent T and B lymphocytes due to *defective stem cell development.*
- *Causes*: Multiple inherited causes:

  1. Deficiency in adenosine deaminase (ADA): *Autosomal recessive.*
  2. MHC class II deficiency.
  3. Defective tyrosine kinase enzyme: *Autosomal recessive.*
  4. Defective IL-2 receptor: *X-linked.*

- *Clinical picture*: Patient is usually *less than 6 months of age* presenting with recurrent bacterial, viral and fungal infections.
- *Prevention and treatment*: Used to be fatal; however, currently early detection and bone marrow transplantation may be curative.

Chronic Granulomatous Disease (CGD)

- *Mechanism*: *X-linked deficiency* of *NADPH oxidase in neutrophils.*
- *Clinical picture*: Recurrent *fungal* and *staphylococcal infections. Suspect it when you see a patient in the USMLE with recurrent oral thrush, diaper rash, abscesses and granulomas.*
- *Diagnosis*: Inability of cells to reduce *nitroblue tetrazolium dye* to *formazan.*
- *Treatment*: *Gamma interferon.*

Chediak-Higashi Syndrome

- *Mechanism*: *Autosomal recessive* disease.
- *Pathology*: Defect in *microtubule polymerization* which leads to failure of chemotaxis and phagocytosis.
- *Clinical picture*: Recurrent staphylococcal and streptococcal infections.
- *Diagnosis*: *Neutropenia* and *prolonged bleeding time.*
- *Association*: Albinism and neurological defects, e.g., ataxia, neuropathy.

Leukocyte Adhesion Deficiency

- *Mechanism*: Defect in the adhesion protein (*LFA-1*) involved in *phagocytosis.*
- *Clinical picture*: Recurrent fungal, staphylococcal and streptococcal infections at a young age.

Transient Hypogammaglobulinemia

- *Mechanism*: Decrease in serum *IgG* after maternal immunity wanes.
- *Age:* Around the age of 6 months.
- *Prognosis*: Spontaneously resolves after 1–2 months to 1–2 years.

Chronic Mucocutaneous Candidiasis

- *Mechanism*: Disorder of *T cell* response to *Candida.*
- *Clinical picture*: Recurrent yeast infections of mucous membranes and skin.

Ataxia-Telangiectasia Syndrome

- *Mechanism*: *Autosomal recessive* disorder.
- *Clinical picture*:

  1. *Combined T and B cell* deficiency: Recurrent infections.
  2. *Cerebellar ataxia* and *oculo-cutaneous telangiectasia.*

- *Complication*: *Stomach cancer* and *non-Hodgkin's lymphoma.*

C1 Estrase Inhibitor Deficiency

- *Mechanism*: *Autosomal dominant* disease causing *hereditary angioedema.*
- *Diagnosis*: Low levels of *C4* and *C1 estrase inhibitor.*

C5–C9 Deficiency

- Complement deficiency associated with increased risk of infection with *meningococcal* and *gonococcal infections.*

Neonatology

Normal Full Term Features

- *Blood pressure*: SBP in *70s–80s*, DBP in *40s–60s.*
- *Pulse*: *100s–150s.*
- *Respiratory rate*: *30s–40s.*
- *Posture*: Partial generalized *flexion.*
- *Skin*: Covered with whitish material known as *Vernix caseosa.*
- *Color*: Purple mottling and *Mongolian spots*, which disappear by *2 years of age.*

- **GI**: First stools are *black*, then turn greenish for 3 or 4 days (*Transitional stools*), after which they become golden yellow in color.
- **GU**:

  1. First urine output occurs *24–48 h after birth*, and is *pink* in color due to high urate content.
  2. Breast enlargement and nipple secretions (*Witch's milk*).
  3. Labial hypertrophy and *bloody vaginal discharge*: Due to *estrogen withdrawal*.

- **Hematology**: Hemoglobin of newborn at birth is 17–18 g/dL, a.k.a. *physiological polycythemia of newborn*, with mild reticulocytosis.
- **Weight**: 10–90% percentile is appropriate for gestational age. *Below 5% is small for age*, and *above 95% is large for age*.
- **Reflexes**:

  1. *Moro's reflex*: Extension and abduction of limbs followed by exactly the opposite, i.e., Flexion and adduction. This reflex disappears by the *3rd month of age*. Persistent Moro's reflex indicates mental injury, e.g., Cerebral palsy or retardation.
  2. Grasp reflex: Also present at birth and disappears by the *3rd month of age*.

- **Care of newborn**: APGAR scoring, *vitamin K injection* and applying *erythromycin eye drops* prophylactically against *Chlamydia's inclusion conjunctivitis*. Note: Inclusion conjunctivitis usually occurs *4–5 days after birth*, while chemical conjunctivitis occurs only in the first 24 h after birth.

Neonatal Sepsis

- **Introduction**: Most common cause of fever in neonates is *dehydration*, so always make sure to assess for dry mucus membranes and sunken fontanelles in any neonate with fever.
- **Most common organisms**: *Group B streptococci*, followed by *E. coli*.
- **Clinical picture**: Lethargy, weak cry, fever or hypothermia and poor feeding.
- **Diagnosis**: CXR, CBC, blood cultures, urine analysis and culture, sputum culture and lumbar puncture.
- **Treatment**: Empirical treatment immediately after cultures are obtained. Best combination used is *Ampgent (Ampicillin + Gentamycin)*. If there is any suspicion for meningitis, a *3rd generation cephalosporin* (e.g., Ceftriaxone) must be added.

Congenital Infections and Drug Induced Disorders

- **Congenital rubella syndrome**:

  1. E.N.T.: *Sensorineural hearing loss*.
  2. Eye: Glaucoma, cataract and *Salt and pepper retinopathy*.
  3. CVS: Patent ductus arteriosus (PDA) and myocardial necrosis.
  4. Bone: Longitudinal radiolucent areas in metaphysis of long bones.

- **Congenital toxoplasmosis syndrome**:

  1. CNS: Hydrocephalus and *scattered intracranial calcifications*.
  2. Eye: Chorioretinitis.

- **Congenital cytomegalovirus syndrome**:

  1. CNS: Hydrocephalus and *periventricular intracranial calcifications*.
  2. Eye: Chorioretinitis.
  3. E.N.T.: Sensorineural hearing loss.

- **Congenital herpes simplex syndrome**: Skin, Eye, Mouth (*SEM syndrome*), presenting with vesicular skin lesions and chorioretinitis. Most infections occur during passage of fetus through an infected birth canal. Prevention: Delivery by *C-section before rupture of membranes*.
- **Congenital varicella zoster syndrome**: Limb hypoplasia and multiple scarring.
- **Fetal alcohol syndrome**:

  1. Microcephaly.
  2. Midfacial hypoplasia.
  3. Short palpebral fissures.
  4. Long philtrum of the lip.

- **Fetal hydantoin syndrome**:

  1. Cleft lip and/or palate, and mental retardation.
  2. Cupid bow: Curved upper lip that looks like the bow of Cupid.
  3. Nail and digits hypoplasia.

- **Medications associated with congenital anomalies**:

  1. Cocaine: *Intestinal atresia* and *limb reduction defects*.
  2. Lithium: *Ebstein anomaly*.
  3. Progesterone: *Virilization and hypospadias*.
  4. Radiation and iodide: *Goiter and hypothyroidism*.
  5. Isotretinoin: *Thymus hypoplasia, microtia and cardiac defects*.
  6. Thalidomide: *Limb defects (Phocomelia)*.
  7. DiethylStilbesterol (D.E.S): *Vaginal clear cell adenocarcinoma and incompetent cervix leading to repeated abortions*.

Hemorrhagic Disease of the Newborn

- **Definition**: It is a physiological self-limited hemorrhage that normally occurs after birth.
- **Onset**: *2–5 days* after delivery; *never in the first day*.
- **Mechanism**: Depletion of vitamin K and vitamin K-dependant clotting factors previously supplied intrauterine through the maternal blood.
- **Clinical picture**:

  1. Prolonged bleeding episodes.
  2. Prolonged *PT and PTT*.

- **Prevention**: All newborns receive vitamin K injection immediately after delivery.
- **Treatment**: Vitamin K, Fresh frozen plasma (FFP) and blood transfusion.

Physiological Anemia of Infancy

- **Definition**: It is a physiological drop in hemoglobin after delivery. The drop starts at the end of the *1st week* and plateaus by the *8th week* to a level of *9–11 g/dL*.
- **Mechanism**: Short life span of *hemoglobin F* and rapid increase in body size and plasma volume.
- **Anemia of prematurity**: Premature infants experience a more severe Hb drop, mainly due to short life span of RBCs caused by *vitamin E deficiency*.

Neonatal Necrotizing Enterocolitis

- **Pathology**: Infection of the intestine leading to necrosis.
- **Most common location**: *Distal ileum and proximal colon*.
- **Most common organisms**: *Clostridium perfringens and E. coli*.
- **Clinical picture**: *Abdominal distention* and *blood in the stools*.
- **Diagnosis**: Abdominal X-ray, which shows gas accumulation in submucosa of intestinal wall *(Pneumatosis intestinalis)*. Air under diaphragm on an upright film indicates intestinal perforation.
- **Treatment**:

  1. Hydration and antibiotics: Best is *antipseudomonas penicillin*, e.g., *Ceftazidime, Cefepime, plus aminoglycoside*.
  2. Surgery: Intestinal resection is reserved for cases with perforation or failure to respond to medical management.

Neonatal Jaundice

- **Definition**: Yellow discoloration of skin and sclera of neonate, due to serum bilirubin elevation beyond *7 mg (Normal = 0.1–0.8 mg)*.
- **Physiological jaundice**:

  1. *Most common form of neonatal jaundice.*
  2. Timing: Starts in the *2nd or 3rd day (Never the first)*, and lasts for a week before resolving spontaneously.
  3. Bilirubin: *Does not exceed 12 mg*, and is mainly *indirect (Unconjugated)*

- **Hemolytic disease of the newborn**:

  1. Occurs mainly due to *Rh incompatibility* in the previous pregnancy, which has led to development of Rh antibodies, or due to *ABO incompatibility*.
  2. Clinical picture: *Jaundice on first day of life*, hydrops fetalis or icterus gravis neonatorum. Discussed in gynecology.

- **Treatment of neonatal jaundice**:

  1. *Phototherapy*:

     - Indicated if cord bilirubin is more than *2.5 mg*, or if serum bilirubin is more than *10 mg. Diarrhea is a common side effect*.
     - Exposure to blue light of *470 nm wavelength*, which leads to formation of a soluble form of indirect bilirubin that can be excreted in the urine. (Remember, *Indirect or unconjugated bilirubin is not allowed to pass in the urine, however, it can* cross the blood brain barrier.)
     - Neonates during phototherapy must wear *dark sun glasses* to protect their retina, and a *metal cover* to protect their genitalia.

  2. *Exchange transfusion*:

     - Indicated if cord bilirubin is more than *5 mg*, or if serum bilirubin is more than *20 mg*. It is done using *type O Rh-ve blood*, and amount given is *double the neonate's plasma volume*.
     - Complications of exchange transfusion: *Neonatal vascular thrombosis or vasospasm, hypocalcemia and hypoglycemia*.

- **Notes**:

  1. *Breast milk jaundice*: *Indirect* hyperbilirubinemia that usually occurs by the *2nd week* after delivery. Mechanism: Inhibition of neonatal conjugation enzyme (Glucuronyl transferase) by 3-alpha-20-beta-pregnandiol in the breast milk. Treatment: *Hold breast feeding for 48 h, then*

resume. Condition resolves spontaneously by *10 weeks* of age.

2. *Congenital biliary atresia*: Mainly *direct* hyperbilirubinemia, causing *dark urine and clay colored stools*. Discussed further in surgery.
3. *Congenital jaundice*: Gilbert, Criggler-najjar and Dubin johnson syndromes. Discussed in internal medicine.

- *Key*:

1. Jaundice on *first day of life*: *Hemolytic disease of the newborn*.
2. Jaundice on *2nd–3rd day of life*: *Physiological jaundice*.
3. Jaundice persistent beyond 1 month of age: Congenital jaundice, biliary atresia or breast milk jaundice.

Kernicterus

- *Definition*: Brain injury due to deposition of *indirect bilirubin*. Main deposition is in the *basal ganglia* and *brain stem's mitochondria*.
- *Clinical picture*:

1. Stage 1: Brain edema causing lethargy, hypotonia and poor feeding.
2. Stage 2 and 3: Rigidity, convulsions and *oculogyric crisis* (Conjugate deviation of eyes).
3. Stage 4: Cerebral palsy and extra-pyramidal manifestations.

- *Prevention and treatment*: Urgent lowering of bilirubin level. Discussed earlier.

Miscellaneous

- *Allergic rhinitis*: Could be seasonal or perennial. *Clinical picture*: Paroxysmal rhinorrhea and nasal stuffiness, dark halos around the eyes (*Allergic shiners*) and a horizontal crease on the nose (*Allergic salute*). *Treatment*: Antihistamines and nasal steroids.
- *Angioedema*: Usually induced by introduction of a foreign substance into the body, e.g., Medication, bee sting. Hereditary angioedema due to deficiency of *C1 estrase inhibitor*. *Clinical picture*: Swelling of eye lids, lips and tongue. *Main concern*: Airway protection. *Treatment*: Epinephrine (*Life saving*), steroids and antihistamines (*H1 and H2 blockers*).
- *Allergic triad* (AAA): *A*llergic rhinitis + *A*topic dermatitis + *A*sthma.
- *Testicular feminization syndrome*: Mechanism: *Mutation of androgen receptors*, through deletion

of the DNA binding protein of the receptors, so *testosterone is produced but it cannot act*. Clinical picture: External female appearance and has a vagina, *but no ovaries or uterus*. Workup reveals *undescended testes* and *46 XY chromosomes*.

- *Male phenotypic genital anomalies*: Mechanisms: *5 alpha-reductase* or *17 beta-hydroxysteroid dehydrogenase* deficiency. Clinical picture: Underdeveloped male genitalia. Diagnosis: High serum *testosterone* or *androstenedione* levels respectively, due to lack of conversion to the active forms.
- *Most common cause of stridor in pediatrics*: *Foreign body aspiration*, and mostly located in the *right main bronchus* (*Wider and more in line with trachea*). Most common foreign body: *Nuts*. Next best step: *Rigid bronchoscopy*.
- *Most common cause* of stridor in someone who uses their voice excessively, e.g., Opera singer: *Laryngeal papilloma*.
- *Infantile microcystic disease*: *Autosomal recessive* disease characterized by cystic dilatation of *PCT*. *Clinical picture*: Edema and proteinuria. *Antenatal diagnosis*: Elevated alpha fetoprotein level.
- *Most common cause of hydronephrosis in children*: *Ureteropelvic junction stricture*. *Treatment*: Pyeloplasty.
- *Most common cause of chronic kidney disease in children*: *Obstructive uropathy*.
- *Most common cause of hemorrhagic cystitis in children*: *Adenovirus infection*.
- *Most common cause of diarrhea in children*: *Viral gastroenteritis*.
- *Most common cause of constipation in children*: *Voluntary (Functional)*.
- *Most common intestinal tumor in children*: *Juvenile colonic polyps*.
- *Most common cause of intracranial hemorrhage in children*: *A-V malformations*.
- *Most common cause of asphyxia in children*: *Choking on food*.
- *Most common cause of epistaxis in children*: *Voluntary nose picking*.
- *Placental insufficiency syndrome*: Affects the fetal weight during the *second half of pregnancy*. Newborn has *big hands, big feet, big head* and *small liver*.
- *Meconium aspiration syndrome*: Asphyxia during labor stimulates fetal breathing, which might lead to aspiration of meconium and respiratory distress for few days after delivery. Complication: Pneumothorax.
- *Beckwith-Wiedemann syndrome*: A chromosomal *deletion* syndrome, resulting in a *macrosomic* neonate with *visceromegaly, polycythemia* and *hypoglycemia*.
- *Sudden infant death syndrome (SIDS)*: Unexplained death during sleep, most common between

2 and 4 months of age. Prevention: Infant should always lie on *their back*.

- **Icthyosis**: *X-linked disease*. Mechanism: *Defective keratinization* of the skin. Location: *Neck and trunk*, sparing the extremities. Clinical picture: Dry scaly skin, frequently compared to *fish scales*. Pathology: Thick *stratum corneum* layer. Treatment: Topical emollients.

- **Toxic epidermal necrolysis**: A subtype of erythema multiforme, and is characterized by *target-like lesions* and *Nikolsky sign* (Easy detachment of mucus membranes and skin lesions upon pressure).

- **Scalded skin syndrome**: Skin infection by *Staphylococci*, and is characterized by *beefy red skin lesions* and *Nikolsky sign*. Treatment: Penicillinase-resistant penicillin.

- **Erythema toxicum neonatorum**: Occurs in *full term neonates*, and disappears by *5 days of age*. *Clinical picture*: Evanescent vesicle, papules and pustules. *Diagnosis*: Gram stain of the fluid in lesions reveals excessive *eosinophils*.

- **Cradle cap**: *Seborrheic dermatitis of the scalp* in newborns. Resolves spontaneously.

- **Pustular melanosis**: Heal with hyperpigmented lesions.

- **Sebaceous nevus**: Yellowish, hair-free lesion on the scalp.

- **Thyroid diseases**: In males and females of the pediatric population occur with the ratio of 1:1.

Congenital hyperthyroidism could occur due to transplacental transfer of TSI or LATS, and it is self resolving in few months without treatment.

- **Polydactyly**: Common among African Americans. *In Caucasians, it is usually associated with cardiovascular anomalies*.

- **Teeth decay**: Bottled sweetened milk causes decay in the *upper central incisors* and *back teeth*.

- **Job Buckley disease**: *Recurrent staph. infections, rash and elevated IgE*.

- **Feil syndrome**: Abnormal fusion of neck vertebrae leading to short neck and high scapula, a.k.a. *Sprengel deformity*.

- **Visual acuity**: At birth it is *20/400*, by the *age of 5 it is 20/20*. Snellen chart can be used to assess visual acuity by the age of *4 years*.

- **Circumcision**: Decreases the risk of penile cancer, *only if done at a young age*.

- **Infant walkers**: Proven to delay the development of walking skills.

- **All congenital infections (Discussed earlier)**: Risk factor for *autism*.

- **Safety measures during car rides**:

  1. Infants must ride in a *rear-facing seat* until they are at least *1 year old* and at least *20 lbs* in weight.
  2. *20 lbs–40 lbs*: Front-facing seat with a harness.
  3. *> 40 lbs*: Belt positioning booster seat until the child is 80 lbs and 4'9'' tall, after which the car seat with seat belt can be safely used.

Chapter 7
Psychiatry

A.W.A. Halim, *Passing the USMLE*, DOI: 10.1007/978-0-387-68984-5_7,
© Springer Science+Business Media, LLC 2009

Introduction

Axes of Mental Disorders

- *I*: Clinical disorder, e.g., Depression.
- *II*: Personality disorder or mental retardation.
- *III*: Medical disease, e.g., Hypothyroidism.
- *IV*: Environmental factors.
- *V*: Global Assessment of Function (*GAF*).

Targets of Doctor-Patient Interview

- *Rapport*: Includes the following techniques:

  1. *Support*, e.g., "That must have been a horrible experience for you."
  2. *Empathy*, e.g., "Oh dear, you must be worried about the complications!"
  3. *Validation*, e.g., "I can understand why you felt the way you did. If I were in your place, I would have felt the same way too."

- *Information*: Obtain information from the patient using the following techniques:

  1. *Silence*: You will get multiple cases in the USMLE about the fact that you should *never interrupt your patient* while he or she is talking. If the patient is very talkative, try to aim for *closed ended questions, but never interrupt the patient.*
  2. *Open-ended questions*, e.g., "What brought you in today?"
  3. *Closed-ended questions*, e.g., "Do you have a cough?"
  4. *Reflection*, e.g., "Okay, so you said you fell and hit your head?"
  5. *Facilitation*, e.g., "What happened after you fell and hit your head?"
  6. *Recapitulation*, e.g., "Now that I have heard the entire story, let me summarize my understanding of what happened."

- *Memory*: 3 types of memory you need to test for:

  1. *Immediate*: Lasts for *5 min*, and is controlled by *mammillary bodies*.
  2. *Recent*: Lasts for *12 h*, and is controlled by *Hippocampus*.
  3. *Remote*: Old concrete information, e.g., Name, place of birth.

Important Definitions

- *Psychosis*: Loss of relation with the real world. Characterized by *hallucinations*.
- *Neurosis*: Mixture of anxiety, worry and irritability.
- *Mood*: Emotion that the patient feels *from within*, e.g., Depressed, happy.
- *Affect*: Emotion that the patient shows *from outside*, e.g., Looks depressed.
- *Concentration*: Tested by asking the patient to start with the number 100 and to count backwards by sevens, i.e., 100, 93, 86, etc....
- *Attention*: Tested by observing the patient during the interview for how easily he/she gets distracted by surrounding stimuli.
- *Cognitive ability*: Tested by asking "How many states are in the US?" or "How much is 5 multiplied by 5?"
- *Spatial ability*: Tested by asking the patient to draw a clock.
- *Abstract reasoning ability*: Ability to understand metaphors, e.g., Proverbs.
- *Perseveration*: Patient thinks or talks about *the same* word or idea over and over again.
- *Flight of ideas*: Patient thinks or talks about *different, unrelated* words or ideas at a fast pace.
- *Delusion*: False perception of *an idea*, e.g., "I think the FBI are watching me" or "I think that my co-workers are trying to set me up."
- *Illusion*: Also false perception of an *actual object*, e.g., A patient would look at a wire on the floor, and tell you "Careful, that snake is too close to your foot."
- *Hallucination*: Seeing, hearing, smelling, or feeling something that *does not exist*, e.g., A patient looks at the floor (*where there is nothing*) and tells you "Careful, there are spiders all over the floor" or "Jesus was talking to me yesterday and told me to try that drug, nobody could hear him, only I did."
- *Idea of reference*: e.g., "I watched that movie on the TV last night, and it was talking about my life, it was full of details of my life, they were telling my story."

Tests

- *Mini-Mental State Examination (MMSE)*: Used to assess *dementia*. Normal is greater than 25 out of 30. *Score 20–25*: Mild dementia. *Score <20*: Advanced dementia.

- **Intelligence Quotient (IQ)**: *IQ = Mental age/Chronological age × 100*. Culture plays a major role in affecting IQ. Scoring:

  1. *Normal*: *90–109*, with standard deviation of *15*.
  2. Borderline: *70–90*.
  3. Mental retardation: *Below 70*.

- **Personality tests**: Multiple, including the Minnesota multiphasic personality inventory (*566 true or false questions*), Rorschach inkblot, sentence completion and Thematic Apperception Test (TAT).
- **Neuropsychological tests**: Multiple, including Halsted battery (*To localize brain lesions*) and Nebraska test (*To determine brain hemispheric dominance*).
- **Others**:

  1. Dexamethasone suppression test: Positive in cases of *depression*.
  2. Serotonin: Low levels in cases of *depression*, *alcoholism* and *aggression*.
  3. Dopamine: Low level in Parkinson's disease and high level in *schizophrenia* and *chorea*.
  4. Na lactate intravenously or CO_2 inhalation: Induce *panic attacks*.
  5. Lie detection test: Done using *Na amobarbital* (*Truth serum*).
  6. Electroencephalogram (EEG): *Normal in dementia and abnormal in delirium. Evoked EEG is used to detect cortical response to stimuli.*

Age

Child Development

- **Infant (0–15 months)**:

  1. Sticks to the mother at all times. If separated from mother at this age, *separation anxiety*, *anaclitic depression* and *failure to thrive* may ensue.
  2. *Stranger anxiety*: Most pronounced during the *first year of life*.

- **Toddler (15 months–2.5 years)**: Show 2 important phenomena:

  1. *Rapprochement*: Separates from mother voluntarily, but returns to her intermittently for reassurance.
  2. *Object permanence*.

- **Pre-schooler (2.5–6 years)**: Show multiple important phenomena:

  1. Control over bowel function: By *age 4*. Encopresis (Loss of control over bowels) could be due to multiple reasons, most common of which is *voluntary retention with overflow*.

  2. Control over bladder function: By *age 5*. Enuresis (Loss of control over bladder) is best treated using a *buzzer* or Imipramine. Functional enuresis is more frequent among *males*, and occurs *just before awakening in the morning*.
  3. *Band-aid phase*: During these few years, the child is so overwhelmed by any minor illness or injury, so *surgery is not preferred during these years*.
  4. They have *no* understanding of the meaning of death.

- **Schooler (6–11 years)**: By that age, the child can:

  1. Understand the meaning of death.
  2. Be taken to surgery and hospitalized if needed, without serious consequences.

- **Adolescents**: By age *11 in females* and *13–14 in males*:
- **Stages of development**: Also been classified as shown in Table 7.1, as follows:
  1. Freud: According to *the organ through which pleasure is achieved*.
  2. Piaget: According to *learning processes* (*Cognitive*).
  3. Erikson: According to *achievement of certain goals* (*Psychosocial*)

Aging

- Average life expectancy for Americans at this time is *75 years*, with more predominance to *Caucasians* compared to African Americans, and to *females* compared to males (*7 years difference*).
- By the year 2020, around *15%* of the people living in the US will be in the elderly age group (*>65 years*).
- Depression is very common among the elderly population, and is commonly misdiagnosed as dementia, hence called *pseudo-dementia*. So when you see any elderly patient in the USMLE with what looks like dementia, make sure to look first for any symptoms indicating depression.

TABLE 7.1 Stages of human development.

Stage	Freud	Piaget	Erikson
Infant	Oral	Sensorimotor	Trust
Toddler	Anal	Sensorimotor	Shame and Doubt
Preschooler	Phallic	Pre-operational	Intent and Guilt
Schooler	Latent	Concrete	Industry and Inferiority
Adolescent	Genital	Abstract (Formal)	Personality, Intimacy and Generosity

- Elderly have low brain weight, increase in the size of ventricles and sulci, along with decreased cerebral blood flow; however, their *IQ does not change*.

Development Disorders

Attention Deficient Hyperactivity Disorder (ADHD)

- *Clinical picture*: As the name implies, the child *cannot pay any attention*, and is *hyperactive*. Classic presentation is for a child who scores poorly in school, cannot follow instructions, is easily distracted and always interrupts his teacher and classmates.
- *Treatment*: *Amphetamine* or *Methylphenidate*. Side effects of these medications include insomnia, tics, night terror and choreiform movements.
- *Notes*:

  1. Incidence of mental retardation in patients with ADHD is *10–20%*.
  2. There is a genetic *component* in ADHD which is strongly associated with *OCD* and *Tourette's* syndrome.

Conduct Disorder

- *Clinical picture*: A child who acts like a "thug". A classic presentation is for a child who *physically assaults other kids*, *destroys property*, *lies* and *steals from others*.
- *Treatment*: Psychotherapy and family therapy.
- *Notes*:

  1. If this disorder persists beyond 18 years of age, it is known as *Anti-social personality disorder*.
  2. Conduct disorder is frequently associated with a history of abuse by addicting parents.

Oppositional Defiant Disorder

- *Clinical picture*: A child who is also acting like a "thug" only *towards authority figures*. A classic presentation is for a child who gets along with his classmates very well, but when it gets to his teachers or parents, he is impolite. Also carries a history of abuse.
- *Treatment*: Psychotherapy and family therapy.

Autistic Disorder

- *Clinical picture*:

  1. A child who *refuses to talk or move*, and is highly nervous and anxious, *especially when anybody tries to help or touch him*.
  2. Characteristic features include *repetitive* and *destructive behavior*, e.g., *Continuous spinning, repetitive head smashing against the wall*.

- *Asperger disorder*: Looks just like autistic disorder, *with the exception that patients communicate and move normally*.
- *Selective mutism*: A disorder that is common in *females*, misdiagnosed as *shyness*. The child is essentially normal, but only in certain situations (e.g., In front of strangers she would not talk).

Rett Disorder

- *Clinical picture*: After a period of normal development, the child starts to *lose already acquired skills*.
- *Note*: Almost always occurs in females. Another form of the disease that presents similarly in males is called *Childhood disintegrative disorder*.

Tourette's Disorder

- *Mechanism*: Dysfunction in the regulation of *dopamine* in *caudate nucleus*.
- *Clinical picture*: More common in *males*, where the child has *multiple motor tics* and *at least one vocal tic*. It could be transient (<1 year) or chronic (>1 year).
- *Treatment*: *Haloperidol. Note that treatment is lifelong*.
- *Note*: There is a strong genetic link between Tourette's, ADHD and OCD syndromes.

Separation Anxiety Disorder

- *Introduction*: Fear of loss of attachment figures.
- *Clinical picture*: Typical presentation is for a child who refuses to leave home right after the family moved to a new house.
- *Prognosis*: These patients usually develop *agoraphobia* later in life.
- *Treatment*: Supportive by gradual acclimatization to the new situation.

Abuse

Child Physical Abuse

- *Clinical picture*: *Shaken baby syndrome*, which is characterized by *retinal hemorrhage and detachment* and *spiral bone fractures*.
- *Treatment*: Hospitalize the patient and *contact social services*.

Child Sexual Abuse

- **Introduction**: Most common age involved is *9–12*.
- **Clinical picture**: Suspect in any child with *recurrent UTIs*, or with *phthirus pubis in eye lashes*.
- **Note**: The abuser is usually a very close family relative or friend.
- **Treatment**: *Contact social services.*

Others

- **Elderly abuse**: The abuser is mostly *the spouse or caregiver*. Treatment: *Contact social services.*
- **Partner abuse**: Whether physical or sexual, starts with *tension* building up, followed by *battery* and ending up with *apology*. Female risk of being physically or sexually abused during their life is around *25%*. Treatment: *Do not contact social services; only advise the patient that abuse is illegal and that she has the right to seek help by contacting social services.*
- **Sexual assault**: It is not a must to have penetration or ejaculation involved to call it an assault. Complication: *Post-traumatic Stress Disorder (PTSD).*
- **Statutory rape**: Any sexual intercourse younger than *18 years* of age falls under this category, regardless whether it was consensual or not.

Drug and Alcohol Abuse

- **Introduction**: Abuse is an abnormal use of a substance that leads to some sort of impairment. *Dependence, on the other hand, is an abuse combined with tolerance and withdrawal symptoms.*
- **Types and features**: Refer to Table 7.2.

TABLE 7.2 Most commonly abused drugs and their effects.

	Transmitter	Clinical picture
Cocaine	Dopamine	- Mechanism: Vasoconstriction - Tactile hallucinations, i.e., Sensation of bugs crawling under your skin - Chest pain: Due to coronary vasospasm - Perforated nasal septum - Sympathetic hyperactivity: Hypertension, tachycardia and dilated pupils - Withdrawal: Crash syndrome (Depression, fatigue and somnolence), followed by dysphoria - Cocaine metabolite: Benzoylecogonine - Note: Cocaine is the only anesthetic that causes vasoconstriction

Opioids	Dopamine	- Analgesia: Due to increase in the pain threshold
		- Euphoria: Due to stimulation of the ventral tegmentum
		- Pin point pupils: Due to stimulation of the Edinger-Westphal oculomotor nucleus
		- Emesis: Due to stimulation of chemoreceptor trigger zone
		- Fluid retention: Due to stimulation of ADH secretion
		- Others: Anti-tussive, increase intracranial pressure and histamine release, and also causes constipation
		- Indications: Pain, diarrhea and cough
		- Elimination: In urine and bile in the form of morphine-6-glucuronide
		- Tolerance: Common to all effects except constipation and pupillary constriction
		- Reversal: Naloxone.
		- Withdrawal (Cold turkey):
		  1. First stage: Lacrimation, rhinorrhea and muscle aches
		  2. Second stage: Excessive sweating
		  3. Third stage: Excessive micturition and defecation, vomiting and diarrhea
		- Treatment of withdrawal: Methadone and clonidine.

Alcohol	GABA	- Euphoria initially, followed by depression. - Wernicke's encephalopathy: Encephalopathy, nystagmus and ataxia. Due to Thiamine (B1) deficiency affecting mammillary bodies. - Korsakoff syndrome: Amnesia (Antero- and retro-grade) and confabulations. Due to Thiamine (B1) deficiency affecting the Hippocampus - Withdrawal: Delirium tremens (DTs) in 2–5 days, where patient has delirium, tremors and possibly seizures. Treatment: BDZ is the first step (Best is Chlordiazepoxide) plus folic acid, thiamine (B1), and pyridoxine (B6) - Alcohol intoxication level: 0.08–0.15% - If patient has blood alcohol level >0.10% and shows no symptoms of intoxication, suspect tolerance - Blood alcohol level >0.4% is fatal - Chronic alcoholism causes impotence, decreased sperm count and testosterone level

TABLE 7.2 (Continued)

	Transmitter	Clinical picture
LSD (Lysergic acid diethylamide)	Serotonin	• Mechanism: An agonist of serotonin 5-HT1 and 5-HT2 receptors • Dream-like state, e.g., Pt thinks he is flying • Visual hallucinations • Bad trips: Panic attacks • Flashbacks: Patient experiences the symptoms he develops in the absence of the drug • Reversal: Haloperidol
Marijuana (Cannabis)	Serotonin	• Depersonalization • Loss of time perception • Conjunctival redness • Increased appetite (The munchies) • Used clinically to treat chemotherapy-induced emesis.
PCP (Angeldust)	Serotonin	• Blocks NMDA receptors, which leads to inhibited uptake of Norepinephrine, serotonin and dopamine. • Hyperthermia, hypersalivation, aggression and violent behavior • Treatment: Phentolamine, diazepam, haloperidol and acidification of urine
Methylxanth-ines (Caffeine)	Dopamine	• Mechanism: Inhibit phosphodiestrase, which in turn leads to elevated cAMP and cGMP levels. This leads to positive inotropic and chronotropic effects • Insomnia, alertness and diuresis • Side effects: Increases gastric HCL production • Precautions: It can cross placenta and is found in breast milk • Withdrawal: Headache, sleepiness and lethargy
Amphetam-ine	Dopamine	• Mechanism: It decreases the appetite and increases alertness • Indications: ADHD and narcolepsy • Side effects: Psychosis, insomnia and GI upset • Reversal: Chlorpromazine
Nicotine	Dopamine	• Mechanism: Inhibits the ganglia after an initial phase of stimulation • Side effects: 1. Low dose: Euphoria and increased alertness 2. High dose: Depression of the respiratory center • Withdrawal: Irritability, headache and craving • Metabolite of nicotine: Cotinine

Sleep

Sleep Waves and Stages

- Patient awake, relaxed and eyes closed: *Alpha waves*.
- Patient awake, concentrating and eyes open: *Beta waves*.
- *Stage 1 of sleep*: *Theta waves*.
- *Stage 2 of sleep*: *Sleep spindles* and *K complexes*. *45% of our sleeping time is spent in stage 2*.
- *Stages 3 and 4 of sleep*: *Delta (Slow) waves. Sleep walking and nocturnal enuresis occur during these 2 stages.*
- *Rapid Eye Movement (REM) sleep*:

  1. Alpha, Beta and Theta waves combined giving a *saw-tooth appearance*.
  2. *Dreams, nightmares, sympathetic stimulation, erection* and *complete skeletal muscles relaxation* occur during this stage.
  3. *REM rebound* to compensate for missed REM on the previous sleep cycle is common.

4. After you fall asleep, the cycle goes as *90 min of normal sleep* alternating with *10 min of REM sleep*, and the cycle keeps repeating itself.
5. REM sleep is regulated by *acetylcholine*, and is suppressed by *MAOI*.

Regulation of Sleep

- *Serotonin and melatonin*: Induce sleep.
- *Dopamine and norepinephrine*: Inhibit sleep. *That is the reason anti-psychotics improve sleep.*

Sleep Disorders

- *Narcolepsy*: Uncontrollable *attacks of falling asleep*. Some key symptoms in these patients are:

  1. *Cataplexy*: Generalized loss of muscle tone. Induced by any form of excitement, e.g., Laughing, cough, orgasm.
  2. *Hallucinations*: Either before falling asleep (*Hypnagogic*), or upon waking up (*Hypnopompic*).

- **Sleep terror**: This disorder occurs during *delta wave sleep* (*Not the REM like all other dreams and nightmares*). Patient is screaming in bed with what looks like a bad nightmare: however, it is *very hard to get him/her to wake up*. After waking up, the patient has *no recollection of the incident*. It is an indicator of possible *temporal lobe epilepsy* later in life.
- **Klein Levin syndrome**: Episodes of *hypersomnia and hyperphagia*, each lasting *1–2 weeks*.
- **Sleep changes during depression**:

  1. *Normal sleep onset.*
  2. Frequent awakenings during the night and in the early morning (*Terminal insomnia*).
  3. REM sleep: *Short latency*, and *high frequency*, which tends to decrease throughout the night.

Delirium

Introduction

- **Definition**: Delirium is a cyclic disorder, where patient fluctuates in and out of *consciousness*, more commonly towards the night time; a.k.a. *sundowning phenomenon*.
- **Population**: Very common to see delirium in elderly patients admitted to the hospital, specifically to the ICU (*ICU psychosis*), where almost *one third* of the patients would suffer some degree of delirium.

Clinical Picture

- Altered level of consciousness.
- Disorientation: *First to time*, then place and finally to person.
- *Visual* hallucinations.
- EEG changes.

Treatment

- **Treat the cause**. Delirium in the elderly is caused by *DIM*; *Drugs, Infections or Metabolic derangement*.
- **Drug of choice**: *Haloperidol*.

Schizophrenia

Introduction

- **Introduction**: Cycle of symptoms that lasts at least *6 months* at a time, more common in the *winter months*, and in *young adults (20–40 years)*.
- **Mechanism**: Unknown, but the fact that it is more prevalent in the cold months suggest a possible link to *viral infection*.

- **Personality**: Most patients already have *borderline personality*; characterized by *splitting, mood swings* and suicidal attempts.
- **Risk**: 50% in monozygotic twins.
- **Forms**: Paranoid, disorganized or *catatonic* (*Waxy flexibility*).
- **Duration**:

  1. Less than 1 month: *Brief psychotic disorder*.
  2. One–6 months: *Schizophreniform disorder*.
  3. More than 6 months: *Schizophrenia*.

Pathology

- **Transmitters**: Decreased GABA neurons in *hippocampus*.
- **Hormones**: Low serum levels of FSH and LH.
- **Positron Emission Tomography (PET) scan**: Shows *decreased glucose uptake* by *frontal lobes*, and *hyperactive dopamine loaded basal ganglia*.
- **EEG**: *Decreased alpha* and *increased Theta and Delta* waves with *epileptiform activity*.

Clinical Picture

- **Prodrome**: Patient is calm, and only shows some change in interests, e.g., Sudden interest in politics, religion or languages.
- **Psychosis**: Characterized by the following:

  1. *Hallucinations*: Mainly *auditory* (*Delirious patients have visual ones*).
  2. *Thought blocking*: Moves his lips frequently without vocalizing.
  3. *Neologism*: Patient uses new non-existing vocabulary.
  4. *Loose association*: Changing subjects quickly while talking.
  5. *Tangentiality*: When you ask the patient a question, he would start the answer in a good organized way, and then slide away from the subject into something else.
  6. *Echolalia*: Increased alertness and response to sounds, often compared to *parrots*.

- **Residual phase**: *Social withdrawal*.

Types of Symptoms

- **Positive**: As above, and *they respond* to *typical antipsychotics* (*Block D2 receptors in the mesolimbic system*).
- **Negative**: Patient does not have typical presentation as discussed above. He is rather blunt and withdrawn at all times. Patients in this category *do not*

respond to typical anti-psychotics; however, they respond only to *atypical anti-psychotics*, e.g., *Clozapine* and *risperidone* (*Both block 5HT-2 receptors*).

Notes

- *Schizophrenia of childhood*: *More common* and *presents at an earlier age* in *males* compared to females.
- *Schizoaffective disorder*: Schizophrenia plus a mood disorder, e.g., Depression.
- *Orbitofrontal syndrome (Pseudo-psychopathic)*: *Disinhibited behavior, emotional lability*, euphoria and *jocular effect*.
- *Side effects of neuroleptics (Anti-psychotics)*:

  1. *Akasthesia*: Subjective feeling of restlessness. *Treatment*: Propranolol.
  2. *Tardive dyskinesia*: Abnormal movements and posturing. *Prevention*: Benztropine. *Treatment*: Discontinue the drug and switch to another neuroleptic.
  3. *Neuroleptic malignant syndrome*: Rigidity and hyperthermia due to severe actin-myosin coupling resulting in excessive ATP production. Treatment: *Dantrolene*.
  4. *Anti-cholinergic effects*, e.g., urinary retention, constipation, xerostomia.
  5. *Drug specific side effects*:

     - Clozapine: *Agranulocytosis*.
     - Chlorpromazine: *Bluish grey skin discoloration*.
     - Thioridazine: *Orthostatic hypotension* and *retinal pigmentation*.

Mood Disorders

Major Depressive Disorder

- *Mechanism*: Depletion of *serotonin and norepinephrine*.
- *Best screening*: Ask the patient if he or she is depressed.
- *Clinical picture*: At least *5* of the following:

  1. S: *S*leeping problems.
  2. I: Loss of *i*nterest, a.k.a. *Anhedonia*, and *"feeling worthless"*.
  3. G: *G*uilt feelings
  4. E: Lack of *e*nergy
  5. C: Lack of *c*oncentration
  6. A: Change in *a*ppetite; increased or decreased
  7. P: *P*sychomotor retardation and agitation
  8. S: *S*uicidal ideation. It occurs in *60–70% of patients*; however, *only 15% actually do it*. *Women are more likely to have suicidal ideas and plans than men; however, men are more likely to be successful in committing suicide than women*.

- *Concordance rate*: 70% in monozygotic twins, 20% in dizygotic twins.
- *Treatment*: SSRIs (*First line*) or TCAs.
- *Notes*:

  1. Most anti-depressants take *3–6 weeks* to be fully effective, so do not make any changes in dosing of medication before 6 weeks from starting the medication.
  2. After initiation of therapy, it is very important to follow up frequently on the patient, as *antidepressants might give the patient enough energy to commit suicide early in the course of their treatment*.
  3. *Electroconvulsive therapy (ECT)* is only indicated for severe depression that is resistant to treatment. *Side effects of ECT*: Retrograde amnesia that resolves gradually over 6 months. *Contraindication to ECT*: High intracranial pressure, e.g., Tumor, bleeding, hydrocephalus.
  4. Patients with suicidal ideation must be admitted (Voluntarily or involuntarily) to a psychiatric ward. Involuntary admission must be certified by *2 physicians*. Risk factors for suicide: Depression, male gender, lack of spouse, alcoholism and most importantly a *previous suicidal attempt*.
  5. Patients with homicidal ideation must be admitted (Voluntarily or involuntarily) to a psychiatric ward. Also the police and the potential victim should be contacted (*Tarasoff decision*).
  6. *Dysthymia*: Patient with depressed mood for at least *2 years* (*Just feels down*), but does not have enough depression criteria to diagnose wih major depressive disorder.
  7. *Double depression*: Major depression episode followed by dysthymia. Treatment: *MAOI*.
  8. *Atypical depression*: Depression with severe anxiety. Treatment: *MAOI*.
  9. Cyclothymia: Patient with *hypomanic mood for at least 2 years*, but does not look manic as described below.
  10. Postpartum blues is a *depressed mood* that occurs during the *first week* after labor; however, postpartum depression is a *major depressive disorder* that does not start till at least *1 month* after labor (*10%* of women suffer from that).

Bipolar Disorder

- *Duration of symptoms*: *At least 3 months*.
- *Types*:

  1. I: Depression alternating with *mania*.
  2. II: Depression alternating with *hypomania*.

- *Clinical picture*: During manic episodes, the patient feels *overjoyed*, *goes out on shopping sprees*, has *flight of ideas* and a strong feeling of *grandiosity*, e.g., "I won't talk to a clerk about my application, people like me talk to CEOs directly."
- *Risk*: 75% in monozygotic twins.
- *Treatment*: *Mood stabilizers*; discussed later. *TCAs and SSRIs are contraindicated in bipolar disorder as they increase the likelihood of suicide*
- *Note*: Theories suggest a link with X chromosome.

Personality and Pain Disorders
Personality Disorders

- *Paranoid*: Multiple delusions and suspicions, e.g., "I think everybody is trying to set me up at work because I am smart."
- *Borderline*: Swinging mood, stormy relationships and *splitting*, e.g., "When I was at the hospital, all nurses on the 7th floor were horrible, but the rest were really good."
- *Passive aggressive*: *Procrastination* is the key finding. They show enthusiasm to whatever you suggest, but then *passively resist* doing it and they end up being aggressive when confronted, e.g., You suggest HIV testing to a patient; he shows enthusiasm that he should have it done, but he comes back one month later without having the test done, and when you ask him, he just gets angry and flustered and tell you "Well, I called the lab and they just did not answer the phone."
- *Histrionic*: Seductive provocative personality. If you see a patient who is dressed and acting like a porn star, you know what to think!
- *Narcissistic*: *Grandiosity*; they believe they are better than everybody else. Do not confuse this with the grandiosity of mania, as the latter is a short term episodic disorder, but narcissism is a life long *personality disorder*.
- *Avoidant*: Avoids getting involved in any activity or relationship for *fear of rejection*.
- *Dependant*: Frequently depends on someone else for decisions and actions.

Pain (Somatoform) Disorders

- *Somatization (Briquet's syndrome)*: Patient presents with at least *4 pain symptoms*, *2 GI related*, *1 sexual* and *1 neurological* complaints. (*And yes, in the exam, you have to count.*)
- *Body dysmorphic disorder*: The patient fixates on one *normal* part of her body with complete belief that it looks wrong, e.g., A model comes to your clinic every week complaining about how big her nose is.

- *Conversion disorder*: Subjective, functional disturbance induced by exposure to a certain emotional event, e.g., A patient who lost her vision for one hour once she found out she failed an exam. These patients don't seem concerned about the functional disturbance; this is known as *La belle indifference*.
- *Hypochondriasis*: The patient exaggerates mild symptoms, insists there is something wrong and demands a work up. He spends his time seeing different doctors, a.k.a. *doctor shopping*, e.g., A patient who has seen 15 doctors in the last 6 months for his headaches. He is convinced he has a brain tumor when the brain imaging and clinical scenario are consistent with typical tension headaches.
- *Pain disorder*: A patient who has *unexplainable pain*, e.g., A patient who complains her arm hurts, but all the work up is normal. *Similarly, if a patient complains of an unexplainable symptom (not pain), it is called "Undifferentiated somatoform disorder"*, e.g., *A patient who complains of shortness of breath, but all the work up is normal.*
- *Factitious disorder (Munchausen's syndrome)*: Patient fakes different symptoms, just for the sake of getting *attention*. These patients *are willing* to take medications or undergo surgeries if you asked them to, e.g., A mother is taking her kid from one clinic to another, and keeps telling the doctor about million complaints that the kid has; however, all the work up comes back normal, this is known as *Munchausen's by proxy*.
- *Malingering*: Patient fakes different symptoms, just for the sake of getting a *certain benefit*, e.g., Time off, financial compensation. These patients *are not willing* to take medications or undergo surgeries if you asked them to.
- *Gain*: When patients complains of pain, they gain 2 things:
  1. *Primary*: They express their emotional problems, but in the form of an illness.
  2. *Secondary*: Getting attention and tender loving care (TLC).
- *Treatment*: Best treatment for all above disorders is *psycho- and group therapy*.

Defense Psychology

Defense Mechanisms

- *Displacement*: Displacing a certain emotion from one unacceptable situation to a more acceptable one, e.g., A lawyer who just had an argument with his domineering wife goes to his office and is rude to his female secretary all day.

- *Acting out*: Irresponsible action induced by a certain emotion, usually done by teenagers, e.g., A 16 year old who just had an argument with her mom goes to her room and destroys the TV set with a baseball bat.
- *Altruism*: Doing good things to avoid certain negative or guilt feelings, e.g., A mafia hit man who just murdered someone last week went to the bank today and gave $1000 to charity.
- *Identification*: Subjectively inheriting a certain behavior, e.g., A person who was mistreated by his parents as a kid insists on mistreating his own kids in the same way.
- *Fixation*: The permanence of a childish attitude, e.g., An adult man watching cartoons every day.
- *Projection*: The projection of certain unacceptable feelings into others, e.g., A person who is angry with his co-worker accuses his co-worker of being angry with him.
- *Rationalization*: Attempting to rethink a certain event to make it seem less serious, e.g., After failing an exam for licensure in Canada, the engineering student says "Well, that's okay, I never really liked Canada that much anyway."
- *Reaction formation*: Attempting to hide certain unacceptable feelings by doing or saying something very acceptable, e.g., A worker is very angry with his boss for messing up his schedule, but when he sees him, he says "Hey boss, I like your tie."
- *Sublimation*: Expressing an unacceptable emotion in an acceptable situation, e.g., A student who is furious after failing his exam goes to practice some boxing.
- *Suppression*: Deliberately not thinking of unacceptable emotions, e.g., A doctor who has phobia from female genitalia puts his feelings aside to examine a female patient who came complaining of vaginal discharge.
- *Repression*: Completely forgetting an unacceptable emotion, e.g., A student who is extremely stressed about the USMLE experiences a period of unconcern and doesn't even recall he's scheduled to take the test.
- *Regression*: Adopting a child's attitude to escape a certain unacceptable emotion, e.g., A 55 year old patient hospitalized for a heart attack wants his mom to stay with him in the room, then he wets the bed during sleep.
- *Intellectualization*: An unconscious avoidance of an unacceptable emotion by using logic or focusing on the minutiae of the situation, e.g., A surgeon explains to his co-workers in details about how he was diagnosed the other day with terminal lung cancer, yet he is talking normally about it without

any emotion, trying to use his case for a routine medical discussion.
- *Isolation of affect*: Failure to express emotions, e.g., The same surgeon as above explains to his co-workers about how his dad died of the same cancer and the details of the days before his death and how much that experience broke his heart, yet not showing any *affect* that fits this dramatic story.

Dissociation

- *Definition*: Group of disorders that occur as a defense mechanism against fear or severe underlying anxiety.
- *Dissociative amnesia*: Patient cannot recall painful events, e.g., A man who does not remember anything about a motor vehicle accident that killed his wife and kids.
- *Dissociative fugue*: Patient cannot recall change in identity and location, e.g., A woman once lived in the UK, then came to Michigan and has been working here for 5 years. She comes to see you in the clinic and she knows she is in Michigan, but has no recollection of having lived in the UK or moved from anywhere to anywhere.
- *Dissociative identity*: A patient who has more than one personality, but none of them is aware of the other, e.g., A conservative librarian received a note in the mail to attend a court trial for stripping in public and attempting prostitution. She shows up to court with the belief that there is a misunderstanding, but they show her pictures showing her naked in the street (which she has no recollection of).
- *Depersonalization*: Patient believes he lives outside of his own body and can watch himself.
- *Treatment*: For all above conditions is *hypnosis and psychotherapy*.

Eating Disorders

Introduction

- Common among *females, adolescents,* and *persons under stress.*
- At least *30%* of the American population falls in the obese range, and *20% in the overweight one.*

Anorexia Nervosa

- *Weight loss*: Loss of at least *15%* of body weight.
- *Eating behavior*: Starvation.
- *Personality*: Perfection seeking person, with good scores in school and *fear of getting fat.*

- *Sexual*: Amenorrhea and absence of any interest in sex.
- *Metabolic*: Metabolic acidosis, hyperlipidemia and osteoporosis.
- *CBC*: Anemia and leucopenia.
- *Skin*: Lanugo (*Downy hair*).
- *GI*: Melanosis coli (Pigmentation of colonic wall), due to *overuse of laxatives*.

Bulimia Nervosa

- *Weight loss*: *Normal body weight or even overweight.*
- *Eating behavior*: Binges of eating followed by induced vomiting.
- *GI*: Esophageal varices, parotid gland swelling and eroded enamel of anterior teeth.
- *Signs of induced gagging*: Scars and marks on the dorsum of hands.

Treatment

- *Anorexia nervosa*: Amitryptiline, Cyproheptadine or SSRIs, *plus behavioral and family psychotherapy.*
- *Bulimia nervosa*: SSRIs, *plus behavioral and family psychotherapy.*

Sex

Gender Identity and Role

- *Gender identity*: When the person can identify his/her gender, i.e., Male vs female. Usually occurs around age *3*.
- *Gender role*: How the person *acts, i.e., Like a male vs female*.

Sex Cycle

- *Excitement*: Characterized by *erection* in males, and *tenting of uterus* in females.
- *Plateau*: Enlarged inner part and contraction of outer part of the vagina.
- *Orgasm*: Characterized by *ejaculation* in males and *uterine contraction* in females. *Contraction of anal sphincter* also occurs during this stage.
- *Resolution*: Muscle relaxation.

Sexual Disorders

- *Sexual disorders*: Multiple; the most common are:

  1. Males: *Secondary impotence*, i.e., Secondary to stress or anxiety.
  2. Females: *Failure to orgasm.*

- *Medically related sexual disorders*: Multiple; the most common are:

  1. Coronary artery disease (CAD): Patients have decreased libido due to *fear* of suffering another heart attack. If the patient can climb *2 flights of stairs* or accommodate a heart rate of *130 bpm* without a problem, he can have sex.
  2. DM: Impotence and retrograde ejaculation.
  3. Spinal cord injury: Retrograde ejaculation.

- *Medication or drug-related sexual disorders*:

  1. Increased sexuality: Anti-depressants, anti-psychotics, marijuana, cocaine, amphetamine and small amounts of alcohol.
  2. Decreased sexuality: Excessive amounts or long duration of alcohol use.

- *Premature ejaculation*: Common sexual problem. Treatment: *SSRI.*
- *Hypoactive sexual desire*: Decreased sexual desire of one partner towards another.
- *Sexual arousal disorder*: Absence of sexual arousal during intercourse.
- *Sexual aversion*: Normal person who is just not so much into sex. Again, the patient is not homosexual or having any psychological problems.
- *Transvestic fetishism*: A man who gets pleasure from wearing women's clothing or vice versa.
- *Frotteurism*: e.g., A man attempting to touch and rub into women in the elevator or the bus without their consent.
- *Voyeurism*: A person enjoying watching other people having sex.
- *Sadism*: A person enjoying *giving* physical pain to his partner during sex.
- *Masochism*: A person enjoying *receiving* physical pain during sex.
- *Vaginismus*: Painful contraction of the outer part of the vagina preventing sexual intercourse.

Important Disorders

Obsessive Compulsive Disorder (OCD)

- *Definition*: Disorder in which patients have recurrent thoughts and repetitive behaviors that *interfere* with the patient's life. They have *strong insight* (Know they have a problem) and *ego dystonia* (Patient views his behavior as inconsistent with the way he sees his own personality).
- *Mechanism*: *Obsessions* with a certain idea, followed by *compulsions* to do something.
- *The most common form*: Obsessions with contamination, e.g., *Frequent hand washing.*

- **Treatment**: *SSRI* are the drugs of choice. Clomipramine (TCA with serotonin activity) is another option.
- **Note**: Ego dystonia of OCD is absent during childhood.

Panic Attacks

- **Mechanism**: Possibly genetic disease; more common in *females*.
- **Common medical association**: *Mitral valve prolapse*.
- **Clinical picture**: At least *2 attacks a week*:

  1. Hyperventilation and tachycardia.
  2. Chest pain, diaphoresis, tremors and sense of *impending death*.
  3. Anxiety and fear of having attacks (*Anticipatory anxiety*), especially when present in an open place (*Agoraphobia*).

- **Treatment**:

  1. Acute attacks: *Benzodiazepine*, e.g., *Alprazolam*.
  2. Maintenance: *SSRI*.

Phobia

- **Definition**: *Irrational fear (Fear without a cause)* of something or a situation.
- **Examples**:

  1. Agoraphobia: Fear of open places. Common in *panic attacks* and *separation anxiety*.
  2. Acrophobia: Fear of *heights*.
  3. Claustrophobia: Fear of *small closed places*.
  4. Social phobia: Fear of social gatherings. Best treatment: *SSRIs*.

- **Treatment**: *Behavioral and cognitive therapy*.

Post-Traumatic Stress Disorder (PTSD)

- **Definition**: Stress disorder that follows a *life threatening event*, e.g., War, motor vehicle accident, rape, assault.
- **Clinical picture**: Anxiety, *nightmares*, *flashbacks* and social withdrawal.
- **Duration of symptoms**:

  1. Longer than 1 month: PTSD.
  2. Shorter than 1 month: *Acute stress disorder*.

- **Note**: If same symptoms develop after a *non-life threatening event*, e.g., A breakup, divorce, death of a pet, it is called *Adjustment disorder* not PTSD.

- **Treatment**: *Behavioral and group therapy* is the treatment of choice. SSRI are also used.

Generalized Anxiety Disorder

- **Definition**: Excessive worry and anxiety about almost everything, which has been lasting for *more than 6 months*.
- **Clinical picture**: Anxiety, nervousness, irritability and muscle tension.
- **Treatment**: Drug of choice is Buspiroue. Benzodiazepines (BDZ) can also be used.

Medically-Induced Psychological Disorders

- **Cancer of tail of the pancreas**: *Depression*.
- **Cushing syndrome**: *Depression*.
- **Wilson's disease**: *Anger and aggression*.
- **Temporal lobe epilepsy**: *OCD* and *paranoia*.
- **Ulcerative colitis and migraine headaches**: *OCD*.
- **Hyperparathyroidism**: *Psychosis*.
- **Asthma**: *Dependency*.
- **Chronic kidney disease and dialysis**: *Depression and suicidal ideation*.

Behavioral and Cognitive Therapy (Refer to Table 7.3)

Extinction

- **Definition**: Gradual decrease of a negative behavior after positive reinforcement is removed.
- **Example**: A kid used to get attention from his family every time his brother took his toys, by claiming that his leg hurt. They rushed him to the doctor many times, and found everything was normal. For the last week, his family stopped paying that much attention, and eventually he stopped claiming that his leg hurts.

Reinforcement

- **Positive reinforcement**: *Giving a reward* to change behavior, e.g., "If you do something good, I will give you a cookie."
- **Negative reinforcement**: *Giving a punishment* to change behavior, e.g., "If you do something bad, I will take away your cookie."
- **Note**: Reinforcement is the most rapid and effective way to adjust a behavior.

TABLE 7.3 Behavioral and cognitive therapy.

Therapy	Process	Explanation scenarios
Aversive conditioning	Classical conditioning	Whenever the dog barks, he gets shocked by an electric device around his neck
Systemic desensitization	Classical conditioning	Patient who is afraid of syringes. First, you show him pictures of syringes and few visits later, you make him touch an actual syringe
Implosion	Habituation	Implosion: Patient who is afraid of needles, you make him close his eyes and imagine living through a scenario where he is getting a blood draw. Flooding: Patient who is afraid of needles, you perform a blood draw on him. Note that flooding is an operant conditioning technique
Token economy	Operant conditioning	Patients are given tokens for desired behavior which they can use for a certain privilege, e.g., making a phone call, watching TV. A common technique in psychiatry wards
Biofeedback	Operant conditioning	Patient can control his organs and functions, e.g., Blood pressure, heart rate
Cognitive therapy	Supportive therapy	Patient trains herself that whenever she gets worried about her exam, she would think about passing it with high scores

Psychopharmacology

Introduction

- *Facts*: Know these two facts well: A patient's mood is regulated by *norepinephrine* and *serotonin,* and mania is the reciprocal of depression.
- *Medications*: TCA, SSRI, MAOI and mood stabilizers.

Tricyclic Antidepressants (TCA)

- *Introduction*: TCAs take *3–4 weeks* to achieve a therapeutic effect.
- *Mechanism*: *Block the reuptake of norepinephrine.*
- *Indications*:

  1. Major depressive disorder.
  2. Imipramine: TCA of choice to treat *enuresis.*
  3. Clomipramine: TCA of choice to treat *Obsessive compulsive disorder (OCD). Note that the drug of choice in general to treat OCD is SSRI.*

- *Side effects*:

  1. *Anti-cholinergic effects*: Urinary retention, constipation, xerostomia.
  2. Toxicity (Low therapeutic index): Hypotension, *prolonged Q-T interval.*

- *Note*: Amoxapine and maprotiline are second generation TCAs.

Selective Serotonin Reuptake Inhibitors (SSRI)

- *Mechanism*:

  1. Inhibit *presynaptic* serotonin reuptake.

  2. *Inhibit cytochrome P450* system, hence increasing free levels of other drugs.

- *Indications*: Major depressive disorder, OCD, anorexia and bulimia nervosa, *premature ejaculation* and panic attacks.
- *Side effects*:

  1. *Delayed ejaculation,* hence used to treat *premature ejaculation.*
  2. Insomnia, tremors and weight loss.

- *Examples*: Fluoxetine, Paroxetine, Sertraline.

Monoamine Oxidase Inhibitors (MAOI)

- *Indications: Atypical* and *resistant depression.*
- *Complications*:

  1. *Tyramine hypertensive crisis*: If given with a tyramine containing substance (Red wine or cheese). Treatment: *Phentolamine plus nifedipine.*
  2. *Serotonin syndrome*: If given with SSRI. Clinical picture: *Muscle rigidity, hyperreflexia* and *clonus.* Treatment: Serotonin antagonist e.g., *Cyproheptadine.*

- *Examples*: Phenelzine, tranylcypromine.

Mood Stabilizers

- *Mechanism*: Lithium acts via the *phosphatidylinositol system.*
- *Indication: Bipolar disorder.*
- *Lithium side effects*:

  1. *Teratogenicity: Ebstein anomaly.*
  2. *Hypothyroidism.*

3. *Nephrogenic diabetes insipidus.*
4. Toxicity: *Vomiting, diarrhea, tremors and nystagmus.* Note: Therapeutic level of lithium: *0.6–1.2* meq/L.

Carbamazepine side effects*: SIADH and Stevens-Johnson syndrome.*
- ***Examples***: Lithium, carbamazepine.

Ethics

Living Will

- ***Definition***: Legal document describing what kind of medical measures should and should not be used.
- ***Rule of thumb***: Simply do what the patient wants, even if it does not make perfect sense to you. If there is a DNR already signed by the patient, *do not ask the family or anybody; just do what the will says.*
- ***Example***: If you see a patient in the USMLE whose will indicate a DNR (Do Not Resuscitate), but the only way to save him is Endotracheal (ET) intubation, *do not intubate.*
- ***Your responsibilities are***:

  1. Make sure the patient understands the advantages and disadvantages of his decision, e.g., "If you do not get intubated, you are going to die."
  2. Do *everything else* you can to save the patient without breaking the DNR limitations, e.g., If it indicates that he does not want to have blood transfusion, but he is losing blood, you can try to give him plasma. If it indicates that he does not want intubation, but now he cannot breathe, try to use a mask or a Bi-level positive airway pressure machine (BiPAP).

Durable Power of Attorney

- ***Introduction***: A patient can choose someone to be the decision maker on his behalf *if he becomes incompetent.* Again, this is a legal document done by a lawyer.
- ***Example***: You see a patient in the USMLE who cannot breath and likely needs intubation, but does not have any living will or DNR, and can't make decisions for himself. If a family member shows up and presents papers that he has durable power of attorney, and asks you not to intubate the patient and to just let him go, *then you do what he says.*
- ***Your responsibilities are***:

  1. Make sure that the decision maker actually does have durable power of attorney *documentation.*

2. Make sure that the patient is actually incompetent to make his own decisions. *The rule of thumb here is that if the patient is competent to make his own decisions, you listen to him and not to the person with the durable power of attorney.* Again, you listen to the latter *only if the patient is incompetent to make his own decisions.*

Surrogate Decision

- ***Introduction***: The idea here is to ask the people who know the patient best what they think *he would have wanted* (Not what the family wants).
- ***Rule of thumb***: What if you get a patient in the USMLE who cannot breathe and needs intubation. He is comatosed, does not have a living will, DNR order or given power of attorney to anyone. Your responsibility is to ask his close family if the patient would have agreed to intubation if he was competent to make his own decision.
- ***To sum up***:

  1. First one to ask for a decision: *The patient.*
  2. If patient is incompetent: *Person with durable power of attorney.*
  3. If no power of attorney: *Surrogates.*
  4. If no surrogates: *Treat the patient fully with no limitations.*

Euthanasia

- ***Passive***: Simply to leave the patient to die and not interfere. The only thing you provide is comfort measures so that the patient would not suffer much. It is legal.
- ***Active***: Speeding up the patient's death, e.g., Using medications, etc.…. *This is illegal and is considered a crime.*

Children

- ***Rule of thumb***: You must get consent before treating or even touching any patient. Any child *below 18 yours* of age is a *minor* who has to be consented for by *his parents or legal guardians* (See exceptions below).
- ***In emergency situations***: Treat the child fully without limitations even if the parents decide otherwise, e.g., A man and his 12 years old son come to the ER after a motor vehicle accident. You find that the kid has intra-abdominal hemorrhage and has to be taken to surgery immediately. The father states that he does not want you to take the kid for surgery even though you explained that he might die if he doesn't go. What you should do: *Take the kid to surgery.*

- *In non-emergency situations*: If the parents refuse to consent to treating their child, what you should do is to *get a court order to treat the child.*
- *Exceptions*: You *do not* need parental consent in the following situations:

  1. Emergency situations: Explained above.
  2. Absence of parents and legal guardian: If a child is brought to the ER by his school teacher because of abdominal pain, but you could not contact his parents and he does not have a legal guardian. Do you take consent from the teacher? Answer: *No, only parents or legal guardian consent; if none is available, you treat the patient without consent.*
  3. Treatment of sexually transmitted diseases (STD).
  4. Contraception.
  5. Care during pregnancy.
  6. Treatment of alcohol or drug dependence.
  7. *Emancipated minors*: Any minor (<18) who has one or more of the following factors: *Self supporting and living on his own, married, has children or in the military.*

Pregnant

- *Introduction*: A pregnant woman has the right to decide for the fetus in her uterus.
- *Example*: A pregnant woman is brought to the ER after a motor vehicle accident, and she is having intra-abdominal hemorrhage, but she tells you that she does not want you to do anything. You explain to her that she will die if you do not act, and she does not change her mind. Then you explain that if you take her to surgery and deliver her baby, he might have a chance of living, and she still refuses. What you should do?: *Do what she says.*

Criminal Law

- *Mental insanity*: Defined as having a mental or severe psychological abnormality, plus one of the following statutory criteria:

  1. *M'Naghten: Most reliable criterion.* Evaluates if the patient understands his actions; what is right and what is wrong at the time of the crime.
  2. *American law institute model penal code*: Reliable. Evaluates whether the patient understands the wrongfulness of his actions at the time of the crime and lacks the capacity to control his actions.
  3. *Durham*: Not reliable. Evaluates if the crime was strictly induced by the mental or psychological abnormality, i.e., No accusation if mentally ill.

- *Mens rea elements*: Evaluates whether or not the crime was based on intent.
- *Irresistible impulse rule*: Defendant unable to refrain from the crime, e.g., Due to a fit of rage.

Miscellaneous Ethics Issues

- *Malpractice*: 4 Ds: *D*ereliction of *d*uty causing *d*irect *d*amage to the patient. It is not a crime; however, it is a *civil wrong* punished *financially (No jail).*
- *Tarasoff decision*: When a patient threatens he has intentions to harm a certain person, you have to *admit the patient involuntarily to the psychiatry ward and contact the authorities and social services*, and *most importantly the potential victim.*
- *Sexual relationships*: Never have a sexual relationship with your patients. What if they give you a patient in the USMLE that sees you regularly, and they ask you what you are going to do if you really like her and want to have a relationship with her? Answer: *Terminate your medical services to her, and ask her to start seeing another doctor.*
- *STDs*: They must be reported to the state health department, which in turn reports them to the Center of Disease and Control (CDC).
- *Confidentiality*: Diagnosis of any patient should not be disclosed to anybody other than the patient himself.
- If the family of a patient asks you to hide a diagnosis from him/her, what should you do?

  1. Inform them that the patient has the right to know his diagnosis.
  2. Inform them that if the patient asks you directly about the diagnosis, you are obligated by the law to disclose the diagnosis.
  3. *Beneficence*: If you believe that the patient will be harmed by knowing his diagnosis at that time, you can withhold that information. However, if the patient asks you directly about his diagnosis, *you must tell him.*
  4. *Nonmaleficience (Do no harm)*: This should be your target at all times.

- *HIV*:

  1. If you have a patient diagnosed with HIV, you (or the Health Department) must inform his wife and/or sexual partners if he/she does not voluntarily do it.
  2. If you have a colleague physician who was diagnosed with HIV, it is okay for him to practice medicine; however, your responsibility is to make sure he/she is taking all the precautions necessary to protect his patients.

- **Alcohol**: If you smell alcohol on the breath of your colleague physician, *talk to him*. If he does not acknowledge your advice, report him to *chief of staff* and to *state boards*.

Health Insurance

- **Private**: Multiple companies and they cover most of the costs depending on the tier, e.g., Blue cross/Blue shield pays for hospitalization (*Blue cross*) and diagnostic tests and physician fees (*Blue shield*).
- **Federal**:

  1. Medicare: Covers the elderly (>65 years of age), and is decided by *federal government*.
  2. Medicaid: Covers the poor (*Aid for the poor*), and is decided by each *state*.

- **Note**: Patients with end-stage renal disease (ESRD) on dialysis are covered by *medicare*.

Miscellaneous

Freud's Theories of the Mind

- **Id**: "*I want.*" Unconscious drives that begin at birth.
- **Superego**: "*You cannot have it.*" The moral compass or conscience that develops by 6 years of age.
- **Ego**: "*Let's find a way.*" Balances the id and super-ego, and it develops *at birth*.
- **Unconscious**: *Primary* thinking, which involves primitive desires with no use of logic or planning.
- **Conscious**: *Secondary* thinking, which involves the use of logic and planning, e.g., Ego.

Kubler Ross Stages of Dying

1. **Denial**: e.g., A patient jumps off the bed right after an MI to do push ups.
2. **Anger**: e.g., "It isn't fair, I didn't deserve this."
3. **Bargaining and undoing**: e.g., "If I make it through this, I'll never smoke again."
4. **Depression**: Discussed earlier.
5. **Acceptance**: Patient accepts reality and shows signs of readiness to face it.

Grief Reactions

- Refer to Table 7.4.

Important Disorders

- **Kleptomania** (*Stealing crazy*): e.g., A rich person walks into a restaurant and cannot resist stealing the silverware.

TABLE 7.4 Grief reactions.

	Normal grief reaction	Abnormal grief reaction
Sleep	Mild disturbance	Major disturbance
Interest	Still enjoys usual habits	Loss of interest
Guilt	Mild guilt feelings	Major guilt feelings
Psychosis	Illusions	Hallucinations
Suicidal	Rare	Common
Treatment	Social support	SSRI

- **Pyromania** (*Fire crazy*): e.g., A person who loves to set things on fire without any purpose.
- **Trichotillomania** (*Hair crazy*): e.g., A person who cannot resist pulling on his hair.

Alcoholism and CAGE Questionnaire

- **CAGE**: Used to screen for alcoholism:

  1. C: Have you ever felt you needed to *C*ut down on drinking?
  2. A: Have you ever felt *A*nnoyed by anyone criticizing your drinking?
  3. G: Have you ever felt *G*uilty about your drinking?
  4. E: Have you ever felt you needed an *E*ye-opener after a night of drinking?

- **Treatment of alcoholism**:

  1. Disulfiram (Antabuse).
  2. Psychotherapy, e.g., Alcohol Anonymous (AA).
  3. DTs: Refer to abuse above. *Neuroleptics are absolutely contraindicated.*

Doctor-Patient Relationship

- **Transference**: Feelings and reactions of the *patient* towards the doctor.
- **Counter-transference**: Feelings and reactions of the *doctor* towards the patient.

Important Theorists

- **Abraham Maslow**: Personality is equal to a group of motivations.
- **Margaret Mahler**: Discussed separation and individualization.
- **Joh Boulby**: Described ethological and psychoanalytical thinking.
- **Rene Spitz**: Isolated kids are at risk of infections and personality disorders.
- **Harry Stack Sullivan**: Described interpersonal relations.

Others

- *Koro*: Delusions of retraction of one's penis into the body.
- *Dhat*: Pathological concern about ejaculation, found in Asian Indian cultures.
- *Nervios*: Attacks of tearfulness, abdominal pain and headache. A term most commonly used by Hispanics.
- *Dormido*: Pathological concern about heart attacks and strokes.
- *Ghost sickness*: Pathological concern about death and the deceased, found in the Navajo culture.
- *Brain fog*: Attacks of neck pain, confusion and headache. Common among students.

- *Nihilism*: The belief that something ceased to exist.
- *Animus*: Masculine part of a female personality.
- *Anima*: Feminine part of a male personality.
- *Universality*: Feeling that everybody else is just like you.
- *Cohesion*: Individuals teaming up to achieve a certain goal.
- *Consensual validation*: Understanding yourself through comparison to others.
- *Idealization*: Perception of yourself as being "Perfect."
- *Asceticism*: Pleasure obtained by refraining from basic pleasures.

Index